T0413738

Genes and Cardiovascular Function

Bohuslav Ostadal • Makoto Nagano
Naranjan S. Dhalla

Editors

Genes and Cardiovascular Function

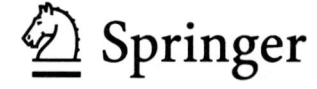 Springer

Editors
Bohuslav Ostadal, MD, DSc
Professor
Institute of Physiology
Academy of Sciences of the Czech
Republic
Prague, Czech Republic
ostadal@biomed.cas.cz

Makoto Nagano, MD, PhD
Professor Emeritus
Jikei University School of Medicine
Tokyo, Japan
naganopr@st.catv.ne.jp

Naranjan S. Dhalla, PhD, MD (Hon)
Institute of Cardiovascular Sciences
St. Boniface General Hospital
Research Centre
University of Manitoba
Winnipeg, Canada
and
Faculty of Medicine
Department of Physiology
University of Manitoba
Winnipeg, Canada
nsdhalla@sbrc.ca

ISBN 978-1-4419-7206-4   e-ISBN 978-1-4419-7207-1
DOI 10.1007/978-1-4419-7207-1
Springer New York Dordrecht Heidelberg London

Library of Congress Control Number: 2011933558

Springer is part of Springer Science+Business Media (www.springer.com)

Preface

We are living in the era of molecular medicine and the influence of basic research on the clinical practice has never been more pronounced. Over the past 15 years, cardiovascular medicine has fully embraced the tools of modern molecular biology creating in effect a bridge between the traditional physiological and clinical discipline of cardiology and genetics, genomics and biotechnology. Moreover, there has been a widespread appreciation of the power of new advances in genetically engineered animal models and novel strategies for rapidly identifying mutations in candidate human genes for diverse cardiovascular diseases, both of which led to an exponential increase in our understanding of the molecular mechanisms that drive disease progression. Gene therapy is then one of the most fascinating consequences of the penetration of molecular biology and genetic engineering into cardiovascular medicine. It is, therefore, understandable that the interest of both experimental and clinical cardiologists in the role of genes in the heart is steadily increasing.

This book is based on the two Mendel symposia "Genes and the Heart", organized in 2003 and 2008 in the Czech Republic as joint meetings of the Japanese and European Sections of the International Academy of Cardiovascular Sciences. The first one took place in Brno, well known for its industry, fairs, technological park, universities and rich cultural life. But this symposium was held in Brno for another reason: it is the birthplace of genetics. Here in the sixties of the nineteenth century an Augustinian friar and later abbot and, at the same time, a mathematician, physicist and biologist, Johann Gregor Mendel, discovered the principal laws of heredity. The abbey, the site of Mendel's activities, has been recently restored and is ready to summon a limited number of scientists for their meetings. Thus, the participants of the first Mendel symposium had a unique opportunity, besides visiting an exhibition concerning Mendel's discovery, to discuss the results of contemporary genetics in the genuine atmosphere of its true father founder.

The scientific and social success of this meeting exceeded the expectations of the organizers; we were repeatedly asked to continue and try to establish a new tradition. This request was strongly supported by our Japanese colleagues, both scientifically and financially. We have decided to invite the participants of the second Mendel symposium to another pleasant place of our country, the beautiful baroque castle Liblice near Prague. It was built between 1699 and 1702 as an aristocratic residence; now it is the property of the Academy of Sciences of the Czech Republic. The recent restoration has transformed the castle into a contemporary conference centre equipped with the latest technology. The castle is surrounded by beautiful French gardens with a ceremonial courtyard and offers exceptional stimulating environment for scientific events.

This book includes chapters which highlight the role of molecular biology and genetics in different areas of cardiovascular research; they are based on the selected contributions from the two Mendel symposia. The book is divided into six sections. The first, introductory, includes the short curriculum of Johann Gregor Mendel and the contemporary view on the possibilities and limitations of the gene therapy. The second section deals with the role of genes in cardiac development; the remaining four sections are devoted to the genetic approach of different cardiovascular disorders: mitochondrial diseases, ischemic heart disease, hypertension and arrhythmias, and cardiac hypertrophy and failure. It should stimulate the curiosity of cardiovascular scientists in gaining insight into the role of genes in the heart function in health and disease.

Twenty-four chapters in this book, written by established investigators, represent a wealth of material to emphasize the role of genetic factors in the genesis of different cardiovascular abnormalities. In addition, changes in gene expression, as a consequence of various pathological stimuli, have been identified to alter the protein content of different subcellular organelles in both cardiac and vascular myocytes and thus result in the development of cardiovascular dysfunction. It appears that a wide variety of gene expressions are excellent targets for gene therapy as well as pharmacological interventions to improve cardiovascular function in the disease state.

We are grateful to Prof. A. Kotyk and Mrs. M. Markova from Prague as well as Dr. Vijayan Elimban and Ms. Eva Little of Winnipeg for their help in the preparation of manuscripts for the purpose of editing. Cordial thanks are also due to Ms. Frances Louie and Mr. Ian Hayes, Springer USA, for their continuous advice and understanding during the editorial process. We hope this book will be of great value to cardiovascular students, fellows, scientists, clinicians and surgeons.

Prague
Tokyo
Winnipeg

Bohuslav Ostadal
Makoto Nagano
Naranjan S. Dhalla

Contents

Contributors

Adriana Adameova Department of Pharmacology and Toxicology, Comenius University, Bratislava, Slovakia

Md. Shahrier Amin University of Ottawa Heart Institute, Ottawa, ON, Canada

Hideo A. Baba Institute of Pathology and Neuropathology, University Hospital of Essen, University of Duisburg-Essen, Germany

Andrea P. Babick Institute of Cardiovascular Sciences, St. Boniface General Hospital Research Centre, Winnipeg, Canada Department of Physiology, University of Manitoba, Winnipeg, Canada

Rushita A. Bagchi St. Boniface Research Centre and Department of Physiology, University of Manitoba, Winnipeg, Canada

Daniel Baumgartner Department of Pathophysiology, Masaryk University, Brno, Czech Republic

Daniel Beckles The Center for Cardiovascular and Muscle Research and Department of Cell Biology, State University of New York Downstate Medical Center, Brooklyn, NY, USA

Jiri Blahak Department of Pathophysiology, Masaryk University, Brno, Czech Republic

Pavel Braveny Faculty of Medicine, Department of Physiology, Masaryk University, Brno, Czech Republic

Wilfried Briest Leibniz Institute for Age Research, Fritz-Lipmann Institute, Jena, Germany

Slavka Carnicka Institute for Heart Research, Slovak Academy of Sciences and Centre of Excellence for Cardiovascular Research of SAS, Bratislava, Slovakia

Lance P. Christensen Department of Anatomy and Cell Biology, Carver College of Medicine, University of Iowa, Iowa City, IA, USA

Michael P. Czubryt St. Boniface Research Centre and Department of Physiology, University of Manitoba, Winnipeg, Canada

Claude Delcayre U942-INSERM, Hôpital Lariboisière Paris, France

Naranjan S. Dhalla Institute of Cardiovascular Sciences,
St. Boniface General Hospital Research Centre, Winnipeg, Canada
Department of Physiology, University of Manitoba, Winnipeg, Canada

Takanori Ebisawa Department of Internal Medicine,
Aoto Hospital, Jikei University, Tokyo, Japan

Jorge Espinoza-Derout The Center for Cardiovascular and Muscle
Research and Department of Cell Biology, State University of New York
Downstate Medical Center, Brooklyn, NY, USA

T. Hisada Graduate School of Frontier Sciences,
The University of Tokyo, Tokyo, Chiba, Japan

Facan Huang The Center for Cardiovascular and Muscle Research
and Department of Cell Biology, State University of New York Downstate
Medical Center, Brooklyn, NY, USA

Jaroslav A. Hubacek Institute for Clinical and Experimental Medicine
and Centre for Cardiovascular Research, Prague, Czech Republic

Cecilia Hurtado Institute of Cardiovascular Sciences,
St. Boniface Hospital Research Centre, Department of Physiology,
University of Manitoba, Winnipeg, MB, Canada

Chian Ju Jong Department of Pharmacology, College of Medicine,
University of South Alabama, Mobile, AB, USA

Michaela Kadlecova Institute of Physiology, Academy of Sciences
of the Czech Republic, Prague, Czech Republic

Tara Kelly School of Biology, Aristotle University of Thessaloniki,
Thessaloniki, Greece

Akinori Kimura Department of Molecular Pathogenesis,
Medical Research Institute, and Laboratory of Genome Diversity,
Graduate School of Biomedical Science, Tokyo Medical
and Dental University, Tokyo, Japan

Jaroslav Kunes Institute of Physiology, Academy of Sciences
of the Czech Republic, Prague, Czech Republic

Antigone Lazou School of Biology, Aristotle University of Thessaloniki,
Thessaloniki, Greece

Frans H.H. Leenen University of Ottawa Heart Institute,
Ottawa, ON, Canada

Thane G. Maddaford Institute of Cardiovascular Sciences,
St. Boniface Hospital Research Centre, and the Department of Physiology,
University of Manitoba, Winnipeg, Manitoba, Canada

Naomasa Makita Department of Molecular Physiology,
Nagasaki University Graduate School of Biomedical Sciences,
Nagasaki, Japan

Eduardo Mascareno The Center for Cardiovascular and Muscle Research
and Department of Cell Biology, State University of New York Downstate
Medical Center, Brooklyn, NY, USA

Jana Matejikova Institute for Heart Research, Slovak Academy
of Sciences and Centre of Excellence for Cardiovascular Research of SAS,
Bratislava, Slovakia

Alison L. Muller Institute of Cardiovascular Sciences, St. Boniface
General Hospital Research Centre, Winnipeg, MB, Canada
Department of Physiology, University of Manitoba, Winnipeg, Canada

Martina Nemcekova Institute for Heart Research, Slovak Academy
of Sciences and Centre of Excellence for Cardiovascular Research of SAS,
Bratislava, Slovakia

Masami Nemoto Department of Internal Medicine, Aoto Hospital,
Jikei University, Tokyo, Japan

Akihiro Nishiyama Department of Internal Medicine, Aoto Hospital,
Jikei University, Tokyo, Japan

J. Okada Graduate School of Frontier Sciences, The University of Tokyo,
Tokyo, Chiba, Japan

Kouichi Ozaki Laboratory for Cardiovascular Diseases,
Center for Genomic Medicine, RIKEN, Yokohama, Japan

Grant N. Pierce Institute of Cardiovascular Sciences,
St. Boniface Hospital Research Centre, and the Department of Physiology,
University of Manitoba, Winnipeg, Manitoba, Canada

Rudolf Poledne Institute for Clinical and Experimental Medicine
and Centre for Cardiovascular Research, Prague, Czech Republic

Tana Ravingerova Institute for Heart Research, Slovak Academy
of Sciences and Centre of Excellence for Cardiovascular
Research of SAS, Bratislava, Slovakia

Jennifer Rueger Department of Cellular and Molecular Medicine,
University of Ottawa, Ottawa, ON, Canada

Jane-Lise Samuel U942-INSERM, Hôpital Lariboisière Paris, France

Stephen W. Schaffer Department of Pharmacology, College of Medicine,
University of South Alabama, Mobile, AB, USA

Chihiro Shikata Department of Internal Medicine,
Aoto Hospital, Jikei University School of Medicine, Tokyo, Japan

M.A.Q. Siddiqui The Center for Cardiovascular and Muscle Research and Department of Cell Biology, State University of New York Downstate Medical Center, Brooklyn, NY, USA

Alexandre F.R. Stewart University of Ottawa Heart Institute, Ottawa, ON, Canada

S. Sugiura Graduate School of Frontier Sciences, The University of Tokyo, Tokyo, Chiba, Japan

Bernard Swynghedauw U942-INSERM, Hôpital Lariboisière Paris, France

Nobuakira Takeda Department of Internal Medicine, Aoto Hospital, Jikei University, Tokyo, Japan

Atsushi Takeda Department of Rehabilitation, University of Tokyo Health Sciences, Tokyo, Japan

Mark I. Talan Laboratory of Cardiovascular Sciences, National Institute on Aging, Baltimore, MD, USA

Toshihiro Tanaka Laboratory for Cardiovascular Diseases, Center for Genomic Medicine, RIKEN, Yokohama, Japan

Frederique Tesson Health Sciences, Ottawa, ON, Canada

Katsushi Tokunaga Department of Human Genetics, Graduate School of Medicine, University of Tokyo, Tokyo, Japan

Robert J. Tomanek Department of Anatomy and Cell Biology, Carver College of Medicine, University of Iowa, Iowa City, IA, USA

Teruhiko Toyo-oka Department of Cardiovascular Medicine, Postgraduate School of Medicine, University of Tokyo, Tokyo, Japan
Department of Molecular Cardiology, Tohoku University Bioengineering Research, Sendai, Japan
Department of Cardioangiology, Postgraduate School of Medicine, Kitasato University, Sagamihara, Japan

Licht Toyo-oka Department of Molecular Cardiology, Tohoku University Bioengineering Research, Sendai, Japan

Balwant S. Tuana Department of Cellular and Molecular Medicine, University of Ottawa, Ottawa, ON, Canada

Anna Vasku Department of Pathophysiology, Faculty of Medicine, Masaryk University, Brno, Czech Republic

Julie Bienertova-Vasku Department of Pathophysiology, Masaryk University, Brno, Czech Republic

Vladimir Vonka Department of Experimental Virology, Institute of Hematology and Blood Transfusion, Prague, Czech Republic

Michael Wagner The Center for Cardiovascular and Muscle Research and Department of Cell Biology, State University of New York Downstate Medical Center, Brooklyn, NY, USA

T. Washio Graduate School of Frontier Sciences, The University of Tokyo, Tokyo, Chiba, Japan

H. Watanabe Graduate School of Frontier Sciences, The University of Tokyo, Tokyo, Chiba, Japan

Jeremias Wohlschlaeger Institute of Pathology and Neuropathology, University Hospital of Essen, University of Duisburg-Essen, Germany

Josef Zicha Institute of Physiology, Academy of Sciences of the Czech Republic, Prague, Czech Republic

Part I

Genes and the Heart

Johann Gregor Mendel: "Father of Modern Genetics"

Pavel Braveny

Abstract

Despite his ecclesiastical career, J. G. Mendel (1822–1884) was early attracted by science, namely mathematics and physics. This inclination fully developed after he appeared as a friar in the Augustinian monastery in Brno. His famous, statistically analyzed experiments on peas, though worldwide recognized only long after his death, became a milestone in modern biology foretelling the era of genetics.

Keywords

Genetics • Heredity • John Mendel

There is hardly any textbook of biology or encyclopedia in the world that would omit Johann Gregor Mendel. Unfortunately, the reality is often wrapped by romantic myths about an eccentric monk who happened to make a discovery due to his queer hobby and good fortune. In fact, there is nothing irrational in Mendel's career and research (Fig. 1).

Johann Mendel was born in 1822 in a small farmer's family in Hynčice, Silesia. The only way to offer a proper education to an obviously talented but poor boy were ecclesiastical schools. Once on such a track, Johann gradually became attracted by science, namely mathematics and physics. In 1843, Mendel suddenly appeared far from his home, in Brno, as friar Gregor of the Augustinian St. Thomas abbey. This location was quite natural. The Augustinian order was known to intentionally support science. Moreover, at that time, an enlightened abbot Napp headed St. Thomas, himself an amateur scientist, in then very popular field of agrology and breeding. Napp observed Mendel's scientific aspirations with sympathy and allowed him to use the rich library of the abbey without restrictions and even to study his favorite disciplines, mathematics and physics, at the University of Vienna (1851–1853). It was a most fortunate decision since his later discovery was based on mathematical analysis, a completely novel approach in biology. Mendel was also kindly offered a piece of land and a greenhouse in the abbey's garden for his experiments (Fig. 2).

The intellectual milieu of the abbey was quite exceptional. It became a meeting point of theologians, philosophers, scientists, and musicians.

P. Braveny (✉)
Faculty of Medicine, Department of Physiology,
Masaryk University, Brno, Czech Republic
e-mail: braveny@med.muni.cz

B. Ostadal et al. (eds.), *Genes and Cardiovascular Function*,
DOI 10.1007/978-1-4419-7207-1_1, © Springer Science+Business Media, LLC 2011

It is well documented that the foremost Czech physiologist J. E. Purkyně, a name certainly familiar to cardiologists, used to be among the guests. For the sake of interest, during Mendel's most intense research, a 10-year-old boy arrived as a choirboy in the affiliated basilica, who became a preeminent, world-famous composer half a century later, Leoš Janáček. Similarly, the academic environment of the rapidly developing city played a role in Mendel's career. He presented a lecture on his results in 1864 at a meeting of a well-established society in Brno, "Gesellschaft für Beförderung des Ackerbaues, der Natur und Landeskunde," and published them in the journal of the society under the title "Versuche über die Pflanzen-Hybride" 1 year later.

It is true that the attempts to verify the rules of heredity on other plant species were a bit disappointing. It may seem that Mendel's original choice of pea was a mere lucky chance. But, more likely, owing to his exceptional observational talent he recognized the distinct features of the pea varieties ready to serve as a model. Obviously this was in the beginning of his idea to analyze these features in successive generations quantitatively, using statistics. This idea may be considered a prelude to currently so popular mathematical modeling in biology.

Johann Gregor Mendel was a remarkably many-sided scholar. Besides his ecclesiastical duties and research activities, Mendel taught physics at the German high school for a couple of years, systematically observed and recorded meteorological data, was a well-informed beekeeper (his beehive still exists), and even sat on the supervisory board of a prominent local bank. When abbot Napp died in 1867, Mendel, as the most revered candidate, became his successor. No wonder that the greenhouse was deserted and the experiments discontinued.

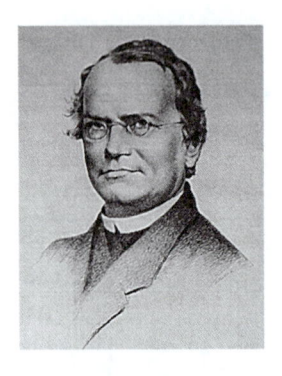

Fig. 1 Johann Gregor Mendel (1822–1884)

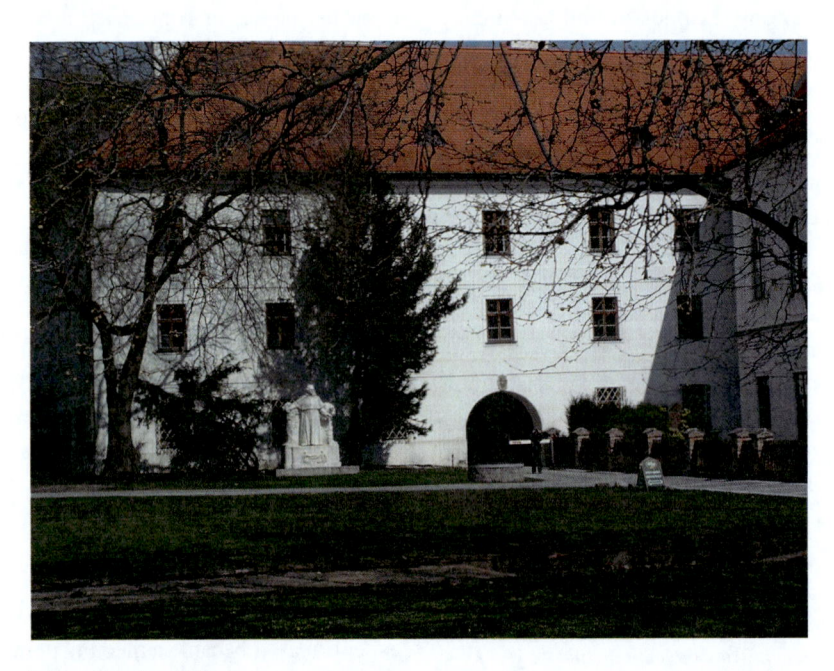

Fig. 2 Augustinian Abbey in old Brno

Mendel's discovery was initially almost completely misunderstood and forgotten, like all premature discoveries used to be. He was aware of its significance and, at the same time, controversial character. He wrote to his friend – and a fierce opponent at the same time – Nägeli in 1867: "I have suspected that it is most difficult to reconcile my results with the current knowledge. With regard to the circumstances which followed the publication of such an unfamiliar experiment, they represent a dual peril: one for the experimenter and another one because of the consequences." He was right. The Mendelian rules of heredity were doomed to unbelievable events to come. They were ignored for the next 35 years to be rediscovered independently by de Vries, Correns, and Tschermak in 1900. They became fully appreciated only gradually and with difficulty. In his homeland and eastward, they were doomed by the communist ideology for nearly two decades.

Johann Gregor Mendel died in 1884 at the age of 62 years. He did not live to see even a hint of recognition of his discovery. Today, he is appreciated as one of the most influential scientists of the nineteenth century, as the very founder of genetics.

Gene Therapy: Hopes and Problems

Vladimír Vonka

Abstract

Gene therapy (GT) is one of the most fascinating consequences of the penetration of molecular biology and genetic engineering into medicine. Originally, it was assumed that monogenic genetic diseases will be the main field of its application. However, a great majority of the GT-based clinical trials in the last decade have dealt with acquired diseases. Still, its introduction into clinical practice is associated with serious problems. The main obstacle preventing a more rapid development in the field of GT is the imperfection of the vectors presently being used for gene transfer. At the present time, GT is predominantly being used in oncology where the barriers against its employment are weaker than in other medical disciplines. Among the acquired diseases, which are now in the focus of interest of GT, are also cardiovascular diseases. A number of different GT strategies have been developed. Their choice primarily depends on the disease to be treated. In addition to technical and strategic problems, ethical issues play a significant role in planning and performance of clinical studies.

Keywords

Cell therapy • DNA • Gene therapy • Oncolytic viruses • Plasmids • Transduction • Transfection • Transgene • Vectors

Introduction

Gene therapy (GT) is a modality whose therapeutic principle is the transfer of sequences of nucleic acids. It can be defined as a transfer of genetic material, which has a therapeutic effect, either because it supplements the cell with a new or missing function or because it suppresses its abnormal, pathological function. It can also be

V. Vonka (✉)
Department of Experimental Virology,
Institute of Hematology and Blood Transfusion,
Prague, Czech Republic
e-mail: Vladimir.Vonka@uhkt.cz

B. Ostadal et al. (eds.), *Genes and Cardiovascular Function*,
DOI 10.1007/978-1-4419-7207-1_2, © Springer Science+Business Media, LLC 2011

Table 1 Reasons for extensive use of gene therapy in oncology

1. It is easier to kill the cell than to repair it.
2. Transitory expression of the transgene may be sufficient for killing the cell.
3. A number of different efficient strategies are available.
4. Because of the nature of the disease, the barriers against its use are weaker than in other medical disciplines.
5. Oncological patients are generally willing to undergo experimental therapies.

employed for increasing the efficacy of other therapeutic modalities and for removing disturbing symptoms of various diseases, like pain. A strong support for GT development is provided by the progress of proteomics and, especially, ever-increasing understanding of the functioning of human genome. GT is definitely one of the most important and most hopeful, but also scientifically most demanding consequence of penetration of molecular biology and genetic engineering into medicine. At the same time GT, together with cell therapy (CT), which is being developed in parallel, represent two of the most controversial therapeutic modalities of contemporary medicine. Both call forth contradictory reactions in the lay and the medical communities alike.

The original aims of GT mainly comprised the treatment of monogenic hereditary diseases, but most of the clinical trials performed till now have dealt with acquired diseases. Among these dominate oncological diseases. The reasons for this are summarized in Table 1. As concerns over the number of clinical trials registered, cardiovascular diseases are on the second place.

The present problems, which GT is facing, are considerable. They can be divided into three categories: technical, methodological (strategic), and ethical. They should be dealt with, at least most of them, before GT can be raised to the level of routine therapy. The author feels that it might be useful to define some of the terms that will be used in the text below and that may not be familiar to some of the readers. A gene, which is being transferred, is a *transgene*. The carriers used for gene transfer are *vectors*, among which an important role is played by *plasmids*; these are small, circular genetic elements of bacterial origin. The term *transfection* describes the transfer of a foreign gene or its portion by means of the "naked" DNA or RNA. The process of transfer of a gene is called *transduction*, and the genetically modified cell is a transduced cell. The genetic material transfected frequently persists in the transduced cell in the form of *episome,* which is a circular, extrachromosomal element, replicating independently of the cell DNA in the transduced cells. *Transposons* are short segments of DNA capable of moving from one genetic location to another in a genome. They can replicate and can be integrated into random sites of the cell genome. *MicroRNAs (miRNAs)* are endogenous, highly conserved, short, non-protein-coding RNA molecules that mediate posttranscriptional gene expression by destabilizing target transcripts. They act by annealing to partly complementary sequences in the 3'-untranslated regions of target mRNA and thereby interfere with translation. It is assumed that miRNAs fine-tune at least 30% of protein-coding genes. Thus, miRNAs play a crucial role in the regulation of biological functions such as cell differentiation [1]. *Ribozymes* are RNA molecules, which possess sequence-specific cleavage activity. They occur naturally but can be synthesized to target-specific nucleic acid sequences.

Technical Problems

When speaking about technical problems in GT, we usually have in mind problems with vectors. Vectors are of principal importance not only for the transduction efficiency and the properties and biological behavior of the transduced cell, but also for the risks associated with GT. The present imperfection of vectors is the main hindrance to rapid progress in GT.

The properties of an ideal vector are shown in Table 2. Vectors fulfilling all these requirements are not available so far. The presently used vectors are shown in Table 3. Extraordinary efforts are being devoted to the development of vectors that would approximate the ideal set down.

Table 2 Properties of an ideal vector

1. It should be easy to prepare.
2. It should penetrate into a large number of target cells.
3. It should not be toxic either for the target cells or for other cells that might be hit unintentionally.
4. The transgene must be transferred in a trancription-ally active state.
5. It should be capable of transferring large genes.
6. The expression of transgene should be sufficiently high and must persist long enough to achieve the effect desired.
7. Its immunogenicity should be low.
8. It should not induce any serious systemic untoward reactions in the recipient.
9. Its administration should not represent any risks for the recipient's contacts.

Many investigators consider this endeavor to be the most important part of contemporary research in GT. The vectors are usually divided into non-viral and viral. The former group is nearly entirely represented by DNA in the form of non-linearized or linearized plasmids, which are introduced into the target cells by physical or chemical means or their combination. A number of different techniques have been developed for this purpose. Plasmids can be introduced into the cell directly, e.g., by microinjection, electroporation, ultra-sound (s.c. sonoporation), bioballistics (by means of the gene gun), hydrodynamic method (based on an increase of intravenous pressure), or in the form of complexes. Especially popular is s.c. *lipofection*, usually based on the connection of DNA with cationic lipids. These lipoplexes fuse with the cell membrane and enter the cell. Another technique making use of the connection of anionic DNA with a variety of cationic polymers is some-times called *polyplexion*. It is the aim of the latter manipulations to increase the stability of DNA and to facilitate the endocytosis mediated by cell receptors. The major advantage of the nonbio-logical methods is the relatively easy preparation of the genetic materials to be administered and their low toxicity and low immunogenicity. Among the disadvantages of the use of the plas-mid-based gene transfer, the dominant are low stability in vivo, low efficiency of uptake by the target tissue, short term expression of the trans-gene, and a rare integration of the foreign DNA into the cell genome. A lot of effort is being exerted to overcome the disadvantages of the present nonviral vectors. The aim is especially to increase their stability outside the cell, their inter-nalization, modification of intracellular traffick-ing from endosome to lysosome, facilitation of their dissociation from the carrier, and their entry into the nucleus. A number of sophisticated approaches are being employed for this purpose [2–4]. One of the most hopeful approaches is the construction of condensed particles of size less than 100 nm. Their preparation pertains to nano-technologies and has been made possible by the recent major progress in the field of mechanics and physics. DNA is condensed and encapsu-lated, making use of the electrostatic interaction between anionic phosphate groups in DNA and the cationic carrier. In this form, DNA is pro-tected against the action of endonucleases, and the cellular uptake is increased. Coupling cell – penetrating peptides and nuclear localization sig-nals to the particle surface – can further facilitate it. Many researchers believe that particles prepared in this way, which are designated as *synthetic virus-like particles* by some of them, might, by their properties, approximate an ideal vector, as has been defined above. Hopes are also associ-ated with the newly introduced transposon-based vectors [5]. Since the transposons present in mammalian genome have been inactivated mil-lions of years ago, the gene carriers used are based on a reconstruction of active elements found in fish and amphibian genomes. Two of them carrying the fairy tale names of Sleeping Beauty [6] and Frog Prince [7] are being used for gene transfer.

In most of the GT clinical studies carried out so far, viral vectors (VV) have been used. The most frequently employed VVs and their basic properties are listed in Table 4. When compared with the nonviral vectors, VVs possess three major advantages. First, their surface structures predetermine their interaction with the cell recep-tors and penetration into the cell. It follows that the uptake of the transgene is much higher than in the case of nonviral vectors. Second, viral genome is equipped with regulation elements easily recog-nizable by mammalian cells. Third, some viruses

Table 3 Vectors used

Vector	Technical demands	Efficacy of Transduction	Integration
1. DNA	Low	Low	Low
2. RNA	Low	Low	-
3. Viruses	High	High	High[a]
4. Synthetic VLP[b]	High	High	?
5. Bacteria	High	High	-
6. Transposons	High	?	High

[a] In the case of some viral vectors
[b] Virus-like particles

(retroviruses, adeno-associated viruses (AAVs)) enable integration of the foreign genetic material into the cell genome, this ensuring a long-term expression of the transgene. On the other hand, VVs also have some disadvantages. First, the construction of VV is a challenging process practicable only in a well-advanced virus laboratory. Second, most of the viruses are strongly immunogenic. Preexisting antibodies may curtail or even block the expression of the gene delivered and the immunity developed after their administration may prevent repeated use of the same VV. Intensive investigations are under way for the preparation of VV with lowered immunogenicity. The "gutless" adenovirus can serve as an example of a significant success [8]. Third, the small size of viruses limits the size of the genetic material to be transferred. Fourth, the broad tissue tropism of some of the VVs is increasing the possibility of untoward off-target effects being induced. Therefore, considerable effort is being directed to such modification of VV as would increase their tissue specificity. There are quite a number of possible solutions [9]. One line of endeavor is to utilize specific receptors, which is attainable by adjusting the viral genome so that the requisite ligand is included in the surface structures of the virus particle. This has been termed *transductional* targeting. Another possibility is the inclusion of a promoter functional only in the target cell. Such targeting is called *transcriptional*. Fifth, there are biological risks associated with the use of VV. These risks are diminished, but not completely eliminated, by modifying the viral genetic material so as to disable the agent for replication.

This is usually achieved by deleting a portion of the virus genome [10]. Specifically genetically modified cell lines that complement the missing virus function are needed for the formation of virus particles from these defective virus particles. Such particles are capable of transferring the genetic material but are unable to replicate in the transduced cells. Still, all of the several tragic events that occurred recently (invariably cases of therapy of hereditary diseases, see below) were caused by virus particles incapable of reproducing in the cells transduced. It should be added that from the iron rule of non-infectivity of VV, two exceptions exist. The first relates to the oncolytic viruses, the effects of which are based on the replication of viruses in the tumor but not in non-tumor cells, this leading to their destruction. The other exception is represented by recombinant viruses, which are being used as experimental therapeutic vaccines.

In addition to the properties of VV shown in Table 4, they also differ by the time and duration of the expression of transgene, which influences the choice of the vector in any particular situation. In the case of adenovirus-based vectors the expression is relatively fast (within 1–4 days), which is of high advantage in situations where prompt expression is important. On the other hand, the expression of the transgene often ceases within a fortnight. If AAVs are used as vectors, the expression of transgene is not very efficient for weeks, but it may be sustained over months or even years. It should be kept in mind, however, that VVs are not the only factors responsible for the duration of transgene expression in vivo. It also depends on the tissue that is targeted and on the host response factors.

There has been an ever-increasing interest in biological vectors other than viruses [11, 12]. These include bacteria genetically modified in such a way to make them nonpathogenic without losing their capability of penetrating into the target cells to be altered. These systems, properly genetically modified, could ensure a long-term expression of transgene without the risk of potent immune reactions against the vector developing. Bactofection might also permit the regulation of the production of the protein of interest, because

Table 4 Basic properties of the viral vectors most frequently used

Virus	Titre[a] (per mL)	Stability	Maximum capacity (kb)	Risks, disadvantages
Retroviruses	10^6	Low	6–7	Oncogenicity, gene silencing
Adenoviruses	$>10^{10}$	High	7.5	Toxicity, immunogenicity
AAV[b]	$>10^{11}$	Very high	4.5	Low capacity
Herpesviruses	10^8	Low	>30	Recombination[c], activation of latent infection, immunogenicity

[a] Titres easily achievable
[b] Adeno-associated viruses
[c] Possible recombination with wild type virus

antibiotics could abolish it. There are two other great advantages of using gene-modified bacteria for GT. Their capacity for foreign genetic material is quite large and their preparation is inexpensive. Biological vectors include also the so-called biological liposomes, which are represented by spherical fragments of erythrocytes or exosomes.

An object of extraordinary interest is the development of vectors with whose aid it would be possible to direct the transgene to a particular position in the human genome. In spite of this aspiration not having been achieved so far, there is no lack of optimism among those who work on this difficult problem, and progress is evident. The mastering of this task would change the face of contemporary GT, in particular the treatment of monogenic hereditary diseases.

Methodical (Strategic) Problems

There exist some general principles for the application of GT. They can be outlined as follows: (1) understanding of the pathogenesis of the particular disease on the molecular level, (2) identification of the causative gene and knowledge of the nature of its aberration, (3) development of a therapeutic gene, (4) development of a vector that will ensure expression of the therapeutic gene over a desired time, (5) consideration of the off-target action of the gene and/or target effects that are different from the anticipated ones. However, these general principles acquire concrete and often very distinct forms, depending on the nature of the disease that is to be treated. Let us illustrate this through the examples of oncological and

cardiovascular diseases (that together are responsible for some 80% of deaths in the developed countries), in whose treatment quite controversial intensions are sometimes involved. This is not surprising. In the case of malignant tumors the object is to destroy life-threatening tissue, while in cardiovascular diseases the aim, in great majority of cases, is to renew the functioning of an impaired organ, the regenerative capacity of which is low.

Still, there exist some general strategies aimed at blocking or tuning the expression of genes. One of the strategies being employed is to use antisense deoxyribonucleotides [13]. These sequences bind directly to the genes to be inactivated, blocking gene transcription, or to their mRNA, blocking gene translation. The latter event results in the formation of an RNA–DNA complex. Owing to the activity of the ubiquitous ribonuclease H, the RNA component of the duplex is destroyed. The antisense molecule remains untouched and can readily bind to another mRNA molecule. A major disadvantage of antisense nucleotides is their low stability. Replacing oxygen atoms with sulfur atoms can increase it. A significant enhancement of stability has been achieved by the introduction of the so-called PNA (protein nucleic acid). PNA is an analogue of the DNA molecule. Its backbone is made up of a peptide to which the individual bases are attached in a sequence, ensuring its binding to the target molecule. Another method of gene silencing, and also its fine-tuning, is based on synthetically prepared small interfering RNAs (siRNAs) mimicking the role of the endogenous double-stranded microRNA (miRNA) (see above). siRNAs, used as GT tools, are represented by synthetically prepared short, double-stranded, noncoding RNA molecules possessing a length of 19–22 ribonucleotides. Within the cell one of the strands is destroyed and the other one binds to complementary mRNA. This results in its degradation [14]. Much interest is devoted to ribozymes, which exhibit a strong antitranslational activity [15]. They can be introduced into cells by transfection or by means of VV.

There are a number of strategies, the value of which is markedly different in oncology and cardiology. Some of the differences will be outlined in the subsequent text.

Oncology

In the treatment of malignancies, GT has at its disposal a large number of different strategies. An attempt will be made to classify the approaches used, although we are aware that this is a task that cannot be fulfilled exactly, because a clear *fundamentum divisionis* is missing. Moreover, the individual strategies can be combined, they may overlap somewhat, and they have their say at different levels.

The strategies of the first group are based on direct modification of tumor cells. In addition to the approaches listed above, which primarily aim at inactivating the activated oncogenes, several others can be put to this group. These include, e.g., the introduction of fully functional tumor-suppressor genes [16]. Their expression may lead to the restoration of cell growth control or result in apoptosis of the tumor cells. Apoptosis can also be induced by the introduction of proapoptotic genes. All of these approaches are successful in the cell-culture systems and in some experimental models. A major problem comes in vivo. It is impossible to introduce the genetic material into all cells of the tumor being treated. The unmodified cells have a growth advantage over those whose malignant phenotype has been altered. They may soon become dominant in the tumor cell population. For successful treatment, combination with other treatment modalities is needed.

Therefore, two other direct modifications of tumor cells deserve more attention. The first one is based on the introduction of genes for immunostimulatory factors into tumor cells [17]. This ensures a high local concentration of such factors without any signs of toxicity that accompany their systemic administration. This raises the probability of a robust immune response that may have a clear therapeutic effect, without it being necessary to genetically modify all cells of the tumor. Similarly, it is not necessary to affect the whole tumor-cell population if the so-called suicide genes (SG) are used [18]. After prodrug treatment the toxic metabolites spread to neighboring cells ("bystander effect"), and the release of large amounts of tumor antigens may stimulate the development of a systemic antitumor immune reaction.

A second major group of GT strategies in the therapy of tumors is the one directed at gene modification of non-tumor cells. It includes, e.g., the introduction of the gene designated MDR-1 (multidrug-resistance-1), the product of which increases resistance of bone-marrow cells to toxic effects of chemotherapy [19] or the creation of conditions for the treatment of the life-threatening graft-versus-host disease by ex vivo introducing SG into donor T-lymphocytes [20].

Another group of GTs in oncology is procedures suppressing neoangiogenesis, a necessary precondition for tumor growth and metastasis formation. Precisely in this strategy, the difference between the GT of malignant tumors and the GT of the heart is the most marked. The introduction of, e.g., the gene for the angiogenesis-suppressing factor endostatin into tumor cells lowers their oncogenic potential and ability of metastasis formation [21]. However, an anti-angiogenetic effect can also be attained by a blockade of the functionality of important proangiogenetic factors, such as members of the families of VEGF (vascular endothelial growth factor) or FGF (fibroblast growth factor), e.g., by means of the corresponding antisense.

Oncolytic viruses, i.e., viruses replicating exclusively or predominantly in tumor cells, are also considered to be agents for tumor GT. Two groups of oncolytic viruses are distinguished: those that are naturally oncolytic and mutants of other viruses. Taken *sensu stricto*, only the latter should be taken as GT agents, because their use was preceded by their genetic adjustment.

The last, viz. the fifth, group consists of genetic therapeutic anticancer vaccines. It is very likely that during the coming decade they will enter medical practice on a large scale. There are several distinct types of vaccines that are at the stage of development. Each of them has some advantages and some disadvantages. Considerable attention is being given to DNA vaccines [22], which are bacterial plasmids into which a gene for a specific tumor antigen has been incorporated. The gene must be in a form that ensures its expression in mammalian cells. Another type of genetic vaccines is recombinant vaccines. They are represented by recombinant proteins with the peptide carrying the immunodominant epitope of the tumor antigen inserted into another protein, known to produce a potent effect on the immune system [23]. A great endeavor is given to recombinant live viruses in which a certain gene that is not essential for replication is replaced by a gene for tumor antigen. Another type of genetic vaccines consists of cellular vaccines. They have a number of advantages. The first is that it is not necessary to know the immunodominant tumor antigens. These vaccines are prepared via modifying tumor cells by the introduction of genes for immunostimulatory factors. Both autologous and allogenic vaccines are under consideration. The development in the recent years rather favors the latter [24].

Cardiovascular Diseases

Interest in the use of GT in cardiology has been growing in the recent past, the reasons being several. The most important has been the gradual but rather fast recognition of the basics of physiological processes and the mechanisms that lead to the development of pathological states at the molecular level. Contributory to its development have been the quickly accruing successes in experimental systems. The growing interest in GT in cardiology has also reflected the slowdown in the development of efficient and safe new drugs.

Similarly as in other medical disciplines, a condition for the use of GT in cardiology is reliable and clinically relevant vectors, with safety aspects being more important than in oncology. The vectors most frequently used so far have been adenoviruses; however, it is probable that their place will gradually be taken over by adeno-associated viruses (AAVs) [25–27]. The recent discovery that some AAV serotypes are highly cardiotropic has been very helpful in this respect. However, a vector is still being sought that could be administered intravenously and that would have specific uptake by cardiomyocytes, with minimal off-target effects [28].

The use of a large spectrum of strategies is being considered and some are already in use. It is much more difficult to classify them in cardiology, because the efforts are less straightforward than in the field of oncology, in which the aim of the interventions is destruction of the unwanted tissue. Possibly the most marked differences are the absence of strategies influencing the immune system (with the exception of transplantations) and no use for SG. Another difference is a closer interconnection of GT and CT in cardiology. The choice of the strategy always depends on the purpose of the intervention. They are necessarily different when the therapy is meant just to serve as bridge to transplantation or bridge to recovery or whether a long-term expression of transgene is required [29]. To find optimal delivery system of the vectors is another important point. Among those which are under investigation is direct needle injection, pericardial delivery, catheter delivery into coronary arteries, and endocardial delivery.

From the literature available, it is apparent that special attention in heart GT is being paid to miRNA. This interest has been ever increasing with the gradual broadening of the recognition of the role played by the different miRNA species in the pathogenesis of cardiovascular diseases such as heart failure, cardiac hypertrophy, ischemia, arrhythmia, and atherosclerosis [30–32], and the recognition of potential approaches for miRNA-based interventions [33]. As has been summarized in a recent review, many cardiac patients can be treated by correcting their miRNA expression [34]. The fact that the involvement of certain miRNAs in several different heart diseases has been experimentally established brings the miRNA-based strategy closer to extensive clinical application.

There have been many applications of GT, with different strategies being used. In the next section some of them will be mentioned, the object not being to cover the entire field and its problems, but rather to document, on several examples, their diversity and the possibilities they offer.

GT is trying to break the classical dogma of heart regeneration, i.e., cardiomyocytes become postmitotic soon after birth. Recent findings of the research on myocardial regeneration suggest that it is possible to induce adult cardiomyocytes to reenter division by means of genes, the products of which are involved in the regulation of the cell cycle or act as pro-mitogenic growth factors, such as VEGF or FGF [35]. However, there seems to be a long way to go before these new observations are fully translated into clinical practice. Although in animal models of ischemic myocardium the administration of plasmids carrying VEGF or FGF have resulted in an increased collateral blood flow [36], similar studies in humans did not provide consistent results. The administration of a plasmid carrying VEGF gene into inoperable heart has been reported to result in increased perfusion and reduced angina symptoms [37], and favorable results have been reported also by another group [38]. However, they have not been confirmed by a more recent study [39].

One of the main topics of GT in cardiovascular diseases is the modification of ion channels. Their aberration is central to many cardiovascular diseases, including hypertension, heart failure, ventricular arrhythmias, or atrial fibrillation [40, 41]. There are also efforts aimed at developing biological pacemakers that might serve as an alternative to electronic devices [42]. A cell therapy approach using gene-modified human mesenchymal stem cells implanted into dog heart produced encouraging results [43].

The last-cited experimental study may serve as an example of interconnection of GT and CT.

It is not the only instance. Quite a few other studies are under way that are based on the same principle, i.e., genetic manipulation of cells using cardiac stem cells, endothelial stem cells, bone-marrow stem cells, and adipose-tissue-derived stem cells, with this resulting in differentiation into cardiomyocytes. Sophisticated techniques for obtaining, for in vitro treatment, for implantation, and for in vivo activation of their growth, differentiation, and migration have been developed (for a review; see Madonna et al. [44]).

Another task for GT in cardiology is the prevention of rejection of heart transplant. In GT the aim is to inactivate genes that code for cytokines and adhesion molecules, the products of which are involved in rejection (for a review; see Suzuki et al. [45]).

To summarize, in spite of considerable efforts having been exerted and in spite of GT clinical trials representing the second largest group (after oncology) of clinical trials registered, the recent progress of GT in cardiology has been rather modest, more modest than anticipated 10 years ago. In their recent fine review Katz et al. [46] summarized the results of the recent experimental studies, described the advantages and disadvantages of the different approaches, and then defined the conditions that would lead to an optimization of the methods to be used. Notwithstanding the existing shortcomings, their conclusion is optimistic "the outlook remains promising."

Ethical Problems

Ethical issues are of paramount importance for GT. Their importance is stressed by some serious events that took place in the past 10 years in the treatment of some genetic diseases. When a group of French scientists reported the successful treatment of children suffering from severe combined immunodeficiency (SCID) with a retrovirus carrying a therapeutic gene, a surge of enthusiasm followed. Unfortunately, 4 of the 11 children treated developed acute T-cell leukemia [47]. One of them died of leukemia. Another case of leukemia was reported in similarly treated British children [48]. The subsequent molecular analysis

Table 5 Guidelines for gene therapy clinical studies

1. Every preparation must be produced in accordance with good manufacturing practice. Its quality and safety must be verified by all the methods specified by the law and must respect the newest achievements of biomedical sciences.

2. The researchers must do their best to inform the patient about both the benefits and possible risks of the therapy. In these interviews they have to respect the education and the intelligence of the patient.

3. Every clinical undertaking should unconditionally respect the rules of good clinical practice. The research group must have extensive experience in testing new pharmaceuticals.

4. The protocol approved must be strictly adhered to. Patients who do not fulfill the criteria specified in the protocol must not be included.

5. Any untoward or unexpected reaction must be reported without delay and thoroughly analyzed.

6. The supervising authority should have enough resources for constant control of the undertaking.

7. All undertakings should be double blind. There are two strong reasons for this. (1) The interest of the researchers in a positive outcome of the study, which may be subconsciously reflected in the process of evaluation. (2) The placebo effect, which is known to be strong in seriously ill patients.

8. At this stage of knowledge, gene therapy should not be performed in patients suffering from diseases which can be successfully treated by other means. On the other hand, gene therapy should not be limited to patients in the terminal phase of their disease.

revealed that in at least four of these children, a similar pathogenic mechanism was involved. The retroviral vector was integrated in close neighborhood of the promoter of LMO2 gene, coding for a transcription factor whose overexpression was apparently involved in the pathogenesis of the disease. The phenomenon, called insertional mutagenesis, resulted in uncontrollable cell proliferation. Such risk is particularly associated with retrovirus integration. Theoretically, a similar risk may be coupled with AAV, the genomes of which are also readily integrated into cell genomes. However, their safety profile seems to be much higher than in the case of retroviruses because AAV DNA preferentially integrates into a certain locus of chromosome 19. Another death was reported from a trial aimed at GT treatment of ornithine-decarboxylase deficiency. It was caused by the use of a disproportionately high concentration of a recombinant adenovirus which produced a deadly toxic shock [49].

Another problem may be caused by the toxicity of siRNAs arising from competition with cellular miRNA processing [50] or from its off-target effects. Yet another possible source of untoward reactions may be chronic overexpression of the gene products, with uncertain consequences [51]. There is also a theoretical possibility that the VV used can recombine with a wild-type strain. The properties of such a recombinant cannot be anticipated.

The warning events call for carefulness in the use of GT and have stimulated a new ethical debate on GT. The result has been considerable toughening of the conditions for performing clinical studies.

Table 5 summarizes the principles that should be respected in all clinical GT studies.

Conclusions

The ongoing development of GT and its gradual introduction into clinical practice embodies some serious problems, which I tried to characterize in the preceding parts of this brief review. However, their existence does not mean that GT reaserch and applications should be calmed down. On the contrary, the breadth of the GT potential – its utility in combating not only genetic diseases but also acquired conditions that are beyond the possibilities of conventional cure – is a great promise for future medicine. Nevertheless, the up-to-now experience signifies that the road from the laboratory bench to the bedside should not be unidirectional. In the years ahead, researchers will be repeatedly returning from clinical studies to the laboratory to clarify the causes of unexpected events. Only in this way will it be possible to fill up the vacancies in our knowledge, reduce the risks involved, and raise the effectiveness of the operations being performed. In the light of what we know at present, it might be expected that in the next decade the progress in the clinical utilization of GT will be faster in oncology than in cardiology.

Acknowledgment The research work of the author is supported by grant no. NS 10 634-3/2009 of the IGA of the Ministry of Health of the Czech Republic and by the Research Project of the Institute of Hematology and Blood Transfusion No. MZOUHKT2005.

References

1. Shivdasani RA. MicroRNAs: regulators of gene expression and cell differentiation. Blood. 2006;108: 3646–53.
2. Li S-D, Huang L. Gene therapy progress and prospects: non-viral gene therapy by systemic delivery. Gene Ther. 2006;13:1313–9.
3. Hattori Y. Development of non-viral vector for cancer gane therapy. Yakugaku Zasshi. 2010;130:917–23.
4. Van den Berg JH, Nuijen B, Schumacher TN, et al. Synthetic vehicles for DNA vaccination. J Drug Target. 2010;18:1–14.
5. Ivics Z, Izsvak Z. Transposons for gene therapy. Curr Gene Ther. 2006;6:493–607.
6. Izsvak Z, Ivics Z. Sleeping beauty transposition: biology: application for molecular therapy. Mol Ther. 2004;9:147–56.
7. Miskey C, Izsvak Z, Plasterk RH, Ivics Z. The frog prince: a reconstructed transposon from *Rana pipiens* with high transpositional activity in vertebrate cells. Nucleic Acids Res. 2003;31:6873–81.
8. Alba R, Bosch A, Cillon M. Gutless adenovirus: last generation adenovirus for gene therapy. Gene Ther. 2005;12:S18–27.
9. Waehler R, Russeli SJ, Curiel DT. Engineering targeted viral vectors for gene therapy. Nat Rev Genet. 2007;8:273–587.
10. Miyoshi H, Biomer U, Takahashi M, Gage FH, Verma IM. Development of self-inactivating lentivirus vector. J Virol. 1998;72:8150–7.
11. Palffy R, Gardlik R, Hodosy J, et al. Bacteria in gene therapy: bactofection versus alternative. Gene Ther. 2006;13:101–5.
12. Seow Y, Wood MJ. Biological gene delivery vehicles: beyond viral vectors. Mol Ther. 2009;17: 767–77.
13. Baker BF, Monia B. Novel mechanism for antisense-mediated regulation of gene expression. Biochim Biophys Acta. 1999;1449:2–18.
14. Bartel DP. MicroRNAs: genomics, biogenesis, mechanism, and function. Cell. 2004;116:281–97.
15. Welch PJ, Barber JR, Wong-Staal F. Expression of ribozymes in gene transfer systems to modulate target RNA levels. Curr Opin Biotechnol. 1998;9:486–96.
16. Anderson SC, Johnson DE, Harris MP, et al. p53 gene therapy in a rat model of hepatocellular carcinoma: intraarterial delivery of recombinant adenovirus. Clin Cancer Res. 1998;4:1649–59.
17. Bubeník J. Gene therapy of cancer by vaccines carrying inserted immunostimulatory genes. Folia Biol. 2007;53:71–3.
18. Altaner C. Prodrug cancer gene therapy. Cancer Lett. 2008;270:191–201.
19. Schiedlmeier B, Schilz AJ, Kuhlcke K, et al. Multidrug resistance 1 gene transfer can confer chemoprotection to human peripheral blood progenitor cells engrafted in immunodeficient mice. Hum Gene Ther. 2002;13: 233–42.
20. Bonini C, Ferrari G, Verzeletti S, et al. HSV-TK gene transfer into donor lymphocytes for control of allogeneic graft-versus-leukemia. Science. 1997;276:1719–24.
21. Lakatosova-Andelova M, Duskova M, Lucansky V, Paral P, Vonka V. Effects of endostatin production on oncogenicity and neoplastic activity of HPV16-transformed mouse cells: role of interleukin 1alpha. Int J Oncol. 2009;35:213–22.
22. Signori E, Iurescia S, Massi E, et al. DNA vaccination strategies for anti-tumor effective gene therapy protocols. Cancer Immunol Immunother. 2010;59:1583–91.
23. Macková J, Stašíková J, Kutinová L, et al. Prime-boost immunotherapy of HPV16-induced tumors with E7 protein delivered by Bordetella adenylate cyclase and modified vaccinia virus Ankara. Cancer Immunol Immunother. 2006;55:39–46.
24. Vonka V. Immunotherapy of chronic myeloid leukemia: present state and future prospects. Immunotherapy. 2010;2:227–41.
25. Wang Z, Zhu T, Qiao C, et al. Adeno-associated virus, serotype 8 efficiently derives genes to muscle and heart. Nat Biotechnol. 2005;23:321–8.
26. Pacak CA, Mah CS, Thattaliyath BD, et al. Recombinant adeno-associated virus serotype 9 leads to preferential cardiac transduction in vivo. Circ Res. 2006;99:e3–9.
27. Asokan A, Conway JC, Phillips JL, et al. Reengineering a receptor footprint of adeno-associated virus enables selective and systemic gene transfer to muscle. Nat Biotechnol. 2010;28:79–82.
28. Grey SJ, Samulski RJ. Optimizing gene delivery vectors for the treatment of heart disease. Expert Opin Biol Ther. 2008;6:911–22.
29. Poller W, Hajjar R, Schultheiss H-P, Fechner H. Cardiac-targeted delivery of regulatory molecules and genes for the treatment of heart failure. Cardiovasc Res. 2010;86:353–64.
30. Divakaran V, Mann DL. The merging role of microRNAs in cardiac remodeling and heart failure. Circ Res. 2008;103:1072–83.
31. Schroen B, Heymans S. MicroRNA and beyond: the hearth reveals its treasure. Hypertension. 2009;54: 1189–94.

32. Mishra PK, Tyagi N, Kumar M, Tyagi SC. MicroRNA as a therapeutic target for cardiovascular diseases. J Cell Mol Ther. 2009;13:778–89.
33. Van Rooij E, Liu N, Olson EN. MicroRNA flex their muscles. Trends Genet. 2008;24:159–66.
34. Pan Z, Lu Y, Yang B. Micro RNAs: a novel class of potential therapeutic targets for cardiovascular diseases. Acta Pharmacol Sin. 2010;31:1–9.
35. Laguens RP, Crottogini AL. Cardiac regeneration: the gene therapy approach. Expert Opin Biol Ther. 2009; 9:411–25.
36. Mack CA, Patel SR, Schwarz EA, et al. Biological bypass with the use of adenovirus-mediated gene transfer of the complementary deoxyribonucleic acid for vascular endothelial growth factor 121 improves myocardial perfusion and function in the ischemic porcine heart. J Thorac Cardiovasc Surg. 1998;115: 168–76.
37. Symes JF, Losordo DW, Vale PR, et al. Gene therapy with vascular endothelial growth factor for inoperable coronary artery disease. Ann Thorac Surg. 1999;68: 830–6.
38. Shintani S, Kusano K, Ii M, et al. Synergistic effect of combined intramyocardial CD34+ cells and VEGF2 gene therapy after MI. Nat Clin Pract Cardiovasc Med. 2006;3(suppl I):S123–8.
39. Stewart DJ, Kutryk MJ, Fitchett D, et al. VEGF therapy fails to improve perfusion of ischemic myocardium in patients with advanced coronary results of the NORTHER Trial. Med Ther. 2009;17:1109–15.
40. Cingolani E, Ramirez-Correra GA, Kizana E, Murata M, Cho HC, Marban E. Gene therapy to inhibit the calcium channel β-subunit: physiological consequences and pathophysiological effects in models of cardiac hypertrophy. Circ Res. 2007;101: 166–75.
41. Telemaque S, Marsh JD. Modification of cardiovascular ion channels by gene therapy. Expert Rev Cardiovasc Ther. 2009;7:939–53.
42. Robinson RB, Brink PR, Cohen IS, Rosen MR. I(f) and the biological pacemaker. Pharmacol Res. 2006;53:407–15.
43. Potapova I, Plotnikov A, Lu Z, et al. Human mesenchymal stem cells as a gene delivery system to create cardiac pacemaker. Circ Res. 2004;94:952–9.
44. Madonna R, Rokosh G, De Caterina R, Bolli R. Hepatocyte growth factor/Met gene transfer in cardiac stem cells-potential for cardiac repair. Basic Res Cardiol. 2010;105:443–52.
45. Suzuki J, Isobe M, Morishita R, Nagai R. Nucleic acid drugs for prevention of cardiac rejection. J Biomed Biotechnol. 2009;2009:916514.
46. Katz MG, Swain JD, White JD, Low D, Stedman H, Bridges CR. Cardiac gene therapy: optimization of gene delivery technique in vivo. Hum Gene Ther. 2010;21:371–80.
47. Cavazzana-Calvo M, Fischer A. Gene therapy for severe combined immunodeficiency: are we there yet? J Clin Invest. 2007;117:1456–65.
48. Porteus MH, Conelly JP, Pruett SM. A look to future direction in gene therapy research for monogenic diseases. PLoS Genet. 2006;2:e133.
49. Raper SE, Chirmule N, Lee FS, et al. Fatal systemic inflammatory response syndrome in an ornithindecarboxylase deficient patient following adenoviral gene transfer. Mol Genet Metab. 2003;80:148–58.
50. Grimm D, Steetz KL, Jopling CL, et al. Fatality in mice due to oversaturation cellular microRNA/short hairpin RNA pathways. Nature. 2006;441:537–41.
51. Fishbein I, Chorny M, Levy RJ. Site-specific gene therapy for cardiovascular diseases. Curr Opin Drug Discov Devel. 2010;13:203–13.

VEGFS, FGFS, and PDGF Coordinate Embryonic Coronary Vascularization

Robert J. Tomanek and Lance P. Christensen

Abstract

The formation of the coronary vasculature during embryonic and fetal life requires many signaling events that involve transcription factors, growth factors, and other molecules. Vascular precursor cells migrate to the heart from the proepicardium, and then differentiate and assemble to form the coronary vasculature. Several growth factors are required for coronary vasculogenesis, angiogenesis, and arteriogenesis, as documented in this chapter, based on both in vitro and in vivo studies in quail, rat, and mouse. Our data reveal that formation of the initial vascular, endothelial-lined channels is regulated by multiple VEGFs (especially VEGF-B), multiple FGFs, and angiopoietins. TGF-β inhibits at least two splice variants of VEGF, thus its expression attenuates endothelial cell proliferation during arteriogenesis. Our findings also document: (1) VEGF-B and VEGFR-1 as the key players in the formation of coronary ostia and stems, and (2) FGF-2 and PDGF as important regulators of coronary arterial formation. These conclusions are based on experiments in which these growth factors were inhibited by injecting neutralizing antibodies into the vitelline vein of quail embryos. Finally, we tested the hypothesis that embryonic mesenchymal stem cells (EMSCs) facilitate coronary tubulogenesis by adding these cells to mouse embryonic heart explants. These experiments revealed an increased tubulogenesis associated with a 22-fold enhancement of stromal-derived factor-1 (SDF-1), most of which was a product of the EMSCs. In conclusion, prenatal coronary vessel development requires temporally and spatially coordinated signaling processes, multiple growth factors, and the influence of progenitor cells.

R.J. Tomanek (✉)
Department of Anatomy and Cell Biology,
Carver College of Medicine, University of Iowa,
Iowa City, IA, USA
e-mail: robrt-tomanek@uiowa.edu

B. Ostadal et al. (eds.), *Genes and Cardiovascular Function*,
DOI 10.1007/978-1-4419-7207-1_3, © Springer Science+Business Media, LLC 2011

Keywords

Angiogenesis • Arteriogenesis • Coronary development • Embryo/fetus • Fibroblast growth factor (FGF) • Platelet-derived growth factor (PDGF) • Progenitor cells • Stromal derived factor-1 • Transforming growth factor-β (TGF-β) • Vascular endothelial growth factor (VEGF) • Vasculogenesis

Introduction

Prenatal myocardial vascularization requires the migration of precursor cells from outside the heart; their differentiation, proliferation, and coalescence; and then further growth by sprouting or partitioning (intussusceptive growth) and remodeling. These events are controlled by a variety of signaling events that are temporally expressed (reviewed in Tomanek 2005). [1] The first key event regarding myocardial vascularization is the formation of the epicardium by proepicardial cells that migrate from the proepicardium located in the dorsal body wall. The proepicardium, a transient, grape-like cluster of cells, develops from the splanchnic mesoderm and is under the control of many transcription factors, e.g., capusulin (epicardin), Is11, NKX2-5. Proepicardial cells migrate via multiple vesicles and cover the myocardium, thus forming the epicardium and sub-epicardium. Epithelial-mesenchymal transformation (EMT) of the epicardial cells results in various cell lineages, as these cells delaminate and change phenotype. This process involves signaling by pathways that include Wnt, Hedgehog, TGF-β, Notch, and the slug/snail family. Myocardial signaling plays an important role in coronary cell specification by expressing Vang12, a cell polarity gene which is required for the migration of epithelial-derived cells. Moreover, the myocardium provides growth factors that regulate the formation of the capillary plexus, formation of the coronary ostia, and development of the arterial hierarchy. This chapter reviews the roles of the key growth factors involved in these events.

Tubulogenesis (Vasculogenesis and Angiogenesis)

Progenitor cells proliferate, migrate, and form vascular tubes (vasculogenesis). These endothelial-lined tubes form branches (angiogenesis) and also coalesce to form larger channels. The regulation of coronary tubulogenesis has been explored in my laboratory by both in vitro and in vivo approaches. That VEGF and FGF-2 induce myocardial vascularization in the embryonic heart was documented by injecting these proteins in ovo into the vitelline vein of chicks [2]. In order to study which growth factors are required for coronary tubulogenesis, we used neutralizing antibodies in embryonic quail heart explants [3–7]. In this system, the tubular network is formed outside the explant in the collagen gel and is identified by antibodies that are specific for endothelial cells. These cells are derived from the epicardium and thus reflect the events that occur in vivo. To test the hypothesis that hypoxia provides a primary stimulus for VEGF expression and tubule formation, we incubated the heart explants in a hypoxic environment [3, 4]. Under this condition, VEGF mRNA was up-regulated; whereas in a hyperoxic environment, it was down-regulated. Although hypoxia stimulated several VEGF-A splice variants, $VEGF_{165}$ was shown to be the main inducer of tubulogenesis. These data support the idea that the myocardium experiences a relative hypoxia as the ventricles develop a compact myocardium [8].

Multiple Growth Factors Regulate Coronary Embryonic Vasculogenesis

Our embryonic quail explant model was employed to test the hypothesis that several tyrosine kinase receptors contribute to vasculogenesis and, therefore, tube formation [5]. This hypothesis was based on our data documenting a total absence of vascular tubes when genestein was added to the explanted hearts in order to negate tyrosine kinase signaling. Tubulogenesis was attenuated

Fig. 1 Immuno-histochemical staining for VEGF. (**a**) The epicardium (*arrows*) and cardiomyocytes stain variably with the greatest intensity of staining near the epicardium in the E7 quail embryo. (**b**) The atrioventricular groove is characterized by a loose network of subepicardial cells. Many of these cells stain intensely for VEGF (*arrows*)

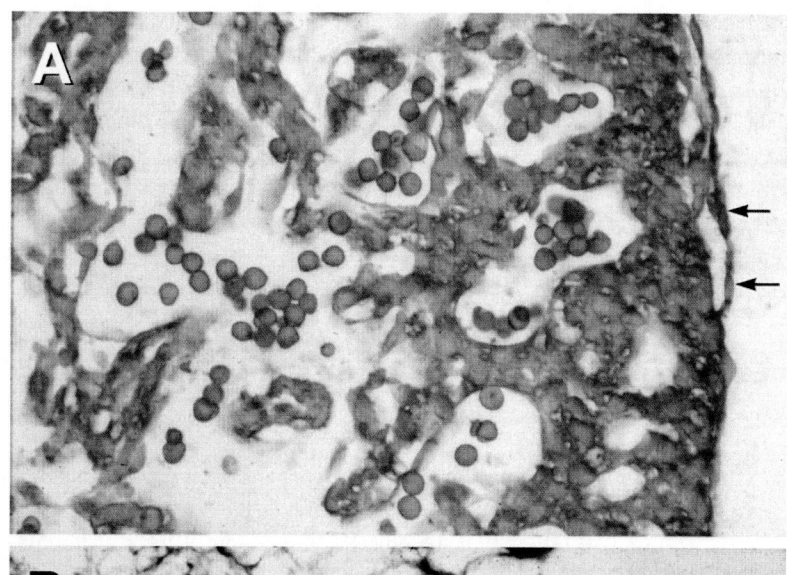

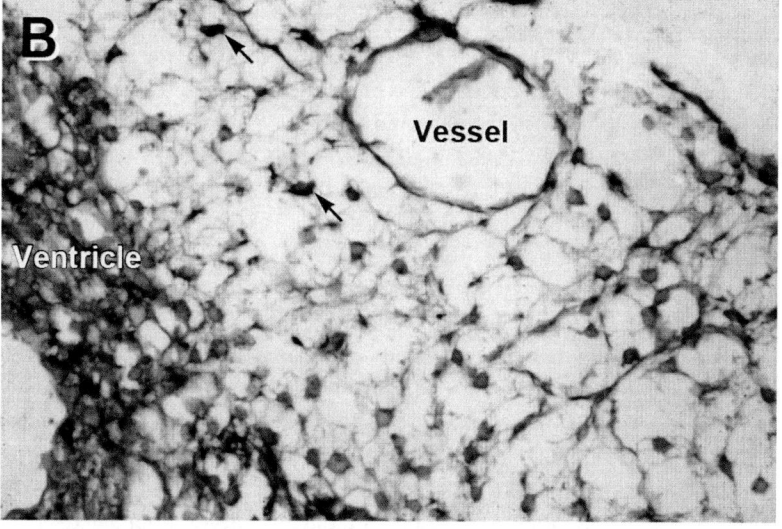

(32–57%) by antibodies to FGF-2 and antibodies to VEGF-A, as well as by soluble Tie-2, a receptor for angiopoietins. When any two growth factors were inhibited, the amount of tubulogenesis was markedly inhibited, i.e., tube formation was only 8–20% of the controls. Additional experiments also documented the interdependence of the growth factors. Stimulation of tubulogenesis by VEGF-A was totally abolished when anti-FGF-2 was also added to the explant cultures. Similarly, soluble Tie-2 also negated VEGF-A induction of tube formation. Finally, the sixfold

increase in tubulogenesis in response to FGF-2 protein was markedly reduced by the presence of anti-VEGF-A. Thus, these experiments provided evidence that at least three growth factors regulate tube formation in this embryonic heart model.

A focus on VEGFs and FGFs was deemed appropriate because these proteins are highly expressed in the developing heart. As seen in Fig. 1a, VEGF transcripts are selectively dense adjacent to the epicardium, the region in which tubulogenesis is first seen [6]. VEGF expression then becomes more pronounced toward the endocardium as tubes form in a gradient in that direction. FGF-2 has also been shown to be abundant in fetal hearts of chick [9] and rat [10, 11]. Its relationship to coronary vascularization is indicated by data that reveal its peak expression at two key time points: early vascularization (embryonic days 14 and 15) and marked microvascular growth (birth) in the rat [11].

VEGF Family Members and Tubulogenesis

VEGF-A has been repeatedly shown to be important for vasculogenesis and angiogenesis. It binds to VEGFR-1 and VEGFR-2. Of the other VEGF family members (B, C, D, and E), the developing heart also contains VEGF-B [12, 13], VEGF-C [12], and VEGF-D [14]. VEGF-B and the related PIGF (placental growth factor) bind only to VEGFR-1, whereas VEGF-C and VEGF-D bind to VEGFR-2 and VEGFR-3. Epicardial and subepicardial cells that function as endothelial cell progenitors are VEGFR-2 positive [15]. VEGF-C and VEGF-A become synergized to enhance plasminogen activator activity in endothelial cell lines [16], a finding that underscores their role in endothelial cell differentiation.

To test the hypothesis that VEGF-B and VEGF-C induce tubulogenesis in the heart, we added neutralizing antibodies in our quail heart explant assay [6]. Inhibition of VEGF-B reduced aggregate tube length in the explanted hearts by nearly 70%. Inhibition of VEGF-C was also effective, in that it attenuated aggregate tube length by 60%. In contrast, VEGF-A inhibition attenuated tubulogenesis by only 30%. Additional experiments were conducted in which soluble VEGFR-1 and soluble VEGFR-2 was added to the culture media. Addition of soluble VEGFR-1 (Flt-1) reduced tube formation to only 23% of controls, whereas in the presence of soluble VEGFR-2 (Flk-1) tube formation was 57% of controls. Thus, when VEGF-B and PIFG are bound, tubulogenesis is markedly inhibited. Subsequent in vivo experiments were conducted on quail embryos in which antibodies to VEGF-A

and VEGF-B were injected into the vitelline vein [17]. These experiments also revealed that anti-VEGF-B is more effective than anti-VEGF-A in reducing embryonic myocardial tubulogenesis. Thus, based on these data, a key role for VEGF-B in embryonic coronary vasculogenesis is documented for the first time. This role is consistent with the high expression of VEGF-B in the embryonic heart.

TGF-β Inhibits VEGF and Tubulogenesis

The three main mammalian TGF-β isoforms, i.e., β_1, β_2, and β_3, have both dissimilar and overlapping effects. Although TGF-β is important for vessel development, its specific effects have been controversial. Its major role is in arteriogenesis, which follows development of the initial vascular plexus consisting only of endothelial cells. We tested the hypothesis that some of the TGF-β isoforms inhibit tubulogenesis, considering the fact that endothelial cell proliferation ceases when the media of the vessel is being developed via smooth muscle recruitment. $TGF-\beta_1$ added to our embryonic heart explants virtually negated tube formation, whereas $anti-TGF-\beta_1$ neutralizing antibodies caused a twofold increase in tubulogenesis [5]. Subsequently, we found that $TGF-\beta_2$ and $TGF-\beta_3$ were similarly effective in negating tube formation [7]. Moreover, the three isoforms also attenuated tubulogenesis induced by VEGF-A or FGF-2. To determine whether anti-TGF-β would enhance tubulogenesis, we added neutralizing antibodies to each of the TGF-β isoforms. Neither $anti-TGF-\beta_1$ nor $anti-TGF-\beta_2$ had such an effect, whereas $anti-TGF-\beta_3$ increased tubulogenesis by 50%. We then examined VEGF-A splice variants in the explants exposed to the three TGF-βs or their neutralizing antibodies. These experiments showed that: (1) $VEGF_{190}$ and $VEGF_{166}$ mRNA were enhanced by anti-TGF-β3 but not by the other anti-TGF-βs and (2) $TGF-\beta_1$, β_2, and β_3 decreased the VEGFs. The data render the conclusion that TGF-βs inhibit embryonic heart tubulogenesis by limiting $VEGF_{190}$ and $VEGF_{166}$ mRNAs.

FGF Family Members and Tubulogenesis

Multiple FGFs, VEGF, and Hedgehog signaling. FGFs and Hedgehog signaling have been documented to drive coronary morphogenesis in an elegant study on engineered mice and organ cultures [18]. The data indicate that FGF signaling to cardiomyocytes regulates Hedgehog signaling, which then influences VEGF and angiopoietin expression. The work also revealed that FGF-9 is essential for coronary vessel formation since FGF-9$^{-/-}$ mice lack a complete vascular plexus. Blood vessel formation requires FGFR-1 signaling [19] and this receptor is over-expressed during epicardial-mesenchymal transformation and epicardial cell delamination [20].

Most recently, we tested several hypotheses that multiple FGF ligands are able to stimulate tubulogenesis and that embryonic mesenchymal stem cells (EMSC) will stimulate tubulogenesis via FGF signaling [21]. Our data, based on both quail and mouse explants, indicate that FGFs 1, 2, 4, 8, 9, and 18 are able to induce tubulogenesis and that FGF-2 is most effective at a lower dose. The effects of each of these FGFs were found to be VEGF dependent. In order to determine the role of FGF signaling in tubulogenesis, we added FGFR1-DN (an adenoviral construct encoding a cytoplasmic domain-deleted FGFR1 that inhibits signaling by all four FGF receptors) or soluble splice variant receptors of FGFR1 and FGFR3. Tubulogenesis and endothelial cell migration were inhibited by FGFR1-DN. Of the receptor splice variants, FGFR1-IIIc, which binds most of the FGF ligands, also decreased endothelial cell migration. Next, we tested the hypothesis that FGF signaling is required for VEGF-induction of tubulogenesis. When FGFR1-DN, FGFR1-IIIc, or FGFR3-IIIc were added to the heart explants, VEGF-induced tubulogenesis was negated. The C (EMSCs) isoforms, noted above, are usually specific for mesenchymal cells.

Embryonic mesenchymal stem cells. Finally, embryonic mesenchymal stem cells were co-cultured with the heart explants to determine their role in tubulogenesis. Endothelial cell density was increased 2.7-fold in the co-cultures compared to cultures containing only the heart explants. This response was completely blocked by the addition of FGFR1-DN, a finding that FGF signaling is required for this EMSC-induced response. ELISA analysis of the culture media revealed that SDF-1α (stromal-derived factor) was 22 times higher when EMSCs were added to the cultures. To determine whether the heart explant or the EMSCs were the source of SDF-1α, media from explants and EMSCs alone were compared. The data indicate that EMSCs provide more than 50 times the amount of SDF-1α than the heart explants. Not finding any evidence that EMSCs incorporate into the vascular tubes, we conclude that their effect is paracrine.

Coronary Arteriogenesis

Coronary ostia are formed when a capillary plexus penetrates the aorta at the left and right coronary cusps (Fig. 2). This phenomenon was first described in quail hearts by Bogers et al. [22]. Subsequent studies confirmed and expanded on this observation using chick-quail chimeras [23] and serial sections of chick [24] and rat [11] hearts. Some peritruncal tubes also enter the aorta at other sites, but fail to form a vascular channel (ostium) in the aorta [25]. The two coronary ostia that form via fusion of the peritruncal tubes require apoptosis of resident cells within the aorta [26]. As the ostia form, the attached vascular plexus concomitantly recruits smooth muscle cells that form the two main coronary stems [25].

The cells of the epicardium and those surrounding the root of the aorta or in the atrioventricular groove stain intensely for VEGF antibodies (Fig. 1). Moreover, VEGF receptors R-2 and R-3 are highly expressed at the base of the aorta, coinciding with the temporal and spatial formation of the coronary arteries [6]. Accordingly, we conducted *in ovo* experiments on quail embryos regarding the role of VEGFs in ostial and coronary artery stem formation [17]. Injection of VEGF-Trap, the VEGFR-1/VEGFR-2 chimera, prior to formation of the

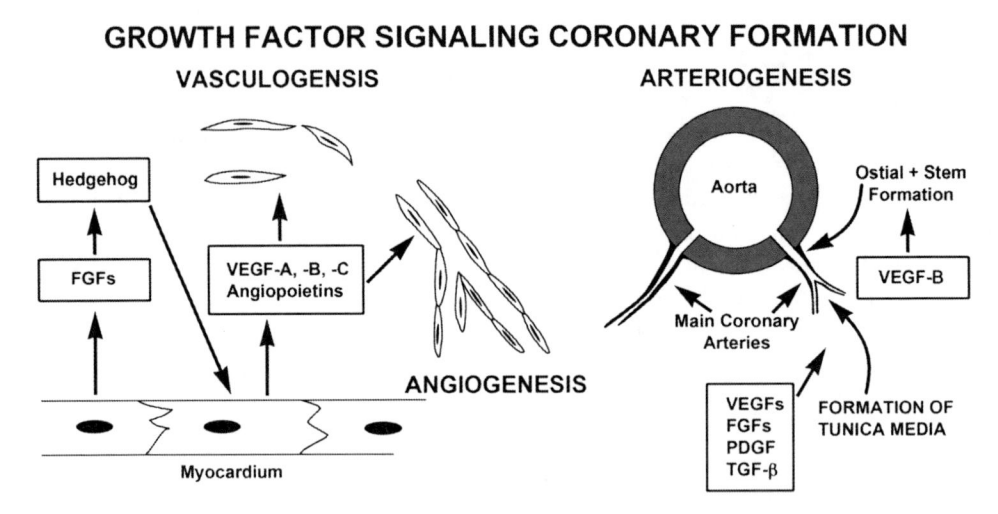

Fig. 2 A summary of growth factors signaling during embryonic/fetal development. Hedgehog signaling plays a key role in vasculogenesis and angiogenesis when activated by FGFs from the myocardium. This causes VEGFs and angiopoietins to be up-regulated and released from the myocardium and to regulate vascular tube formation and growth. The subsequent ostial and stem formation is VEGF-B dependent. Several growth factors contribute to medial formation of the coronary arteries

main coronary arteries at E9 prevented formation of the coronary arteries in 11 of 13 embryos; the remaining two embryos had only one coronary artery. Injections of soluble VEGFR-1 or soluble VEGFR-2 usually limited coronary formation to one artery or prevented coronary artery formation. Antibodies to VEGF-A had little effect. In contrast, anti-VEGF-B most often prevented coronary artery stem formation or limited formation to one artery. These experiments established that VEGF-B and VEGFR-1 signaling are key regulators of coronary ostial and stem formation. This finding underscores the importance of VEGF-B and VEGFR-1 signaling in coronary arteriogenesis, as well as vasculogenesis and angiogenesis.

Based on the well-established roles of FGFs and PDGF in arteriogenesis, we tested the hypothesis that these growth factors regulate: (1) ostial, (2) stem, and (3) downstream development of coronary arteries by injecting quail embryos *in ovo* at embryonic (E) days E6, E7, or E8. Neutralizing antibodies to either FGF-2 or PDGF-limited coronary artery stem formation, especially when injected 2 days (at E6) before stem formation is under way. Anti-FGF-2 was more effective in this regard. If the neutralizing antibodies were administered when coronary artery stem formation may already be under way, the main effect was a delay in artery stem formation.

Muscularization of the endothelial-lined channels that form the coronary arteries proceeds in a base to apex direction. To study this process, we used serial sections to determine the extent of tunica media formation and the distance from the aorta that it progressed. The data revealed that when a coronary stem forms, despite being subjected to neutralizing antibodies, the process of muscularization is limited, compared to the controls. Thus, both FGF-2 and PDGF play a role in downstream development of the tunica media. Moreover, even in muscularized arteries, the tunica media is less developed compared to controls. We also showed that VEGF, in addition to its role in ostial and stem formation, is important in the development of the tunica media downstream from the coronary stems. These data are based on embryos injected with VEGF-Trap after the formation of the coronary stems. In conclusion, at least three growth factors (i.e., VEGF, FGF-2, and PDGF) regulate coronary artery formation and growth.

Conclusions

All three of VEGF, FGF-2, and PDGF antibodies produced some common phenotypes. First, the sinusoidal area of the ventricles persisted, whereas the growth of the compact region was limited. Other anomalies included: (1) persistence of isolated multiple channels in the aorta, (2) occasional failure of the coronary ostia to enlarge sufficiently, and (3) massive accumulations of blood cells in the subepicardium or in the middle of the interventricular septum. In the study using VEGF-Trap [17], we found that the erythrocytes in the ventricular walls and blood islands of treated embryos were derived from the proepicardium, as documented by retroviral cell tagging. Thus, limitations in VEGF signaling induce proepicardial-derived hemangioblasts to differentiate into erythrocytes.

References

1. Tomanek RJ. Formation of the coronary vasculature during development. Angiogenesis. 2005;8:273–84.
2. Tomanek RJ, Lotun K, Clark EB, et al. VEGF and bFGF stimulate myocardial vascularization in embryonic chick. Am J Physiol. 1998;274:H1620–6.
3. Yue X, Tomanek RJ. Stimulation of coronary vasculogenesis/angiogenesis by hypoxia in cultured embryonic hearts. Dev Dyn. 1999;216:28–36.
4. Yue X, Tomanek RJ. Effects of VEGF(165) and VEGF(121) on vasculogenesis and angiogenesis in cultured embryonic quail hearts. Am J Physiol Heart Circ Physiol. 2001;280:H2240–7.
5. Tomanek RJ, Zheng W, Peters KG, et al. Multiple growth factors regulate coronary embryonic vasculogenesis. Dev Dyn. 2001;221:265–73.
6. Tomanek RJ, Holifield JS, Reiter RS, et al. Role of VEGF family members and receptors in coronary vessel formation. Dev Dyn. 2002;225:233–40.
7. Holifield JS, Arlen AM, Runyan RB, et al. TGF-beta(1), -beta(2) and -beta(3) cooperate to facilitate tubulogenesis in the explanted quail heart. J Vasc Res. 2004;41:491–8.
8. Nanka O, Valasek P, Dvorakova M, et al. Experimental hypoxia and embryonic angiogenesis. Dev Dyn. 2006;235:723–33.
9. Joseph-Silverstein J, Consigli SA, Lyser KM, et al. Basic fibroblast growth factor in the chick embryo: immunolocalization to striated muscle cells and their precursors. J Cell Biol. 1989;108:2459–66.
10. Spirito P, Fu YM, Yu ZX, et al. Immunohistochemical localization of basic and acidic fibroblast growth factors in the developing rat heart. Circulation. 1991;84:322–32.
11. Tomanek RJ, Haung L, Suvarna PR, et al. Coronary vascularization during development in the rat and its relationship to basic fibroblast growth factor. Cardiovasc Res. 1996;31:E116–26.
12. Lagercrantz J, Farnebo F, Larsson C, et al. A comparative study of the expression patterns for vegf, vegf-b/vrf and vegf-c in the developing and adult mouse. Biochim Biophys Acta. 1998;1398:157–63.
13. Ikuta T, Ariga H, Matsumoto KI. Effect of tenascin-X together with vascular endothelial growth factor A on cell proliferation in cultured embryonic hearts. Biol Pharm Bull. 2001;24:1320–3.
14. Achen MG, Jeltsch M, Kukk E, et al. Vascular endothelial growth factor D (VEGF-D) is a ligand for the tyrosine kinases VEGF receptor 2 (Flk1) and VEGF receptor 3 (Flt4). Proc Natl Acad Sci USA. 1998;95:548–53.
15. Perez-Pomares JM, Macias D, Garcia-Garrido L, et al. The origin of the subepicardial mesenchyme in the avian embryo: an immunohistochemical and quail-chick chimera study. Dev Biol. 1998;200:57–68.
16. Pepper M, Mandriota S, Jeltsch M, et al. Vascular endothelial growth factor (VEGF)-C synergizes with basic fibroblast growth factor and VEGF in the induction of angiogenesis in vitro and alters endothelial cell extracellular proteolytic activity. J Cell Physiol. 1998;177:439–52.
17. Tomanek RJ, Ishii Y, Holifield JS, et al. VEGF family members regulate myocardial tubulogenesis and coronary artery formation in the embryo. Circ Res. 2006;98:947–53.
18. Lavine KJ, White AC, Park C, et al. Fibroblast growth factor signals regulate a wave of Hedgehog activation that is essential for coronary vascular development. Genes Dev. 2006;20:1651–66.
19. Lee SH, Schloss DJ, Swain JL. Maintenance of vascular integrity in the embryo requires signaling through the fibroblast growth factor receptor. J Biol Chem. 2000;275:33679–87.
20. Pennisi DJ, Mikawa T. FGFR-1 is required by epicardium-derived cells for myocardial invasion and correct coronary vascular lineage differentiation. Dev Biol. 2009;328:148–59.
21. Tomanek R, Christensen L, Simons M, et al. Embryonic coronary vasculogenesis and angiogenesis are regulated by interactions between multiple FGFs and VEGF and are influenced by mesenchymal stem cells. Dev Dyn. In press.
22. Bogers AJ, Gittenberger-de Groot AC, Poelmann RE, et al. Development of the origin of the coronary arteries, a matter of ingrowth or outgrowth? Anat Embryol Berl. 1989;180:437–41.
23. Poelmann RE, Gittenberger-de Groot AC, Mentink MM, et al. Development of the cardiac coronary

vascular endothelium, studied with antiendothelial antibodies, in chicken-quail chimeras. Circ Res. 1993;73:559–68.

24. Waldo KL, Willner W, Kirby ML. Origin of the proximal coronary artery stems and a review of ventricular vascularization in the chick embryo. Am J Anat. 1990;188:109–20.

25. Ando K, Nakajima Y, Yamagishi T, et al. Development of proximal coronary arteries in quail embryonic heart: multiple capillaries penetrating the aortic sinus fuse to form main coronary trunk. Circ Res. 2004;94:346–52.

26. Velkey JM, Bernanke DH. Apoptosis during coronary artery orifice development in the chick embryo. Anat Rec. 2001;262:310–7.

The E2F Pathway in Cardiac Development and Disease

Jennifer Rueger and Balwant S. Tuana

Abstract

Regulation of the cardiac cell cycle is an important and unique process in myocardial development. During embryonic growth cardiomyocytes rapidly proliferate, but shortly after birth they enter a final round of the cell cycle after which they permanently withdraw and cardiac growth depends on physiological hypertrophy. When the heart becomes stressed, it undergoes pathological hypertrophy to compensate for increased load on the heart. This process appears to involve the induction of genes involved in regulating the fetal gene program as well as the cell cycle which is largely controlled by the E2F family of transcription factors. In this review we summarize the current understanding of the E2F pathway and its contribution to normal and pathological cardiac development and growth.

Keywords

Cardiac growth • Cell cycle • E2Fs • Gene expression

Introduction

Proper cardiac development requires tight and coordinated expression of genes controlling both the cell cycle and differentiation. During embryonic development cardiomyocytes divide very rapidly, and thus approximately 70% of cells are synthesizing DNA. As cardiac precursor cells begin to differentiate they lose their proliferative capacity, resulting in only about 45% of cardiomyocytes synthesizing DNA [1]. Several days after birth cardiomyocytes undergo a final round of DNA synthesis without cell division, called acytokinetic mitosis, leaving many cardiomyocytes binucleated. Cardiomyocytes then permanently withdraw from the cell cycle and all postnatal cardiac growth depends on physiological hypertrophy. As the heart ages and is exposed to stressors and damage, this triggers abnormal or pathological cardiac hypertrophy often leading to heart failure. This abnormal growth is associated with a reactivation of the fetal gene program as well as the expression of genes involved in cell cycle reentry [2, 3]. Thus it appears that proper

B.S. Tuana (✉)
Department of Cellular and Molecular Medicine,
University of Ottawa, Ottawa, ON, Canada
e-mail: btuana@uottawa.ca

B. Ostadal et al. (eds.), *Genes and Cardiovascular Function*,
DOI 10.1007/978-1-4419-7207-1_4, © Springer Science+Business Media, LLC 2011

regulation of the cell cycle is the key for both embryonic and postnatal cardiac development.

The Cell Cycle

The cell cycle is a complex and tightly regulated process which exists in five distinct phases and has numerous checkpoints to inhibit abnormal cell cycle entry and proliferation. The cell cycle begins in Gap 1 (G_1) in which the cell grows and prepares to enter the cell cycle. Cells which remain in G_1 for extended periods of time can exit the cell cycle and are said to be in a quiescent stage termed G_0. They may reenter the cell cycle or express genes necessary for terminal differentiation and become senescent. When the appropriate growth signals are received, cells can pass through a restriction point in G_1, after which they are committed to the cell cycle. The next stage is the synthesis (S) phase in which DNA is duplicated, followed by a second preparatory phase Gap 2 (G_2). Cells then enter mitosis (M) in which chromatin is condensed and assembled at the mitotic plate. DNA and cellular components are separated into two daughter cells which divide in a process called cytokinesis.

Cell cycle regulation is managed in large by cyclin-dependent kinases (CDKs) that, in association with cyclins, phosphorylate a wide range of proteins leading to the appropriate expression of genes for coordinated induction and passage through the cycle. Cyclin type and expression fluctuates throughout the cycle and different cyclins positively regulate CDKs which remain at stable levels throughout the cell cycle. Cyclin D associates with CDK4 and CDK6 during G_1 and is important for passage through the G_1/S restriction point. Cyclin E or A associates with CDK2 to create the S-phase-promoting factor (SPF). Cyclin B or A associates with CDK1 to promote mitosis by creating the M-phase-promoting factor (MPF). While the embryonic heart contains large amounts of cyclins and CDKs, they are down-regulated in quiescent adult cardiomyocytes [4].

In contrast to cyclins, CDK inhibitors (CDKIs) negatively regulate CDKs by competitive binding with cyclins to CDKs, thus blocking cell cycle progression. They exist in two groups: Cip/Kip (p21, p27, and p57) which broadly inhibit CDK4/6 and CDK1/2, and Ink4 (p15, p16, p18, and p19) which selectively inhibit CDK4/6 [5, 6]. In contrast to cyclins, Cip members are highly expressed in adult cardiomyocytes which have permanently withdrawn from the cell cycle [7].

Together cyclins and CDKIs respond to signaling pathways and mitogens to activate or inactivate the appropriate CDK complexes throughout the cell cycle which appears to be crucial for cardiac development. Deletion of CDK2 and CDK4 is embryonically lethal due to cardiac defects [8], and hyperplasia is observed in mice which overexpress cyclin D [9] and CDK2 [10]. These defects have been attributed to hypophosphorylation of the pocket protein pRb and consequently the activation of E2F-responsive genes. In fact, the pocket protein and E2F families are among the most widely studied targets of CDK complexes. This is because the E2F/pocket protein families play a pivotal role in the cell cycle by controlling the expression and repression of genes involved in cellular proliferation, differentiation, and death by apoptosis [11–13].

E2F Family Member Structure

The E2F family consists of nine transcription factors: E2F1, E2F2, E2F3a, E2F3b, E2F4, E2F5, E2F6, E2F7, E2F8 (Fig. 1). Each member shares a DNA-binding domain in common, consisting of a winged helix motif. In order to form functional DNA-binding complexes, E2F1–6 also share a dimerization domain containing a leucine zipper which allows them to heterodimerize with differentiation proteins DP1 and DP2 [14, 15]. DPs also share regions of homology to the E2F family in their DNA binding and dimerization domains. E2F7 and E2F8 lack a dimerization domain and instead have two DNA-binding domains and form homo and/or heterodimers with one another [16, 17].

E2F1–5 also share homology at their C-termini termed a transactivation domain, which is thought to recruit basal transcriptional machinery

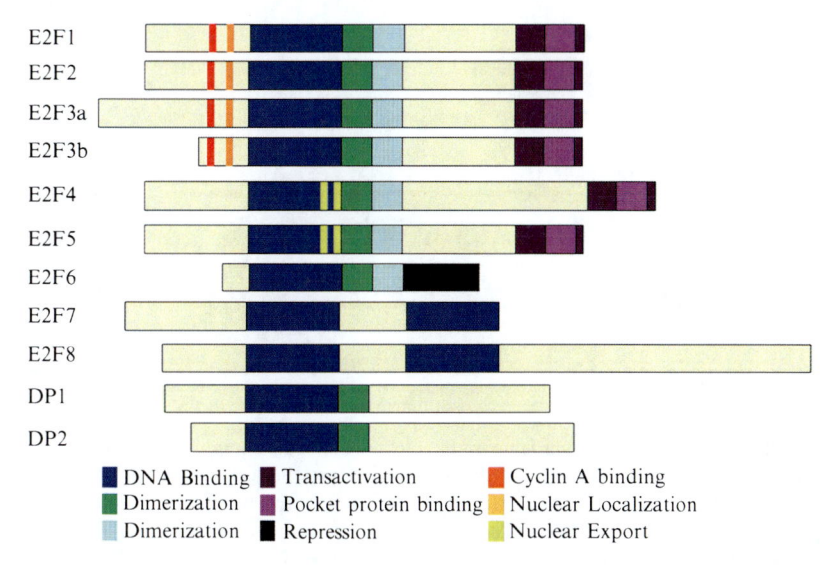

Fig. 1 Schematic of the E2F and DP family members. All members share a DNA-binding domain and E2F1–6 dimerize with DPs through their dimerization domain in order to form functional DNA-binding heterodimers. E2F7 and E2F8 do not bind to DPs and instead have two DNA-binding domains. E2F1–5 share a C-terminal domain that is responsible for transcriptional transactivation which also contains a pocket-protein-binding domain. E2F1–3 share a cyclin-A-binding motif as well as a nuclear localization signal in their amino-terminal while E2F4 and E2F5 share nuclear export signals embedded in the DNA-binding domain. The C-terminus of E2F6 contains a domain important for the recruitment of polycomb proteins for gene repression

to promote transcription [18]. Embedded within this domain is a pocket protein-binding motif which, when bound by pocket proteins, inhibits transactivation and forms a repression complex [19]. Additionally, E2F1–3 share regions of homology in their N-termini, including a domain which binds cyclin A [20, 21] and a nuclear localization signal [22, 23]. E2F4 and E2F5 instead share a nuclear export signal within their DNA-binding domains, while E2F6–8 lack any recognizable nuclear import or export signals. E2F6 contains a region at its C-terminus termed a "repression" domain which has been shown to interact with a variety of different proteins which form gene repression complexes [24, 25].

E2F/Pocket Protein Pathway

Underscoring the importance of the E2F-RB pathway is its evolutionary conservation in *Drosophila melanogaster* [26], *Caenorhabditis elegans* [27], and *Arabidopsis thaliana* [28]. In more primitive animals, there exists only a single E2F activator and repressor and one pocket protein: pRb. The mammalian pocket proteins include pRb, p130, and p107, which interact with the "classical" E2Fs (1–5). E2F1–3 interact primarily with pRb [29], E2F5 with p130 and p107, and E2F4 interacts with all members [30]. Although the mammalian E2F/pocket protein family is much more diverse, E2F1–5 are regulated by pocket proteins in a fashion similar to that of invertebrates.

During G_0 and early G_1 stages of the cell cycle hypophosphorylated pocket proteins bind to E2Fs, masking the transactivation domain at their C-terminus leading to transcriptional repression [31]. Pocket proteins can recruit a number of histone-modifying enzymes including histone deacetylases (HDACs), histone methyl transferases (HMETs), and heterochromatin proteins (HP1) which recruit HMETs, in order to form heterochromatin and maintain gene repression [32, 33]. As cells receive growth signals CDK4 (in association with cyclin D) phosphorylates pocket proteins, causing them to become hyperphosphorylated and release the E2Fs (Fig. 2).

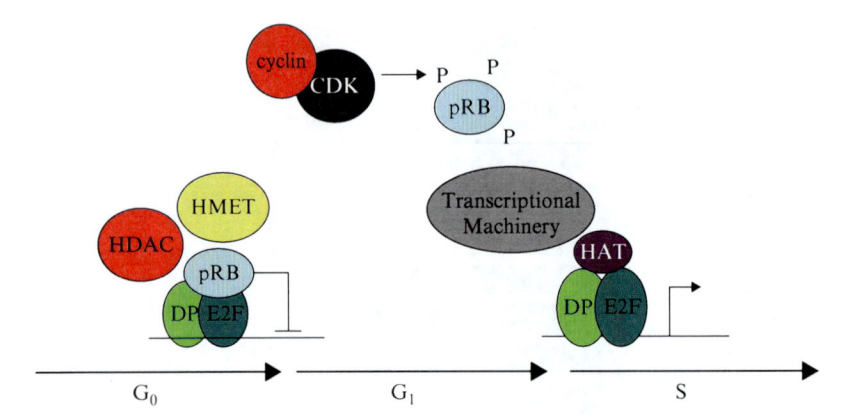

Fig. 2 The E2F/RB pathway is regulated throughout the cell cycle. During G_0 E2F's transactivation domain is masked by pocket protein binding, resulting in E2F-responsive gene repression. Pocket proteins can recruit histone deacetylases (HDACs) and histone methyltransferases (HMETs) to actively repress gene activity by chromatin remodeling. As cells transition into G1/S phase, pocket proteins become phosphorylated by cyclin/CDK complexes freeing E2F/DP complexes. Histone acetyl transferases (HATs) are recruited to open chromatin architecture and the basal transcriptional machinery activates the E2F-responsive genes necessary for cell cycle progression

Subsequently, E2Fs can recruit chromatin-modifying enzymes, such as the histone acetyl transferases (HAT) p300 and Tip60, in order to relax chromatin architecture and activate gene expression [34, 35].

E2F Family Member Function

E2F family members are generally separated into two categories based on their capacity to drive quiescent cells into S phase and their presence at E2F-responsive promoters during the cell cycle. E2F1–3a are described as activators of transcription while E2F3b–8 are gene repressors. The "repressors" are usually subdivided into those that interact with pocket proteins (E2F3b–5) and those whose mechanism of repression is pocket protein independent (E2F6–8). These categories appear to be oversimplistic as increasing evidence suggests that repressor E2Fs can activate and activator E2Fs can repress transcription (discussed in the next section). Further complicating the understanding of individual E2Fs is their large family size. When an individual member is deleted, other members have the capacity to compensate highlighting their redundancies [36]. In addition, over-expression and knockout of individual E2Fs will shift the balance of activating and repressing E2Fs as well as the availability of DP and pocket proteins; thus these types of studies should be interpreted with caution. Despite this, knockout and double knockout (DKO) mouse models have aided in determining some of the tissue- and temporal-specific functions of particular E2Fs and have contributed overall to our understanding and the importance of proper regulation of this pathway.

Activating E2Fs

E2F1–3a represent the activator E2Fs which appear to have some overlapping and specific functions. When over-expressed, each member induced activation of E2F-responsive genes and had the capacity to cause cell cycle reentry in quiescent cells [29, 37]. Deletion of individual activators did not affect fibroblast proliferative capacity, but deletion of all three inhibited proliferation, suggesting a redundancy between members [38]. In spite of this their temporal- and tissue-specific expression points at nonredundant roles as well. E2F1 and E2F2 are up-regulated at the G_1/S boundary of the cell cycle [39], while E2F3 is expressed very highly during mid G_1 and remains stable through the S phase [40]. In addition, E2F1 is the only activator expressed in the brain after early embryonic development [15], while E2F1 and E2F3 are expressed in the heart as E2F2 is not [41].

E2F1 was the first E2F member to be identified and its function is the best described. E2F1[-/-] mice are viable and their isolated fibroblasts have a normal proliferative capacity, but adult mice have a higher incidence of tumor development [42–44]. In support of its role in cancer, elevated levels of E2F1 have been found in breast [45], ovarian [46], and gastric [47] cancers. Furthermore, mutations of its inhibitor pRb have been implicated in dozens of cancers, and DKO of pRb and an activating E2F can reverse tumor incidence [48].

In addition to cancer, E2F1 has been demonstrated to participate in both p53-dependent and -independent apoptotic pathways. E2F1 can directly activate the expression of the CDKI p14^{ARF} which in turn inhibits MDM2, an inhibitor of p53, resulting in the stabilization of p53 and activation of apoptotic pathways [49, 50]. It has also been suggested that E2F1 can directly interact with p53 through its cyclin-A-binding domain [51]. Thus, E2F1's ability to activate p53 would depend on competitive binding between cyclin A and p53 [52].

Like E2F1 null mice, E2F2[-/-] mice are also viable and fibroblasts proliferate at a normal rate [53]. Adult E2F2[-/-] mice are more susceptible to infection and develop late-onset autoimmune disease. Although E2F2 is usually described as an activator and driver of cellular proliferation, its ablation also resulted in hyperproliferation in T-lymphocytes suggesting a repressive function in T-cell proliferation [53].

E2F3 has also been widely researched and its ablation is the only individual E2F knockout which appears to affect embryonic viability. E2F3 KO leads to partial embryonic lethality which has been attributed to defects in proliferation [54]. The lethality of E2F3[-/-] appears to be dependent on mouse strain. Pure strain 129/Sv mice have 100% embryonic lethality, while in mixed background mice (C57BL/6 × 129/Sv) 30% die in utero, 45% die within 24 h after birth, and 25% survive to adulthood, although 85% of these mice eventually die of congestive heart failure [44].

Interestingly, the authors noted that the major time points of death correlate with major proliferative events in embryonic development as well as perinatally during the final round of the cell cycle suggestive of a proliferation defect [55]. Upon histological analysis of E2F3 KO mice, several cardiac defects were discovered including hypoplastic septal walls and defects in septal development. A decrease in the proliferative index (measured by BRDU incorporation) in the embryonic heart of KO mice was observed. Thus it appears that E2F3 is necessary for proliferation and embryonic cardiac development. Additionally, autopsy of mice which lived into adulthood revealed dilated hearts and atrial thrombi in E2F3 knockouts [55]. The late-onset dilated cardiomyopathy is potentially due to the progressive accumulation of stress on the heart due to defects in sarcomere organization which were observed. Thus it appears that E2F3 is crucial for both embryonic and postnatal cardiac development and function.

Despite the array of studies depicting specific roles for individual activator E2Fs, in 2008 Tsai [56] provided evidence suggesting that, like *Drosophila*, mammals can survive with a single activating E2F. The authors created different combinations of compound knockout mice in order to more closely evaluate the individual and redundant roles of activator E2Fs. Their studies confirmed many previously published results with respect to adult phenotypes of individual E2F members, such as increased incidence of tumor development in E2F1[-/-] mice. They also took a closer look at E2F3's role by creating separate E2F3a and E2F3b KOs. Although mice with deletion of E2F1, E2F2, E2F3b were viable, deletion of E2F1, E2F2, E2F3a was lethal, suggesting that the crucial role of E2F3 in cardiac development can be attributed to E2F3a. Most interestingly, when E2F3b or E2F1 was expressed from the same genetic locus as the deleted E2F3a mice were rescued from the phenotype of E2F3a[-/-] [56]. This suggests that the specificity of activating E2Fs has more to do with genetic context which controls spatial and temporal expression than a specific function of an individual family member.

Repressor E2Fs

E2F4 and E2F5

E2F4 and E2F5 represent the E2F class of repressors governed by pocket proteins. Both members are nuclear during early stages of the cell cycle and are thought to be necessary to repress cell cycle gene activity, but become exported from the nucleus as the cell cycle continues and cell cycle genes should be expressed [57, 58]. E2F4 is constitutively expressed throughout the cell cycle, while E2F5 is expressed more highly during mid-G_1 [30]. Over-expression of E2F4 and E2F5 revealed that they did not have a similar capacity as activator E2Fs to drive cell cycle reentry in quiescent cells, and instead they tended to act as repressors of E2F-responsive genes [24]. This repressor effect may be tissue specific as other groups have found that E2F4 over-expression drove neonatal cardiomyocytes into S phase [59] and promoted cellular proliferation during fetal erythropoiesis [60].

Knockout mouse models of E2F4 and E2F5 are in agreement with early studies, depicting them as negative regulators of the cell cycle important in terminal differentiation. MEFs lacking E2F4 and E2F5 are unable to exit the cell cycle [61], and DKO mice die late in embryogenesis due to defects in differentiation [62]. E2F4$^{-/-}$ mice display defects in differentiation of erythrocytes as well as gut epithelial cells and die very early due to increased susceptibility to infections [63, 64]. E2F5$^{-/-}$ mice develop a nonlethal hydrocephalus due to excess cerebrospinal fluid production attributed to a defect in choroid plexus differentiation [57]. Like E2F1, E2F5 also appears to play a role in the development of cancer [65, 66].

E2F6

E2F6 was the first E2F family member identified which did not have a C-terminal activation domain and was a strong repressor of E2F activity [67]. When over-expressed, E2F6 has been demonstrated to inhibit cell cycle progression and cell cycle reentry in quiescent cells [67, 68]. The truncated C-terminus of E2F6 alluded to the fact that its mechanisms of regulation and its manner of repression are independent of the classical pocket protein pathway. Although not regulated by the cell cycle in the same manner as activating E2Fs, E2F6 expression does change throughout the cell cycle. Its expression is up-regulated at both the mRNA and protein level at the G_1/S phase boundary. Our laboratory has shown that E2F6's promoter contains two E2F-binding elements which when bound by other E2Fs, activates E2F6 expression [69]. This implies that when activating E2Fs are expressed early in the cell cycle, they up-regulate E2F6 expression to ensure there is no improper passage through the G_1/S checkpoint. In support of this, ChIP studies demonstrated that E2F6 could be found bound to E2F-responsive gene promoters during G_1 and S phase but not other phases of the cell cycle [22].

E2F6's capacity to repress gene expression appears to involve the recruitment of polycomb group proteins (PcGs). PcGs include a wide variety of chromatin-modifying enzymes found in two distinct types of complexes which are epigenetic gene silencers during development [70]. The polycomb repressive complex 2 (PRC2) is important for the definition and trimethylation of genes to be repressed at histone 3 lysine 27 (H3K27). This marker recruits the PRC1 complex for long-term silencing marked by trimethylation at histone 3 lysine 9 (H3K9). E2F6 has been identified in complexes containing proteins from both types of complexes including Bmi1, Ring and YY1 binding protein (RYBP), EPC1, and EZH2 [24, 25].

Complimenting E2F6's interaction with PcG proteins, deletion of E2F6 has a similar phenotype to the deletion of the PcG protein Bmi1, including posterior homeotic transformations of the axial skeleton [71]. Interestingly, MEFs from these mice did not display any defect in proliferative capacity. The authors have attributed this to functional compensation by E2F4. A similar effect was observed previously in ChIP experiments in which E2F4 replaced missing E2F6 at responsive genes in E2F6 KOs [36].

E2F6 has also been described in a unique complex in HeLa cells capable of binding to E2F sites during G_0 [72]. This E2F6 complex includes DP1, HMET, HP1, various PcGs, as well as the transcription factors Max and Mga. This complex was capable of binding and repressing E2F, as well as Max and Mga-responsive genes (E-box and T-box sites), thereby implicating E2F6 in a complex which could be important for the repression of an expansive array of genes during cell-cycle arrest. Although this study differs with other studies suggesting only E2F4 is expressed and bound to promoters during G_0 [22], the authors have attributed the observed differences to the use of different cell types and mechanisms of cell-cycle arrest. This appears plausible since ChIP studies done by Xu [73] and colleagues found that E2F1, E2F4, and E2F6 could be found bound to the same promoters in various cell types, yet E2F6 appeared to have some specific functions in Ntera2 cells in which it bound to its own set of genes. This suggests that E2Fs can share interchangeable roles, yet in specific cells and settings E2F6 (as well as other E2Fs) could play some unique roles in gene expression. These special roles probably involve interactions with other transcription factors and chromatin-modifying enzymes.

E2F7 and E2F8

E2F7 and E2F8 represent the last group of E2Fs that have been identified. Like E2F6 they are not regulated by pocket proteins and unlike all other E2Fs, they do not dimerize with DPs. They appear to be strong repressors of E2F activity which, unlike other E2Fs, are capable of inhibiting cellular proliferation when over-expressed [74, 75]. The two proteins appear to have overlapping roles in development since individual KO mice develop normally but DKO mice die very early during embryonic development due to mass apoptosis in various cell lineages [75]. Their redundancy is supported by their capacity to form heterodimers to repress gene expression.

Moon and Dyson [76] review a feedback loop, similar to what we described for E2F6 [69] in which E2F1 expression activates the transcription of E2F7 and E2F8 which, in turn, represses E2F-responsive genes including E2F1 itself. In fact, the lethal apoptosis in E2F7/E2F8 DKO mice has been attributed to elevated levels of both E2F1 and p53 [75]. Interestingly the mice also exhibit severe dilation of blood vessels which is not yet understood but may represent a specific function for these outlier E2Fs outside of repressing E2F1.

Counterintuitive to its role as a repressor of proliferation and E2F1-mediated apoptosis, E2F8 is up-regulated in human hepatocarcinoma (HCC) specimens [77]. Furthermore, its knockdown is sufficient to inhibit colony formation of HCC-derived cell lines and decrease tumorogenicity in vivo. The authors found that E2F8 over-expression caused an increase in DNA synthesis and cyclin D1 expression, which has been previously linked to HCC [78] while knockdown had the opposite effect. The authors have attributed this unexpected up-regulation of cyclin D1 (an E2F target) to excess E2F8, outcompeting E2F1 which would normally bind in association with pRb leading to gene repression [77].

This study is a perfect example of how E2Fs cannot be restricted to activators and repressors of gene expression and cellular proliferation, but the outcome of E2F activity will depend on the regulation of a delicate balance in E2F activity. Although not all E2F members are necessary for viability, the size of the family not only safeguards against mutation but also allows the tight regulation of development and function in complex mammalian tissues and organisms. E2F activity will depend on a variety of different factors including genetic context of E2Fs as well as their responsive genes, subcellular localization, tissue expression, and cell-cycle stage/signals.

E2Fs in Cardiac Growth and Pathology

Since proper cardiac development requires a very tight regulation of the cell cycle, it is likely that the E2F pathway will play a pivotal role in cardiac development and pathology, as demonstrated in

Table 1 E2F pathway function in the heart. Knockout mouse models of E2F and partner proteins

Gene	Phenotype	Reference
E2F1	Cardiac apoptosis.	[42, 43]
E2F3	Partial penetrant embryonic lethality due to cardiac developmental defects. Young adults develop congestive heart failure.	[44, 54, 55]
E2F1, E2F2, E2F3a	Partial embryonic lethal, perinatal lethal. Reduction in white adipose tissue deposits.	[56]
E2F1, E2F2, E2F3b	Viable, but have reduced body weight.	[56]
E2F7, E2F8	Embryonic lethal. Excess apoptosis (due to increased E2F1 and p53) and blood vessel dilation.	[75]
Rb[a], p130	Cardiac hyperplasia.	[90]
Rb[a], p107	Embryonic lethal. Increased proliferation in central nervous system, blood vessel endothelial cells, and heart defects (double-outlet right ventricle).	[91]

[a] Cardiac restricted deletion

the E2F3 KO studies described earlier (summarized in Table 1). E2F1 was the first of the E2F family to display a role in cardiomyocyte cell-cycle control. When neonatal cardiomyocytes were transfected with E2F1, they displayed a marked increase in DNA synthesis accompanied by a high rate of apoptosis, thereby demonstrating for the first time the capacity of E2Fs to control cardiomyocyte cell cycle and death [79, 80]. Since neonatal cardiomyocytes still retain some proliferative capacity and differ greatly from post-mitotic adult cardiomyocytes, adult rat ventricular myocytes were transfected with E2F1 which induced DNA synthesis, but to a lesser extent (19% vs. 47%) which again was accompanied by apoptosis [80]. The effects of ectopic expression of E2F1 were also explored in vivo by injecting adenoviral-E2F1 into the myocardium of adult mice. Similar to the cardiomyocytes, an increase in DNA synthesis was observed and cardiomyocytes accumulated in G2/M but none were capable of overcoming the G2/M checkpoint to proliferate. Since E2F1 interacts with the p53 pathway, Agah [80] and colleagues tried transfecting E2F1 into the myocardium of p53 null mice. Surprisingly this did not alleviate the rate of apoptosis, indicating that E2F1 can induce cell death in a p53-independent pathway.

In addition to the p53 pathway of apoptosis, the mitochondria play an important role in programmed cell death. During hypoxic injury the mitochondrial permeability pore opens, causing a loss of membrane potential and cytotoxic protein release which activates apoptotic pathways leading to ventricular myocyte death [81]. It has previously been shown that the mitochondrial death protein Bnip3 plays a role as a sensor of oxidative stress during MI [82] and its induced expression leads to ventricular myocyte death [83]. Yurkova [84] showed that ectopic E2F1 directly activates the transcription of this death factor *Bnip3*. Protein levels of Bnip3 were not confirmed, but two inhibitors of Bnip rescued cells from the apoptosis incurred by E2F1 in cardiomyocytes [84]. Thus it appears that E2F not only plays a role in apoptosis by interacting with p53 but in cardiomyocytes also by directly controlling the levels of hypoxia-inducible pro-apoptotic factors.

In addition to regulating apoptosis in cardiomyocytes, it appears that the E2F family also plays a central role in regulating cell growth, a very important aspect of cardiomyopathic heart failure. Upon hypertrophic stimulation with phenylephrine (PE) E2F1–4 and E2F6 become up-regulated in neonatal cardiomyocytes [85, 86]. Vara and colleagues further demonstrated the importance of the E2F pathway in cardiac hypertrophy by inhibiting the pathway with specific inhibitors for E2F/DP heterodimerization, which resulted in a decrease in the intensity of hypertrophy as well as blocked the expression of hypertrophic markers ANP and BNP [85].

A few years later the capacity of E2Fs to induce cell cycle reentry in the heart was evaluated and indeed over-expression of E2F1–4 induced S phase in neonatal cardiomyocytes by inducing transcription of cyclins A and E [59]. In this study only E2F2 and E2F4 induced S phase without also causing apoptosis and only E2F2 over-expression resulted in mitosis. In order to determine if this was relevant in the adult heart, Ebelt and colleagues stably over-expressed E2F2 and E2F4 in adult mouse hearts by adenoviral infection [87]. Similar to what was observed in the neonatal cardiomyocytes, over-expression of both E2F2 and E2F4 resulted in the reentry of cardiomyocytes into S phase and cardiomyocyte hypertrophy. More importantly, expression of E2F2 also resulted in a modest increase in the number of mitotic adult cardiomyocytes. This is especially interesting since E2F2 is not normally expressed in the heart [41, 88]. Perhaps a lack of E2F2 hints at a protective mechanism against excess proliferation in the heart in order to maintain postnatal cardiac function. It also points to a therapy to stimulate cardiac regeneration post-myocardial infarction.

Recently van Amerongen [89] and colleagues demonstrated a specific function for E2F4 during cardiomyocyte mitosis. In this study E2F4 over-expression did not induce cell-cycle entry in cardiomyocytes. Although this differs from earlier work in which Ebelt [59] found that E2F4 over-expression induces DNA synthesis, different time points of cardiomyocyte isolation were used in each experimental study. In Ebelt's [59] study cardiomyocytes were isolated from newborn rats, while in van Amerongen's [89] study cardiomyocytes were isolated from 3-day-old rat hearts. At day 3 cardiomyocytes may have lost some proliferative capacity when taking into consideration that they permanently exit the cell cycle within a few days after birth. In this study both the expression and nuclear localization of E2F4 were correlated to cardiac development and the proliferative potential of cardiomyocytes, supporting its role in normal cardiac growth and development [89]. Unexpectedly, the authors found that E2F4 co-localized with kinetochores in cardiomyocytes and when knocked down by siRNA-restricted mitosis, suggesting a potential novel role for E2F4 in cell cycle regulation

outside of transcriptional control. The relevance of these results in the adult myocardium is unknown as this was tested in postnatal cardiomyocytes which were artificially stimulated to proliferate (using FGF1 and a p38 inhibitor), but may be a useful tool in cardiac regeneration studies.

Pocket-Protein-Mediated E2F Regulation in the Heart

In addition to a balance in levels of individual E2F family members, appropriate regulation of the E2F pathway by pocket proteins is crucial for normal cardiac development. Although cardiac-specific deletion of individual pocket proteins does not lead to specific cardiac defects, compound knockouts tell a different story. Since pRb$^{-/-}$ mice are not viable cardiac-restricted knockouts of pRb in conjunction with p130 or p107 knockouts have been utilized. Ablation of p130 and cardiac pRb led to a threefold increase in heart weight: body weight ratio due to abnormal hyperplasia [90]. In this model an increase in Myc, E2F1, and G$_1$ CDK activity was observed, indicating that indeed the E2F pathway and cell cycle had been activated.

The importance of p107 in the heart was also highlighted in a study in which an embryonic lethal double knockout of pRb and p107 developed cardiac defects [91]. Mice lacking the two proteins developed a double outlet right ventricle (pulmonary artery and aorta exit from the right ventricle) and many embryos also displayed thinner myocardium, dilated atria, and septal defects [91]. Thus it appears that all three pocket proteins play an important role in cardiac development although, much like the E2Fs, they have the capacity to compensate for each other's loss.

Clinical Relevance and Conclusions

Accumulating evidence suggests that appropriate regulation of the E2F/pocket protein pathway is crucial to normal cardiac development. Highlighting this is the developmental regulation of individual E2F and pocket protein members within the heart [4, 86, 90]. Recently, a direct link between E2Fs and congestive heart failure was demonstrated in humans. In this study patients with CHF displayed up-regulated levels of E2F1, pRb, p107, and p130 in comparison with control patients [92]. A positive correlation between pRb and p130 with cardiomyocyte diameter was also found, suggestive of their role in cardiomyocyte hypertrophy. Following unloading by left ventricular assistance device, a significant decrease in expression of E2F1 and pocket proteins was observed, indicating that ventricular unloading can reverse the process. Thus it appears that similar to studies in cultured cardiomyocytes and mouse models, the E2F/pocket protein pathway is a pivotal player in pathological cardiac hypertrophy. This fits well with recent studies which correlate an up-regulation of genes involved in cell cycle reentry (which are controlled by E2Fs) with cardiac hypertrophy and heart failure [2, 3].

In addition to playing an important role in regulating cardiac hypertrophy, the capacity of E2Fs to regulate cell cycle entry and exit may prove to be very important tools in cardiac regeneration. The capacity of E2F2 to induce proliferation in vivo is sufficient to warrant further investigation. Furthermore, the expression and role of the pocket-protein-independent E2Fs in the heart has yet to be addressed. The mechanisms of E2F6–8 are still quite poorly understood and will probably also prove important in cardiac development and disease.

Acknowledgments Funded by CIHR.

References

1. Pasumarthi KBS, Field LJ. Cardiomyocyte cell cycle regulation. Circ Res. 2002;90:1044–54.
2. Frey N, Olson EN. Cardiac hypertrophy: the good, the bad, and the ugly. Annu Rev Physiol. 2003;65:45–79.
3. Li JM, Poolman RA, Brooks G. Role of G1 phase cyclins and cyclin-dependent kinases during cardiomyocyte hypertrophic growth in rats. J Phys. 1998;275:H814–22.
4. Ahuga P, Sdek P, Maclellan R. Cardiac myocyte cell cycle control in development, disease, and regeneration. Physiol Rev. 2007;87:521–44.
5. Sherr CJ. G1 phase progression: cycling on cue. Cell. 1994;79:551–5.
6. Sherr CJ, Roberts JM. Inhibitors of mammalian G1 cyclin-dependent kinases. Genes Dev. 1995;9:149–1163.
7. Lim JM, Brooks G. Downregulation of cyclin dependant kinase inhibitors p21 and p27 in pressure-overload hypertrophy. Am J Physiol Heart Circ Physiol. 1997;273:H1358–67.
8. Berthet C, Klarmann KD, Hilton MB, et al. Combined loss of Cdk2 and Cdk4 results in embryonic lethality and Rb hypophosphorylation. Dev Cell. 2006;10:563–73.
9. Soonpa MH, Koh GY, Pajak L, et al. Cyclin D1 overexpression promotes cardiomyocyte DNA synthesis and multinucleation in transgenic mice. J Clin Invest. 1997;99:2644–54.
10. Liao HS, Kang PM, Nagashima H, et al. Cardiac-specific overexpression of cyclin- dependent kinase 2 increases smaller mononuclear cardiomyocytes. Circ Res. 2001;88:443.
11. Ishida S, Huang E, Zuzan H, et al. Role for E2F in control of both DNA replication and mitotic functions as revealed from DNA microarray analysis. Mol Cell Biol. 2001;21:4684–99.
12. Muller H, Bracken A, Vernell R, et al. E2Fs regulate the expression of genes involved in differentiation, development, proliferation, and apoptosis. Genes Dev. 2008;15:267–85.
13. Ren B, Cam H, Takahashi Y, et al. E2F integrates cell cycle progression with DNA repair, replication, and G(2)/M checkpoints. Genes Dev. 2002;16:245–56.
14. Tao Y, Kasszatly RF, Cress WD, et al. Subunit composition determines E2F DNA binding site specificity. Mol Cell Biol. 1997;17:6994–7007.
15. Helin K, Wu CL, Fattaey AR, et al. Heterodimerization of the transcription factors E2F-1 and DP-1 leads to cooperative trans-activation. Genes Dev. 1993;7:1850–61.
16. Di Stefano L, Rugaard Jensen M, Helin K. E2F7, a novel E2F featuring DP-independent repression of a subset of E2F-regulated genes. EMBO J. 2003;22:6289–98.
17. Baidehi M, Jing L, de Bruin A, et al. Cloning and characterization of mouse *E2F8*, a novel mammalian *E2F* family member capable of blocking cellular proliferation. J Biol Chem. 2005;280:18211–20.
18. Johnson DG, Schneider-Broussard R. Identification of E2F-3B, an alternative form of E2F-3 lacking a conserved N-terminal region. Front Biosci. 1998;3:447–58.
19. Flemington EK, Speck SH, Kaelin Jr WG. E2F-1 mediated transactivation is inhibited by complex formation with the retinoblastoma susceptibility gene product. Proc Natl Acad Sci USA. 1993;90:6914–8.
20. Kitagawa M, Higashi H, Suzuki-Takahashi I, et al. Phosphorylation of E2F-1 by cyclin A-cdk2. Oncogene. 1995;10:229–36.
21. Krek W, Ewen ME, Shirodkar S, et al. Negative regulation of the growth-promoting transcription factor E2F-1 by a stably bound cyclin-A dependant protein kinase. Cell. 1994;78:161–72.

22. Takahashi Y, Rayman J, Dynlacht B. Analysis of promoter binding by the E2F and pRB families in vivo: distinct E2F proteins mediate activation and repression. Genes Dev. 2000;14:804–16.
23. Mariconti L, Pellegrini B, Cantoni R, et al. The E2F family of transcription factors from Arabidopsis thaliana. Novel and conserved components of the retinoblastoma/E2F pathway in plants. J Biol Chem. 2002;277:9911–19.
24. Trimarchi JM, Fairchild B, Wen J, et al. The E2F6 transcription factor is a component of the mammalian Bmi1-containing polycomb complex. Proc Natl Acad Sci USA. 2001;98:1519–24.
25. Attwooll C, Oddi S, Cartwright P, et al. A novel repressive E2F6 complex containing the polycomb group protein, EPC1, that interacts with EZH2 in a proliferation-specific manner. J Biol Chem. 2005;280: 1199–208.
26. Ohtani K, Nevins JR. Functional properties of a Drosophila homolog of the E2F1 gene. Mol Cell Biol. 1994;14:1603–12.
27. Ceol C, Horvitz H. dpl-1 DP and efl-1 E2F act with lin-35 Rb to antagonize ras signaling in C. elegans vulval development. Mol Cell. 2001;7:461–73.
28. Ramirrez P, Xie Q, Boniotti M, et al. The cloning of plant E2F, a retinoblastoma-binding protein, reveals unique and conserved features with animal G(1)/S regulators. Nucleic Acids Res. 1999;27:3527–33.
29. Lees JA, Saito M, Vidal M, et al. The retinoblastoma protein binds to an E2F family of transcription factors. Mol Cell Biol. 1993;13:7813–25.
30. Moberg K, Starz MA, Lees JA. E2F-4 switches from p130 to p107 and pRb in response to cell cycle reentry. Mol Cell Biol. 1996;16:1436–49.
31. Ginsberg D, Vairo G, Chittenden T, et al. E2F-4, a new member of the E2F transcription factor family, interacts with p107. Genes Dev. 1994;8:2665–79.
32. Brehm A, Miska EA, McCance DJ, et al. Retinoblastoma protein recruits histone deacetylase to repress transcription. Nature. 1998;391:597–601.
33. Ferreira R, Magnaghi-Jaulin L, Robin P, et al. The three members of the pocket proteins family share the ability to repress E2F activity through recruitment of a histone deacetylase. Proc Natl Acad Sci USA. 1998;95:10493–8.
34. Marzio G, Wagener C, Gutirrez MA, et al. E2F family members are differentially regulated by reversible acetylation. J Biol Chem. 2000;275:10887–92.
35. Taubert S, Forrini C, Frank SR, et al. E2D-dependent histone acetylation and recruitment of the Tip60 acetyltransferase complex to chromatin in late G_1. Mol Cell Biol. 2004;24:4546–56.
36. Giangrande PH, Zhu W, Schlisio S, et al. A role for E2F6 in distinguishing G1/S- and G2/M-specific transcription. Genes Dev. 2004;18:2941–51.
37. Lukas J, Petersen BO, Holm K, et al. Deregulated expression of E2F family members induces S-phase entry and overcomes p16INK4A-mediated growth suppression. Mol Cell Biol. 1996;16:1047–57.
38. Wu L, Timmers C, Maiti B, et al. The E2F1-3 transcription factors are essential for cellular proliferation. Nature. 2003;414:457–62.
39. Johnson Ohanti K, Nevins JR. Autoregulatory control of E2F1 expression in response to positive and negative regulators of cell cycle progression. Genes Dev. 1994;8:1514–25.
40. Leone G, DeGregori J, Yan Z, et al. E2F3 activity is regulated during the cell cycle and is required for the induction of S phase. Genes Dev. 1998;12:2120–30.
41. Slansky JE, Farnham PJ. Introduction to the E2F family: protein structure and gene regulation. Curr Top Microbiol Immunol. 1996;208:1–30.
42. Field SJ, Tsai F, Kuo F, et al. E2F-1 functions in mice to promote apoptosis and suppress proliferation. Cell. 1996;85:549–61.
43. Yamasaki L, Jacks T, Bronson R, et al. Tumor induction and tissue atrophy in mice lacking E2F-1. Cell. 1996;85:537–48.
44. Cloud JE, Rogers C, Reza TL, et al. Mutant mouse models reveal the relative roles of E2F1 and E2F3 in vivo. Mol Cell Biol. 2002;22:2663–72.
45. Han S, Park K, Bae BN, et al. E2F1 expression is related with the poor survival of lymph node-positive breast cancer patients treated with fluorouracil, doxorubicin and cyclophosphamide. Breast Cancer Res Treat. 2003;82:11–6.
46. Reimer D, Sadr S, Wiedemair A, et al. Expression of the E2F family of transcription factors and its clinical relevance in ovarian cancer. Ann NY Acad Sci. 2006; 1091:270–81.
47. Xiao Q, Li L, Xie Y, et al. Transcription factor E2F-1 is upregulated in human gastric cancer tissues and its overexpression suppresses gastric tumor cell proliferation. Cell Oncl. 2007;29:335–49.
48. Yamasaki L, Bronson R, Williams BO, et al. Loss of E2F-1 reduces tumorigenesis and extends the lifespan of Rb (+/−) mice. Nat Genet. 1998;18:360–4.
49. Haupt Y, Maya R, Kazaz A, et al. Mdm2 promotes the rapid degradation of p53. Nature. 1997;387: 296–9.
50. Hiebart SW, Packham G, Strom DK, et al. E2F1:Dp1 induces p53 and overrides survival factors to trigger apoptosis. Mol Cell Biol. 1995;5:6864–74.
51. Hsieh J, Yap D, O'Connor DJ, et al. Novel function of the cyclin A binding site of E2F in Regulating p-53 induced apoptosis in response to DNA Damage. Mol Cell Biol. 2002;22:78–93.
52. Rogers Kt, Higgons PDR, Milla MM, et al. DP-2, a heterodimeric partner of E2F: identification and characterization ofn DP-2 proteins expressed in vivo. Proc Nat Acad Sci USA. 1996;93:7594–9.
53. Murga M, Fernandez-Capetillo O, Field SJ, et al. Mutation of E2F2 in mice causes enhanced T lymphocyte proliferation, leading to the development of autoimmunity. Immunity. 2001;15:959–70.
54. Humbert PO, Verona R, Trimarchi JM, et al. E2F3 is critical for normal cellular proliferation. Genes Dev. 2000;14:690–703.

55. King JJ, Moskowitz I, Burgon P, et al. E2F3 plays an essential role in cardiac development and function. Cell Cycle. 2008;7:3775–37780.

56. Tsai SY, Opavsky R, Sharma N, et al. Mouse development with a single E2F activator. Nature. 2008;458:137–1142.

57. Lindeman GJ, Dagnino L, Gaubatz S, et al. A specific, non-proliferative role for e2F-5 in choroid plexus function revealed by gene targeting. Genes Dev. 1998;12:1092–8.

58. Verona R, Moberg K, Estes S, et al. E2F activity is regulated by cell cycle-dependent changes in subcellular localization. Mol Cell Biol. 1997;17:7268–82.

59. Ebelt H, Hufnagel N, Neuhaus P, et al. Divergent siblings: E2F2 and E2F4 but not E2F1 and E2F3 induce DNA synthesis in cardiomyocytes without activation of apoptosis. Circ Res. 2005;96:509–17.

60. Kinross KM, Clark AJ, Iazzolino RM, et al. E2f4 regulates fetal erythropoiesis through the promotion of cellular proliferation. Blood. 2006;108:886–95.

61. Bruce JL, Hurford RK, Classon M, et al. Requirements for cell cycle arrest by p16(INK4A). Mol Cell. 2000;6:737–42.

62. Gaubatz S, Lindeman GJ, Ishida S, et al. E2F4 and E2F5 play an essential role in pocket protein-mediated G1 control. Mol Cell. 2000;6:729–35.

63. Humbert PO, Rogers C, Ganiastas S, et al. E2F4 is essential for normal erythrocyte maturation and neonate viability. Mol Cell. 2004;6:281–91.

64. Rempel R, Saenz-Robels M, Storms R, et al. Loss of E2F4 activity leads to abnormal development of multiple cellular lineages. Mol Cell. 2000;6:293–306.

65. Kothandaraman N, Bajic VB, Brendan PNK, et al. E2F5 status significantly improves malignancy diagnosis of epithelial ovarian cancer. BMC Cancer. 2010;10:1–13.

66. Polanowska J, Le Cam L, Orsetti B, et al. Human E2F5 gene is oncogenic in primary rodent cells and is amplified in human breast tumors. Gen Chromo Cancer. 2000;28:126–30.

67. Gaubatz S, Wood JG, Livingston JM. Unusual proliferation arrest and transcriptional control properties of a newly discovered E2F family member, E2F-6. Proc Natl Acad Sci USA. 1998;95:9190–5.

68. Cartwright P, Muller H, Wagner C, et al. E2F-6: a novel member of the E2F family is an inhibitor of E2F-dependent transcription. Oncogene. 1998;17:611–23.

69. Lyons T, Salih M, Tuana BS. Activatings E2Fs mediate transcriptional regulation of human E2F6 repressor. Am J Physiol Cell Physiol. 2006;290:C189–99.

70. Sparmann A, van Lohuizen M. Polycomb silencers control cell fate, development and cancer. Nat Rev Cancer. 2006;6:846–56.

71. Storre J, Elsasser H, Fuchs M, et al. Homeotic transformations of the axial skeleton that accompany a targeted deletion of E2f6. EMBO Rep. 2002;3:695–700.

72. Ogawa H, Ishiguro K, Gaubatz S, Livingston DM, Nakatani Y. A complex with chromatin modifiers that occupies E2F- and myc-responsive genes in G0 cells. Science. 2002;296:1132–6.

73. Xu X, Bedia M, Jin V, et al. A comprehensive ChIP-chip analysis of E2F1, E2F4, and E2F6 in normal and tumor cells reveals interchangeable roles of E2F family members. Genome Res. 2007;17:1550–61.

74. Christensen J, Cloos P, Toftegaard U. Characterization of E2F8, a novel E2F-like cell-cycle regulated repressor of E2F-activated transcription. Nucleic Acids Res. 2005;33:5458–70.

75. Li J, Ran C, Li E, Gordon F, et al. Synergistic function of E2F7 and E2F8 is essential for cell survival and embryonic development. Dev Cell. 2007;14:62–75.

76. Moon NS, Dyson N. E2F7 and E2F8 keep the E2F family in balance. Dev Cell. 2008;14:1–3.

77. Deng Q, Wang Q, Zong WY. E2F8 Contributes to human hepatocellular carcinoma via regulating cell proliferation. Cancer Res. 2010;70:782–91.

78. Tashiro E, Tsuchiya A, Imoto M. Functions of cyclin D1 as an oncogene and regulation of cyclin D1 expression. Cancer Sci. 2007;98:629–35.

79. Kirshenbaum LA, Abdellatif M, Chakraborty S, et al. Human E2F-1 reactivates cell cycle progression in ventricular myocytes and represses cardiac gene transcription. Dev Biol. 1996;179:402–11.

80. Agah R, Kirschebaum LA, Abdellatif M, et al. Adenoviral delivery of E2F-1 directs cell cycle reentry and p53-independent apoptosis in post mitotic adult myocardium In Vivo. J Clin Invest. 1997;100:2722–8.

81. Wang C, Youle RJ. The role of mitochondria in apoptosis. Annu Rev Genet. 2009;43:95–118.

82. Kubli DA, Quinsay MN, Huang C, et al. Bnip3 functions as a mitochondrial sensor of oxidative stress during myocardial ischemia and reperfusion. Am J Physiol Heart Circ Physiol. 2008;295:H2025–31.

83. Regula KM, Ens K, Kirschenbaum LA. Inducible expression of BNIP3 provokes mitochondrial defects and hypoxia mediated cell death of ventricular myocytes. Circ Res. 2002;91:226–31.

84. Yurkova N, Shaw J, Blackie K, et al. The cell cycle factor E2F-1 activates Bnip3 and the intrinsic death pathway in ventricular myocytes. Circ Res. 2008;102:472–9.

85. Vara D, Bicknell KA, Coxon CH, et al. Inhibition of E2F abrogates the development of cardiac myocyte hypertrophy. J Biol Chem. 2003;278:21388–94.

86. Movassagh M, Bicknell KA, Brooks G. Characterization and regulation of E2F-6 and E2F-6b in the rat heart: a potential target for myocardial regeneration? J Pharm Pharmacol. 2006;58:73–82.

87. Ebelt H, Zhang Y, Kampke A, et al. E2F2 expression induces proliferation of terminally differentiated cardiomyocytes in vivo. Cardiovasc Res. 2008;80:219–26.

88. Dirlam A, Spike BT, MaCleod KF. Deregulated E2f-2 underlies cell cycle and maturation defects in retino-

blastoma null erythroblasts. Mol Cell Biol. 2007;27: 8713–28.

89. van Amerongen MJ, Diehl F, Novoyatleva T, et al. E2F4 is required for cardiomyocytes proliferation. Cardiovasc Res. 2010;86:92–102.

90. MacLellan WR, Garcia A, Oh H, et al. Overlapping roles of pocket proteins in the myocardium are unmasked by germline specific deletion of p130 plus heart specific deletion of Rb. Mol Cell Biol. 2005; 25:2486–97.

91. Berman SD, West JC, Danielian PS, et al. Mutation of p107 exacerbates the consequences of Rb loss in embryonic tissues and causes cardiac and blood vessel defects. Proc Nat Acad Sci USA. 2009;106: 14932–6.

92. Wohlschlaeger J, Jurgen Smitz K, Takeda A, et al. Reversible regulation of the retinoblastoma protein/ E2F-1 pathway during "reverse cardiac remodeling" after ventricular unloading. J Heart Lung Transplant. 2010;29:117–24.

Cardiac Sodium–Calcium Exchanger Expression

Cecilia Hurtado, Thane G. Maddaford, and Grant N. Pierce

Abstract

The sodium–calcium exchanger (NCX) is thought to be a critical protein in excitation-contraction (E-C) coupling in the heart through its regulation of intracellular $[Ca^{2+}]$. The exchanger removes Ca^{2+} from the cell in exchange for extracellular Na^+ in the "forward mode" to induce cardiac relaxation. Although still controversial, NCX may also participate in cardiomyocyte contractile activity in a "reverse mode" by bringing Ca^{2+} into the cell in exchange for intracellular Na^+. In addition to its important physiological role, the NCX has been associated with the pathology of ischemia-reperfusion injury, hypertension, cardiac hypertrophy, and heart failure. Therefore, it has the potential of being a valuable therapeutic target in the treatment of heart disease.

A limitation in the study of the exchanger has been the dearth of pharmacological blockers that specifically inhibit the NCX. Initially, therefore, the role of NCX in ischemic injury was elucidated with the use of blockers of the Na^+-H^+ exchanger, an upstream component of the NCX in the ischemia-reperfusion pathway. These drugs effectively inhibited the Na^+-H^+ exchange-NCX cascade during ischemia and early reperfusion to provide cardioprotection in isolated hearts and cardiomyocytes. Alternatively, the development of new genetic tools to increase or down-regulate the expression of the NCX has effectively characterized the role of the NCX in contractile activity and during ischemic injury. Compared to alternative molecular approaches to alter gene expression, the adenovirally delivered shRNA has been the most efficient method to alter gene expression in vitro. Cardiomyocytes with significantly depleted NCX through adenovirally delivered shRNA can still contract but are cardioprotected from ischemic

G.N. Pierce (✉)
Institute of Cardiovascular Sciences, St. Boniface
Hospital Research Centre, and the Department of
Physiology, University of Manitoba, Winnipeg,
Manitoba, Canada
e-mail: gpierce@sbrc.ca

B. Ostadal et al. (eds.), *Genes and Cardiovascular Function*,
DOI 10.1007/978-1-4419-7207-1_5, © Springer Science+Business Media, LLC 2011

insult. Furthermore, the cardiac isoform NCX1.1 causes more severe Ca^{2+} overload during ischemia-reperfusion injury and glycoside toxicity than the renal NCX1.3 isoform of the exchanger when they are expressed in neonatal cardiomyocytes and HEK-293 cells. In summary, the data support an important but not a critical role for NCX in excitation-contraction coupling in the heart but an important, possibly critical role, for the NCX in ischemic reperfusion injury and drug-induced challenges. Overall, these results identify NCX as an important molecule to target to develop new strategies to influence heart function and dysfunction.

Keywords

Ca^{2+}-transport • Ischemia/reperfusion injury • Myocardium • Na^+-Ca^{2+} exchanger • Na^+-H^+ exchanger

Introduction

Calcium is used within the cells as an intracellular messenger. Local and temporal changes in Ca^{2+} concentration activate a wide variety of cellular functions. Intracellular Ca^{2+} concentration, therefore, needs to be tightly regulated. A number of channels and transporters maintain calcium homeostasis. The sodium–calcium exchanger (NCX) is one of the transporters that is particularly important in the heart because of its involvement in the mechanism of excitation-contraction coupling. The NCX is a plasmalemmal protein. It is found in almost all cell types and is abundant in excitable tissues, like the brain and the heart. It transports Ca^{2+} in exchange for Na^+ and is able to remove Ca^{2+} from the cell or transport it into the cell. The direction of this movement depends on the concentration gradient across the membrane for Ca^{2+} and Na^+, and also on the membrane potential. Generally, in the heart, the NCX plays an important role in Ca^{2+} removal from the cell during relaxation and may also contribute to Ca^{2+} influx during the peak of an action potential.

In addition to its important physiological role, the NCX has been associated with the pathology of ischemia-reperfusion injury, hypertension, cardiac hypertrophy, and heart failure. Therefore, it has the potential of being a valuable therapeutic target in the treatment of heart disease. Intensive study of the NCX would be of great value not only to advance our understanding of the function of the heart during normal healthy conditions but also to devise strategies to improve cardiac performance under pathological challenge as well.

NCX Structure

The 938 amino acids that form the mature cardiac NCX protein are arranged in 9 transmembrane segments (Fig. 1) [1]. Five transmembrane segments are present in the amino part of the protein and are separated from the other four by a large intracellular loop. A leader peptide, corresponding to the first amino acids of the protein, is removed during processing of the protein [2]. Once the leader peptide is removed, the resulting amino end is extracellular and glycosylated [3]. Two regions with homologous sequences are found within the protein: α-1 is located between transmembrane segments 2 and 3, and α-2, between transmembrane segments 7 and 8. The α-1 and α-2 sequences form reentrant loops that are involved in ion translocation [4–7]. These regions of homology are believed to have originated by gene duplication and can be found in other proteins of the NCX superfamily [8]. The large intracellular loop is involved in regulation of NCX activity. It contains the XIP (eXchanger

Fig. 1 Topological model of the cardiac NCX. Regulatory regions of the intracellular loop are indicated with boxes. Numbers indicate the amino acids positions. TM, transmembrane segments; $\alpha 1$ and $\alpha 2$, regions of intramolecular homology; XIP, exchanger inhibitory peptide region. From [1] with modifications

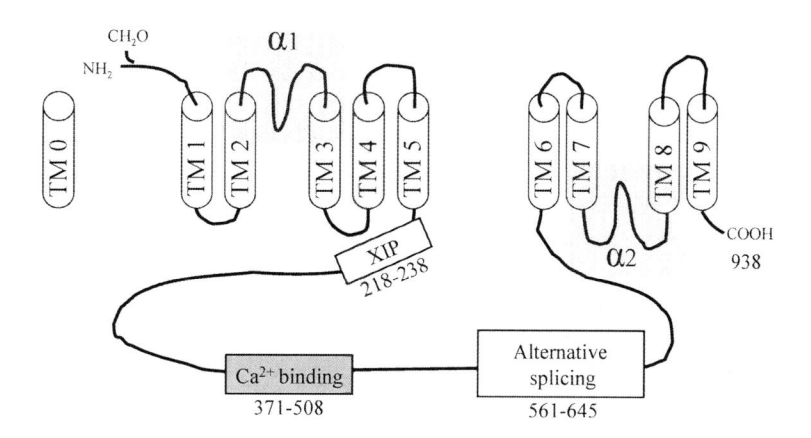

Inhibitory Peptide) region, the regulatory Ca^{2+} binding site, and the region of alternative splicing. The region of alternative splicing will be discussed in the "NCX isoforms" section. The C-terminus is found on the cytoplasmic side of the protein.

The topology of the NCX that is currently accepted was determined by studying the ability of cysteine residues at different locations to form disulfide bonds [1, 9]. These studies indicated that the α repeats are located on opposite sides of the membrane and close to each other in the folded protein. A previous model, based on hydropathy analysis of the cloned NCX, had established that the exchanger was composed of 12 transmembrane segments [10].

The XIP region corresponds to amino acids 218–238, and is located close to the N-terminus of the intracellular loop. The sequence of this region was found to be similar to a calmodulin-binding site [11]. It is rich in hydrophobic and basic amino acids. To test its regulatory properties, a peptide containing the sequence of this region was synthesized (XIP) and was found to inhibit the exchanger (see NCX inhibitors). Mutational analysis of the endogenous XIP region indicated that it is involved in Na_i^+ regulation of the exchanger [12].

Two calcium-binding domains exist within the intracellular loop: one spans amino acids 371–509 and binds calcium with high affinity [13] and another is located between amino acids 501–560 with lower calcium affinity. Calcium binding to these regions causes conformational changes that activate the protein, and mutations within these sequences affect the calcium regulatory properties of the exchanger [14]. The different calcium sensitivity would allow the exchanger to function over a wide range of intracellular calcium concentrations.

The variable region of the gene *NCX1* corresponds in the cardiac exchanger protein to amino acids 561–681, located toward the C-terminus of the intracellular loop. This region of the gene undergoes alternative splicing.

NCX Localization

In cardiomyocytes, NCX is found on the cell surface, t-tubules, and intercalated discs [15]. Thomas et al., using confocal laser scanning microscopy, showed NCX staining in adult cardiomyocytes in the vertical t-tubules, but not in the longitudinal t-tubules. NCX was co-localized with the ryanodine receptor [16]. A previous study using the same technique had failed to show any co-localization of NCX with either the Na^+ channel or ryanodine receptors but did show co-localization of ryanodine receptors with L-type Ca^{2+} channels [17]. Thomas et al. [16], looking for further resolution, used electron microscopy differential gold labeling and measured the distance that exists between the different transporters. They found that the distance separating the NCX from ryanodine receptors or L-type Ca^{2+} channels was the same as the distance between these latter two transporters (which were previously found to co-localize). It would be important to resolve this discrepancy in the future because the activity of the NCX in the Ca^{2+} entry mode would require physical proximity between these transporters to become physiologically important in excitation-contraction coupling.

NCX Isoforms

Variability in NCX isoforms and their degree of expression and tissue distribution is, in mammals, under three levels of regulation: the existence of different genes, the use of alternative promoters, and, finally, alternative splicing of the RNA transcript.

NCX Genes

Three genes code for the NCX in mammals: *NCX1* [10], *NCX2* [18], and *NCX3* [19]. The three genes were probably generated by three duplication events and one deletion: only one gene has been found in invertebrates and four (NCX1–NCX4) are found in fish, amphibians, and reptiles. In mammals, whereas *NCX1* is expressed in several tissues, *NCX2* and *NCX3* are both expressed mainly in brain and skeletal muscle [20]

Alternative Promoters

The NCX1 gene contains three alternative promoters [21–23]. Depending on the promoter, three alternative exons 1 could be incorporated, creating transcripts that are: cardiac specific, kidney specific, and one that is ubiquitous. This third transcript has highest expression in brain. The alternative exon 1 is spliced to a common exon 2. Exon 2 starts at position −31 from the translational start codon (upstream). Because exon 1 is present in the 5′UTR (untranslated terminal

repeat), its sequence will not affect protein sequence. The functional importance of the different promoters is, therefore, related to the level of expression of the protein (either constitutive or regulated by tissue-specific factors [24]). NCX gene expression has been reported to be regulated at the chromatin remodeling level by histone deacetylases.

Alternative Splicing

Variations in the structure of the protein are generated by alternative splicing of the mRNA. *NCX1* and *NCX3* undergo alternative splicing of the primary transcript. The region that undergoes splicing corresponds to the carboxyl terminus of the intracellular loop of the protein. In NCX1, the part of the gene that codes for this region is composed of six exons (A, B, C, D, E, and F, corresponding to exons number 3–8 of the 12 exons that compose NCX1) [25]. NCX3 codes for exons A, B, and D. Exons A and B are mutually exclusive (only one of them has to be present). Inclusion of both exons A and B would produce a shift in the reading frame of the message. Exons A and B are followed by a combination of the other four cassette exons. Combinations of the different exons could lead to 32 isoforms. Up to now, 12 different isoforms of NCX1 have been identified. The isoforms are expressed in a tissue-specific manner [20, 21]. In general, excitable tissues contain isoforms with exon A, and all other tissues contain isoforms with exon B. The isoforms that relate to this study are NCX1.1 (ACDEF) and NCX1.3 (BD) (Fig. 2). The former is the only isoform found in the heart and is also present in skeletal muscle [26]. NCX1.3 is the most abundant isoform in the kidney and is expressed together with NCX1.7 in arterial smooth muscle cells [27]. Inclusion of exon B, for example, in NCX1.3 and 1.7, confers the exchanger forward mode (calcium efflux) inactivation and sensitivity to the NCX blocker KBR-7943.

The origin of the different genes and splice variants was discussed by Quednau et al. [20]. NCX1 and NCX3 contain mutually exclusive

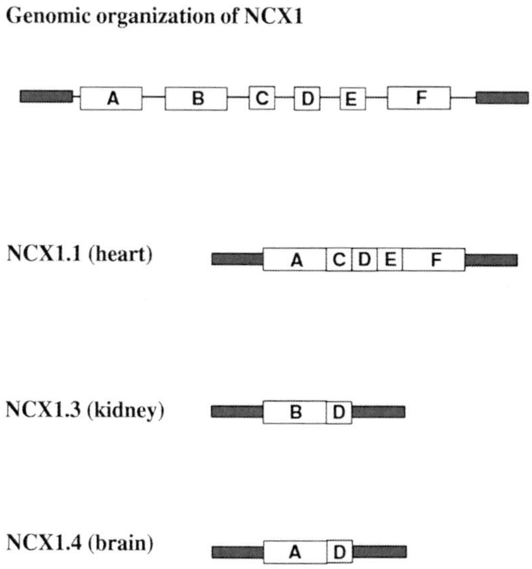

Genomic organization of NCX1

Fig. 2 NCX1 genomic organization and exon composition of NCX1.1, NCX1.3, and NCX1.4 isoforms

exons A and B, and these two exons contain a certain degree of homology. Since it is unlikely that intragenic events creating the exons occurred independently in the different NCX genes, it is probable that the alternative exons were created first followed by the new genes (by gene duplication). Furthermore, closer homology exists between exon A in NCX1 compared to exon A in NCX3, than exon A with B in either gene.

The sequence corresponding to the splicing variants is located in the region corresponding to amino acids 561–645, overlapping with part of the exchanger known to be important for regulation (the region of the intracellular loop involved in regulation was determined by deletion mutants to be between amino acids 562–685 [28]). These observations lead to the idea that the diversity of splice isoforms is related to the regulation of exchanger activity.

Activities of the different isoforms are regulated by different factors as well. For example, significant differences between the NCX1.1, NCX1.3, and NCX1.4 isoforms regarding ionic regulation were detected in excised giant patch studies on exchanger protein expressed in Xenopus oocytes [14, 29]. In addition, Ruknudin et al. showed that NCX1.1, but not NCX1.3, was affected by PKA phosphorylation [30].

Changes in NCX During Development

The SR is not well developed at the time of birth. SERCA expression starts in the rat embryo at day 9 of development [31] and increases after birth [32]. Ryanodine receptor density is also relatively low at the end of gestation. Some authors found that ryanodine (a compound that blocks SR Ca^{2+} release) had no effect in neonatal cardiomyocytes [33, 34], whereas others found a minor effect [35, 36] and still others have reported a more significant effect [37, 38]. Ca^{2+}-induced Ca^{2+} release (CICR) is less important early in development. Mature CICR is reached 3–4 weeks after birth in the rat [39, 40]. Before that time, the heart is more dependent on transsarcolemmal Ca^{2+} fluxes to induce contraction.

Ca^{2+} influx in the neonate is mediated primarily by L-type Ca^{2+} channels ([41, 42], T-type Ca^{2+} channels [43], and NCX [44, 45]. The changes in NCX expression during development oppose those of SERCA [46]. NCX mRNA and protein levels peak at birth and then decline [44, 47, 48]. Relaxation in newborn myocytes may occur predominantly through Ca^{2+} extrusion through NCX as opposed to Ca^{2+} uptake by the SR.

Another difference in E-C coupling between adults and neonates is that T-tubules are absent at birth. They develop around 10 days after birth in the rat. Previous to that time the smaller volume/surface relation is enough to provide Ca^{2+} to the myofilaments for contraction.

Models of NCX Over-expression and Down-regulation

Over-expression

To clarify the role played by the NCX in the regulation of Ca^{2+} homeostasis in the heart and to observe the changes in its expression in disease states, alternative approaches have been used to modify its expression level. NCX expression has been up-regulated by the use of transgenic mice and adenoviral vectors and has been down-regulated in knockout mice and through the use of antisense technology.

Philipson's group developed a transgenic mouse for cardiac-specific expression of the exchanger. The canine NCX1.1 gene was expressed under the α-myosin heavy chain promoter in this model [8]. In heterozygous mice, 1.5–3-fold higher NCX activity was measured using isotope uptake and electrophysiological methods, respectively. No changes in intracellular Na^+ concentration, resting Ca^{2+}, Ca^{2+} transient amplitude, or adaptations in other Ca^{2+} regulatory proteins were observed [49, 50]. Increased NCX activity, however, accelerated relaxation and the decay of the caffeine-released Ca^{2+} transients (in intact cells and under voltage clamp). These observations support the role of the exchanger in Ca^{2+} efflux. One study showed higher SR Ca^{2+} content in NCX over-expressing cells [49]. To sustain an increase in Ca^{2+} efflux via the exchanger without a depletion of Ca_i^{2+} (since no changes in Ca^{2+} current were observed), an increase in Ca^{2+} entry through the same exchanger has been proposed. The importance of the reverse mode exchanger was shown in experiments where depolarization of the membrane to positive potentials caused SR Ca^{2+} release in some cells. It was also shown that Ca^{2+} entering the cell through NCX can be buffered by the SR. In Yao's study, myocytes from heterozygous animals could maintain Ca^{2+} transients at a low frequency of stimulation after blockade of the L-type Ca^{2+} channel, showing that increased levels of NCX (working in reverse mode) can contribute to Ca^{2+}-induced Ca^{2+} release from the SR [50]. In this last situation, SR function was required indicating that NCX can induce Ca^{2+} release from the SR but not in enough quantities to support contraction.

Heterozygous NCX transgenic mice did not show a cardiac disease phenotype. On the contrary, homozygous NCX over-expressors were found to exhibit mild hypertrophy by 3.5 months of age (22% increase in heart weight to tibia length ratio) [51]. Homozygous postpartum females and mice from both sexes showed more severe hypertrophy under stress conditions that resulted in heart failure [52–55]. The characterization of excitation-contraction coupling in ventricular myocytes from homozygous mice showed a decrease in gain. In other words, an increased L-type Ca^{2+} channel current activated a smaller Ca^{2+} transient without changes in SR Ca^{2+} content. The mechanism for increased and slower inactivation of the L-type Ca^{2+} channel current could not be completely explained by the authors, because no changes were observed in channel density and, in addition, NCX was shown to have no direct effect on channel activity (when NCX activity was transiently blocked, an enhanced L-type current was maintained).

NCX transgenic mice were shown to be more susceptible to ischemia/reperfusion injury [56]. The effect was observed only in males, probably due to the protective effect of estrogen in females. Estrogen prevented the rise of $[Na^+]_i$ that drives NCX in males [57]. The mechanism responsible for the gender difference in Na_i^+ is not known. In this last study, after 30 min of ischemia, $[Ca^{2+}]_i$ in myocytes from transgenic mice was 1.5-fold higher than in cells from wild-type mice. However, another study using the same transgenic mice showed that increased NCX expression had a protective effect. Transgenic hearts showed preserved Ca^{2+} transients during ischemia and hypoxia [58]. This surprising result probably is due to the short periods of ischemia or hypoxia used in the study.

The other approach to induce increased expression of the exchanger has been to use NCX adenoviral transfection vectors. The effects observed have varied with the species of myocyte studied. Adenoviral transduction of the exchanger in rabbit ventricular myocytes showed that Ca^{2+} efflux through the exchanger was dominant in this species. The changes observed included a depletion of SR Ca^{2+} content and a reduction of the amplitude of the Ca^{2+} transient [59]. In this case, relaxation and decay of the Ca^{2+} transient were prolonged. Conversely, in adult rat ventricular myocytes, the effect of increasing the NCX expression depended upon the extracellular Ca^{2+} concentration. SR Ca^{2+} content and Ca^{2+} transients decreased at low $[Ca^{2+}]_o$ and increased at high $[Ca^{2+}]_o$ [60].

Down-regulation

The first approach that was used to decrease the expression of the NCX was to employ antisense oligodeoxynucleotides (ODN). ODNs are synthetic DNA molecules with a complementary nucleotide sequence to a specific mRNA. RNA–DNA duplexes, formed by base-pairing between the mRNA and the ODN, activate cleavage of the corresponding mRNA by RNAse [61]. ODNs may also interfere with the ability of the mRNA to access the ribosomes for translation. A limitation for this methodology is the low efficiency of transfection that can be achieved in cardiomyocytes. ODNs when modified, for example, as phosphorothioated ODN, are relatively stable molecules.

For the study of the effects of ODNs on NCX expression, 19 nucleotide long phosphorothioate ODNs targeting the 3' untranslated region of the RNA were initially used at a concentration of 3 μM in neonatal cardiomyocytes [62]. In this first study, ODNs nearly abolished NCX activity within 48 h. Another group used 0.5 μM of a pair of ODN sequences targeting the region around the start codon for the NCX [63]. These ODNs exhibited a significant effect after 4 days of treatment. NCX half-life was measured as 33 h [64]. This would indicate that when effects were observed just 24–48 h after treatment and using high concentrations of ODNs, these effects were probably due to a nonspecific action of the ODNs [62, 65]. The most recent study used 2 μM ODN to target one specific sequence near the NCX start site. This technique was used to demonstrate that decreased expression of NCX prevents Ca^{2+} overload in adult cardiomyocytes upon reoxygenation after anoxia [66].

To complement the data examining the effects of down-regulation of NCX expression using the ODN approach, transgenic NCX1 knockout mice have also been generated. Ablation of the NCX1 gene was performed independently by four laboratories [52–55]. Even though some differences were observed between the four knockout mice models, all of the mouse lines resulted in embryonic lethality.

The most significant characteristics of the knockouts were as follows: Homozygous NCX−/− mice died at 9.5–10 dpc [52, 55, 67] or 11.5 dpc [53]. Prior to death, the embryos were found to be smaller, with signs of necrosis in tissues other than the heart. The heart itself was also smaller in size, with an increased number of apoptotic cells [52, 55]. In one case, however, the incidence of apoptosis was normal and the heart was normal [53]. Spontaneous contractions of the heart and Ca^{2+} transients could be observed only in 30% of the embryos and at significantly lower frequency [55], or in one study they were not observed at all [53]. The heart tubes, however, responded to electrical stimulation, and surprisingly, Ca^{2+} transients and contractions were very similar to control responses [67]. The cardiomyocytes, therefore, appeared to be able to remove Ca^{2+} in the absence of NCX. However diastolic Ca^{2+} was significantly elevated when the stimulation frequency was increased [67]. The cardiomyocytes also showed myofibrillar disorganization. Reuter et al. observed almost complete depletion of SERCA protein without changes in PMCA in the homozygous null mouse [67]. The ability of the cells to extrude Ca^{2+} in the absence of NCX and without upregulation of PMCA expression (the other Ca^{2+} extrusion mechanism) would suggest that the activity or efficiency of the PMCA might be able to increase. Despite the decrease in SERCA protein, SR Ca^{2+} content was not altered [67].

The NCX1 −/+ heterozygous showed no cardiac defects. NCX protein expression in the heart and other tissues was 50% of wild type [52, 67], or was the same as in control [53]. NCX1 expression was restricted in only the heart before and at the time of lethality [68]. Consequently, lethality must have been due to the lack of NCX1 in the heart. The lack of heart contractile function would limit the perfusion of nutrients in the developing embryo to maintain growth. It is not clear what causes the lack of spontaneous contractions. It could be either a consequence of the myofibril disorganization, or an effect of the absence of NCX on the pacemaker activity of the heart. Reintroduction of cardiac expression of the NCX1 did not rescue the NCX knockout mouse [69].

Philipson and coworkers developed a cardiac-specific knockout of the NCX1 using the Cre-lox system [70]. Cre recombinase activity is under the MLCv2 promoter. Therefore, ablation of the gene occurs in ventricular cardiomyocytes during development. The MLCv2 promoter activates at 8 dpc in mouse [71]. As opposed to the global knockout, the cardiac-specific NCX1 knockout survived to adulthood. Cardiac function was depressed 20–30% despite the NCX expression being inhibited by ~90%. However, the animals could not withstand stress (breeding). Animals also died at a younger age, probably due to heart failure. Approximately 90% of the cardiomyocytes in the knockout animal showed no NCX1 expression, whereas the remaining cells expressed normal levels of NCX1. No compensatory changes were observed in the other Ca^{2+} regulatory proteins. SR Ca^{2+} content was not affected and interestingly, no differences in the shape and magnitude of the Ca^{2+} transients were observed. The L-type Ca^{2+} current, however, was significantly decreased. Therefore, the authors hypothesized that the hearts were able to maintain Ca^{2+} fluxes by a combination of up-regulating the activity of the PMCA and decreasing the amount of Ca^{2+} that enters the cell through the Ca^{2+} channels. However, PMCA expression was not altered and PMCA activity was not measured.

The Use of RNA Interference (RNAi) to Alter NCX Expression

RNAi is the process of sequence-specific posttranscriptional gene silencing initiated by double-stranded RNA that is homologous in sequence to the silenced gene. This phenomenon was first observed in *Caenorhabditis elegans* by Drs. Fire, Mello, and coworkers in 1998 [72]. The impact of their discovery in biology and medicine was recognized a few years later with the 2006 Nobel Prize in Medicine. In plants and lower animals [73–78], RNAi serves as a natural mechanism of defense against viral infection and transposon elements. In vertebrates, it is a mechanism of gene regulation [79, 80]. In addition, RNAi is now being used as a powerful tool to study gene function.

Double-stranded RNA is processed within the cell by the ribonuclease III Dicer into 21–22

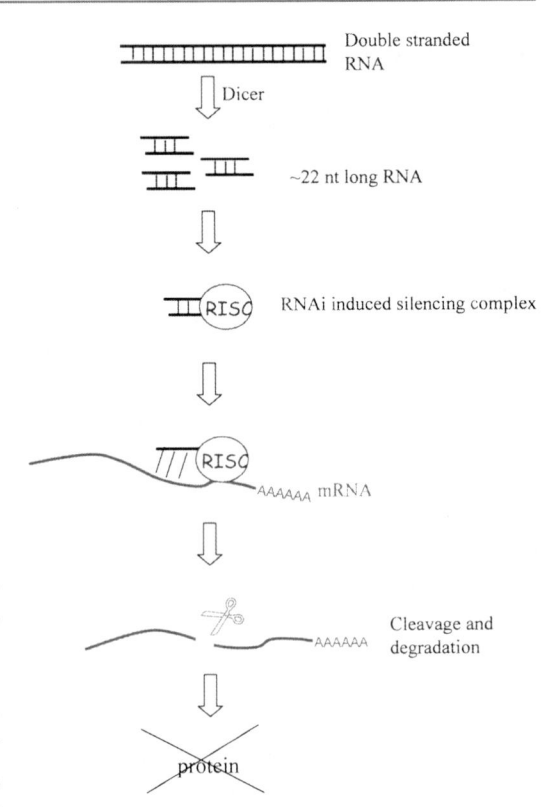

Fig. 3 Mechanism of RNA interference

nucleotides long RNA duplexes (siRNA or small interfering RNAs) [79, 80]. siRNAs contain a phosphate group on the 5′ end, and 2 nucleotides overhang on the 3′ end. These characteristics are necessary for siRNA to be recognized by the next component of the RNAi pathway: the multinuclease complex RISC (RNAi-induced silencing complex). RISC unwinds the short duplex RNA and uses it to find mRNAs of homologous sequence (through base-pairing of the antisense sequence of the duplex with the mRNA). RISC then proceeds to cleave the mRNA (at the midpoint of the homologous sequence), preventing its translation (Fig. 3) [79, 80].

Double-stranded RNAs introduced into invertebrate cells (and also in mammalian embryonic cells) are processed by DICER to induce the RNAi pathway. In all other mammalian cells, however, long dsRNAs activate a nonspecific mechanism that leads to apoptosis. Double-stranded RNAs of more than 30 nucleotides long trigger the synthesis of interferon. Interferon activates protein kinase R (PKR) and 2′–5′ oligoadenylate synthase that halts all protein synthesis and induces the degradation of all mRNAs in the cell, respectively.

Elbashir et al. [81] showed for the first time that RNAi can indeed be achieved in mammalian cell lines. They were able to bypass the interferon response by transfecting the cells with synthetic siRNAs. Today, siRNAs are widely used to down-regulate the expression of target genes. Multiple siRNAs have been pre-designed, some even pre-validated, and are commercially available from different sources.

An alternative approach to transfection of naked siRNA exists with the transfection of mammalian cells with DNA expression plasmids that code for RNA duplexes of 30 or less nucleotides long [82]. The RNA duplexes synthesized within the cell are also processed by DICER to form siRNA that induces gene silencing. The method could be achieved by placing the sense and antisense sequences under separate promoters (either on the same or on two separate plasmids), or by using a sequence that codes for a self-complementary short RNA hairpin (shRNA), where the sense and antisense sequences are separated by a loop of nucleotides (Fig. 4). In our laboratory, we utilized the shRNA approach, and to achieve high efficiency of transfection in cardiomyocytes, the shRNA construct was introduced into a replication-deficient recombinant adenovirus vector.

Adenovirus vectors are the vectors of choice for high efficiency of transfection in vitro for non-dividing cells. The advantage of adenoviral transfection vectors is that they remain episomal. They do not cause insertion mutations that could disrupt or alter the expression of important genes.

We employed adenoviral-shRNA in both neonatal and adult cardiomyocytes to effectively deplete NCX [83–86]. Other groups have utilized siRNA to target NCX expression in neurons and osteoclasts. In neonatal cardiomyocytes, ~95% of the NCX can be effectively depleted [84] whereas only ~60% can be depleted from adult cardiomyocytes through the use of shRNA delivered by adenoviruses. This is due to the limited time available to expose isolated adult cells to any intervention

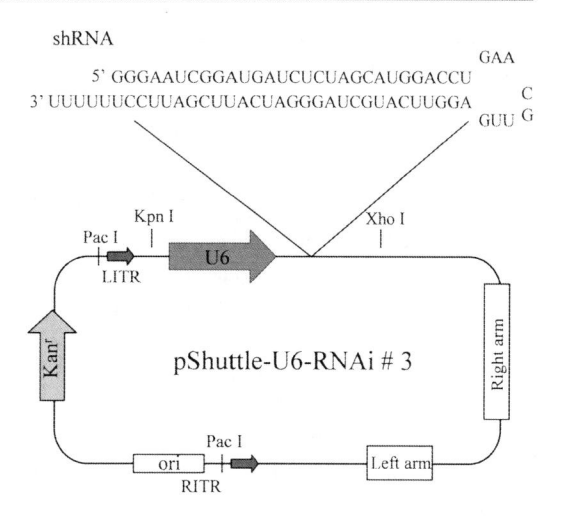

Fig. 4 Example of RNAi construct and hairpin. Diagram of pShuttle-U6-RNAi #3 used to generate one of the adenoviruses for RNAi against NCX. Sequence of the shRNA coded by this vector is shown on top of the figure. RNAi #3 targets nucleotides 142–171 of the NCX1. U6, U6 promoter; Kan^r, kanamycin resistance; ori, origin of replication; right and left arms for recombination with AdEasy-1; LITR and RITR, left and right internal terminal repeats

in a cell culture environment. Adult cardiomyocytes tend to change their morphology and functional characteristics after >48 h in culture. Neonatal cardiomyocytes do not and can then be exposed to interventions in culture for longer periods. Thus, the shorter exposure time to the Ad-shRNA and the relatively slow turnover time of the NCX (a half-time for turnover of 33 h) limits the depletion of the NCX that can be achieved in the adult cells before their morphological changes compromise the experimental results.

We have found that RNAi is one of the most effective methods available to inhibit NCX expression and activity [84, 86]. Despite ~95% depletion of NCX protein in the neonatal cardiomyocytes, only a few alterations in their contractile activity were observed [84]. Similar conclusions had been reached earlier from data obtained from knockout mice depleted of cardiac NCX by ~80% [87]. A large increase in PMCA expression appeared to compensate for the depletion in NCX [84]. This has brought into question the critical role of NCX in excitation-contraction coupling [84]. However, the role of the NCX in ischemic/reperfusion injury does not appear to be in question. Over-expression of NCX in cardiomyocytes has resulted in augmented damage when cells were subjected to an ischemic insult [56, 85] and, conversely, cells survived better when the NCX expression was depressed [85, 87–89].

Unfortunately, some of these experiments [84, 85] have been conducted in neonatal cardiomyocytes, and adult and neonatal cardiomyocytes differ significantly in their excitation-contraction coupling process, activity, and expression levels of NCX [48, 89–91] and in their response to ischemic reperfusion challenge [92]. Although genetically modified mice provide excellent models to examine the effects of changes in NCX expression, the use of single cells can avoid potential influences from extra-cardiac factors (hemodynamic, hormonal, etc.). NCX expression was inhibited ~60% in comparison to the scrambled control infection in the adult cardiomyocytes. This degree of depletion of NCX protein over the 48-h incubation time was sufficient to induce a significant depression in NCX function. The adult cardiomyocytes that had a depressed NCX expression and activity maintained normal Ca^{2+} homeostasis upon electrical stimulation of contraction. This is consistent with studies in neonatal cardiomyocytes and transgenic mouse models where no dramatic loss of contractile activity and Ca^{2+} homeostasis was observed despite severe NCX depletion [84, 87]. There was, however, a slowing of cardiac contractile activity and Ca^{2+} homeostasis [84, 87].

Adult cardiomyocytes that have a depressed NCX expression and activity are less sensitive to ischemic/reperfusion challenge. NCX-depleted cells were significantly protected from the rise in cytoplasmic Ca^{2+}, and this resulted in less damage than was observed in control cells during ischemia and reperfusion. This is consistent with previous work that has shown that increased expression results in greater damage [56] and, conversely, blocking NCX activity with drugs or reducing NCX expression protects the heart from ischemic/reperfusion injury [12, 85, 87, 88, 93] in both neonatal and adult heart preparations.

Blocking the Na^+/H^+ exchanger or the Na^+ channels has been shown to lower intracellular Na^+ levels and protects the heart from ischemic/

reperfusion injury [93]. The advantage of blocking the NCX instead of these two alternative Na^+ transport pathways is twofold. First, it likely allows the transsarcolemmal H^+ gradient to dissipate more quickly because the Na^+/H^+ exchanger should still be very active. This would allow the Na^+ pump to activate faster as well and reduce the intracellular Na^+ concentrations. Second, NCX inhibition is directly blocking the primary cause of ischemic damage – intracellular Ca^{2+} overload. It should be mentioned that NCX not only plays a critical role in ischemia/reperfusion injury but different forms of its isoforms are regulated by various pathophysiological conditions such as diabetes, hypertension, neurodegeneration, and bone resorption [94–104].

Conclusions

We can now conclude on the basis of increasingly persuasive evidence that NCX is extremely important in the Ca^{2+} overload and damage that accompanies ischemic/reperfusion insult in the heart. This protection is afforded to both neonatal cells and adult preparations as well. The strength of these conclusions about the role of NCX in ischemic injury is not transferred to its role in excitation-contraction coupling. Significant depletion of the NCX does not induce a loss of contractile activity in heart preparations. It would appear it is critical for modulating characteristics of the contraction/relaxation event but not for its maintenance.

Acknowledgments This work was supported by the Heart and Stroke Foundation of Manitoba. Indirect research support was provided by St Boniface Hospital Research Foundation.

References

1. Nicoll DA, Ottolia M, Lu L, et al. A new topological model of the cardiac sarcolemmal Na^+-Ca^{2+} exchanger. J Biol Chem. 1999;274:910–7.
2. Durkin JT, Ahrens DC, Pan YC, et al. Purification and amino-terminal sequence of the bovine cardiac sodium-calcium exchanger: evidence for the presence of a signal sequence. Arch Biochem Biophys. 1991;290:369–75.

3. Hryshko LV, Nicoll DA, Weiss JN, et al. Biosynthesis and initial processing of the cardiac sarcolemmal Na$^+$–Ca^{2+} exchanger. Biochim Biophys Acta. 1993; 1151:35–42.

4. Nicoll DA, Hryshko LV, Matsuoka S, et al. Mutation of amino acid residues in the putative transmembrane segments of the cardiac sarcolemmal Na$^+$-Ca^{2+} exchanger. J Biol Chem. 1996;271:13385–91.

5. Doering AE, Nicoll DA, Lu Y, et al. Topology of a functionally important region of the cardiac Na$^+$/Ca^{2+} exchanger. J Biol Chem. 1998;273:778–83.

6. Iwamoto T, Nakamura TY, Pan Y, et al. Unique topology of the internal repeats in the cardiac Na$^+$/Ca^{2+} exchanger. FEBS Lett. 1999;446:264–8.

7. Iwamoto T, Kita S, Uehara A, et al. Structural domains influencing sensitivity to isothiourea derivative inhibitor KB-R7943 in cardiac Na$^+$/Ca^{2+} exchanger. Mol Pharmacol. 2001;59:524–31.

8. Adachi-Akahane S, Lu L, Li Z, et al. Calcium signaling in transgenic mice overexpressing cardiac Na$^+$-Ca^{2+} exchanger. J Gen Physiol. 1997;109: 717–29.

9. Iwamoto T, Uehara A, Imanaga I, et al. The Na$^+$/Ca^{2+} exchanger NCX1 has oppositely oriented reentrant loop domains that contain conserved aspartic acids whose mutation alters its apparent Ca^{2+} affinity. J Biol Chem. 2000;275:38571–80.

10. Nicoll DA, Longoni S, Philipson KD. Molecular cloning and functional expression of the cardiac sarcolemmal Na$^+$-Ca^{2+} exchanger. Science. 1990;250:562–5.

11. Li Z, Nicoll DA, Collins A, et al. Identification of a peptide inhibitor of the cardiac sarcolemmal Na$^+$-Ca^{2+} exchanger. J Biol Chem. 1991;266:1014–20.

12. Matsuoka S, Nicoll DA, He Z, et al. Regulation of cardiac Na$^+$-Ca^{2+} exchanger by the endogenous XIP region. J Gen Physiol. 1997;109:273–86.

13. Levitsky DO, Nicoll DA, Philipson KD. Identification of the high affinity Ca^{2+}-binding domain of the cardiac Na$^+$-Ca^{2+} exchanger. J Biol Chem. 1994;269: 22847–52.

14. Matsuoka S, Nicoll DA, Hryshko LV, et al. Regulation of the cardiac Na$^+$-Ca^{2+} exchanger by Ca^{2+}. Mutational analysis of the Ca^{2+}-binding domain. J Gen Physiol. 1995;105:403–20.

15. Kieval RS, Bloch RJ, Lindenmayer GE, et al. Immunofluorescence localization of the Na-Ca exchanger in heart cells. Am J Physiol. 1992;263: C545–50.

16. Thomas MJ, Sjaastad I, Andersen K, et al. Localization and function of the Na$^+$/Ca^{2+}-exchanger in normal and detubulated rat cardiomyocytes. J Mol Cell Cardiol. 2003;35:1325–37.

17. Frank JS, Mottino G, Reid D, et al. Distribution of the Na$^+$-Ca^{2+} exchange protein in mammalian cardiac myocytes: an immunofluorescence and immunocolloidal gold-labeling study. J Cell Biol. 1992;117:337–45.

18. Li Z, Matsuoka S, Hryshko LV, et al. Cloning of the NCX2 isoform of the plasma membrane Na$^+$-Ca^{2+} exchanger. J Biol Chem. 1994;269:17434–9.

19. Nicoll DA, Quednau BD, Qui Z, et al. Cloning of a third mammalian Na$^+$-Ca2$^+$ exchanger, NCX3. J Biol Chem. 1996;271:24914–21.

20. Quednau BD, Nicoll DA, Philipson KD. Tissue specificity and alternative splicing of the Na$^+$/Ca^{2+} exchanger isoforms NCX1, NCX2, and NCX3 in rat. Am J Physiol. 1997;272:C1250–61.

21. Lee SL, Yu AS, Lytton J. Tissue-specific expression of Na$^+$-Ca^{2+} exchanger isoforms. J Biol Chem. 1994; 269:14849–52.

22. Barnes KV, Cheng G, Dawson MM, et al. Cloning of cardiac, kidney, and brain promoters of the feline ncx1 gene. J Biol Chem. 1997;272:11510–7.

23. Scheller T, Kraev A, Skinner S, et al. Cloning of the multipartite promoter of the sodium-calcium exchanger gene NCX1 and characterization of its activity in vascular smooth muscle cells. J Biol Chem. 1998;273:7643–9.

24. Nicholas SB, Philipson KD. Cardiac expression of the Na$^+$/Ca^{2+} exchanger NCX1 is GATA factor dependent. Am J Physiol. 1999;277:H324–30.

25. Kofuji P, Lederer WJ, Schulze DH. Mutually exclusive and cassette exons underlie alternatively spliced isoforms of the Na/Ca exchanger. J Biol Chem. 1994;269:5145–9.

26. Reilly RF, Lattanzi D. Identification of a novel alternatively spliced isoform of the Na$^+$-Ca^{2+} exchanger (NACA8) in heart. Ann NY Acad Sci. 1996;779: 129–31.

27. White KE, Gesek FA, Friedman PA. Structural and functional analysis of Na$^+$/Ca^{2+} exchange in distal convoluted tubule cells. Am J Physiol. 1996;271: F560–70.

28. Matsuoka S, Nicoll DA, Reilly RF, et al. Initial localization of regulatory regions of the cardiac sarcolemmal Na$^+$-Ca^{2+} exchanger. Proc Natl Acad Sci USA. 1993;90:3870–4.

29. Dyck C, Omelchenko A, Elias CL, et al. Ionic regulatory properties of brain and kidney splice variants of the NCX1 Na$^+$-Ca^{2+} exchanger. J Gen Physiol. 1999;114:701–11.

30. Ruknudin A, He S, Lederer WJ, et al. Functional differences between cardiac and renal isoforms of the rat Na$^+$-Ca^{2+} exchanger NCX1 expressed in Xenopus oocytes. J Physiol. 2000;529(Pt 3):599–610.

31. Moorman A, Vermeulen J, Koban M, et al. Patterns of expression of sarcoplasmic reticulum Ca^{2+}-ATPase and phospholamban mRNAs during rat heart development. Circ Res. 1995;76:616–25.

32. Lompre A, Lambert F, Lakatta E, et al. Expression of sarcoplasmic reticulum Ca^{2+}-ATPase and calsequestrin genes in rat heart during ontogenic development and aging. Circ Res. 1991;69:1380–8.

33. Nakanishi T, Seguchi M, Takao A. Development of the myocardial contractile system. Experientia. 1988;44:936–44.

34. Tanaka H, Shigenobu K. Effect of ryanodine on neonatal and adult rat heart: developmental increase in sarcoplasmic reticulum function. J Mol Cell Cardiol. 1989;21:1305–13.

35. Escobar A, Ribeiro-Costa R, Villalba-Galea C, et al. Developmental changes of intracellular Ca^{2+} transients in beating rat hearts. Am J Physiol. 2004;286:H971–8.

36. Agata N, Tanaka H, Shigenobu K. Possible action of cyclopiazonic acid on myocardial sarcoplasmic reticulum: inotropic effects on neonatal and adult rat heart. Br J Pharmacol. 1993;108:571–2.

37. Seki S, Nagashima M, Yamada Y, et al. Fetal and postnatal development of Ca^{2+} transients and Ca^{2+} sparks in rat cardiomyocytes. Cardiovasc Res. 2003;58:535–48.

38. Wibo M, Bravo G, Godfraind T. Postnatal maturation of excitation-contraction coupling in rat ventricle in relation to the subcellular localization and surface density of 1,4-dihydropyridine and ryanodine receptors. Circ Res. 1991;68:662–73.

39. Fabiato A. Calcium release in skinned cardiac cells: variations with species, tissues, and development. Fed Proc. 1982;41:2238–44.

40. Vornanen M. Activation of contractility and sarcolemmal Ca^{2+}-ATPase by Ca^{2+} during postnatal development of the rat heart. Comp Biochem Physiol A. 1984;78:691–5.

41. Cohen N, Lederer W. Changes in the calcium current of rat heart ventricular myocytes during development. J Physiol. 1988;406:115–46.

42. Vornanen M. Contribution of sarcolemmal calcium current to total cellular calcium in postnatally developing rat heart. Cardiovasc Res. 1996;32:400–10.

43. Xu X, Best P. Postnatal changes in T-type calcium current density in rat atrial myocytes. J Physiol. 1992;454:657–72.

44. Artman M. Sarcolemmal Na^+-Ca^{2+} exchange activity and exchanger immunoreactivity in developing rabbit hearts. Am J Physiol. 1992;263:H1506–13.

45. Nabauer M, Morad M. Modulation of contraction by intracellular Na^+ via Na^+-Ca^{2+} exchange in single shark (Squalus acanthias) ventricular myocytes. J Physiol. 1992;457:627–37.

46. Reed TD, Babu GJ, Ji Y, et al. The expression of SR calcium transport ATPase and the Na^+/Ca^{2+} Exchanger are antithetically regulated during mouse cardiac development and in Hypo/hyperthyroidism. J Mol Cell Cardiol. 2000;32:453–64.

47. Boerth SR, Zimmer DB, Artman M. Steady-state mRNA levels of the sarcolemmal Na^+-Ca^{2+} exchanger peak near birth in developing rabbit and rat hearts. Circ Res. 1994;74:354–9.

48. Vetter R, Studer R, Reinecke H, et al. Reciprocal changes in the postnatal expression of the sarcolemmal Na^+-Ca^{2+}-exchanger and SERCA2 in rat heart. J Mol Cell Cardiol. 1995;27:1689–701.

49. Terracciano CM, Souza AI, Philipson KD, et al. Na^+-Ca^{2+} exchange and sarcoplasmic reticular Ca2+ regulation in ventricular myocytes from transgenic mice overexpressing the Na+−Ca2+ exchanger. J Physiol. 1998;512(Pt 3):651–67.

50. Yao A, Su Z, Nonaka A, et al. Effects of overexpression of the Na^+-Ca^{2+} exchanger on $[Ca^{2+}]_i$ transients in murine ventricular myocytes. Circ Res. 1998;82: 657–65.

51. Reuter H, Han T, Motter C, et al. Mice overexpressing the cardiac sodium-calcium exchanger: defects in excitation-contraction coupling. J Physiol. 2004; 554:779–89.

52. Wakimoto K, Kobayashi K, Kuro OM, et al. Targeted disruption of Na^+/Ca^{2+} exchanger gene leads to cardiomyocyte apoptosis and defects in heartbeat. J Biol Chem. 2000;275:36991–8.

53. Koushik SV, Wang J, Rogers R, et al. Targeted inactivation of the sodium-calcium exchanger Ncx1 results in the lack of a heartbeat and abnormal myofibrillar organization. FASEB J. 2001;15:1209–11.

54. Reuter H, Henderson SA, Han T, et al. The Na^+-Ca^{2+} exchanger is essential for the action of cardiac glycosides. Circ Res. 2002;90:305–8.

55. Cho CH, Kim SS, Jeong MJ, et al. The Na^+ -Ca^{2+} exchanger is essential for embryonic heart development in mice. Mol Cells. 2000;10:712–22.

56. Cross HR, Lu L, Steenbergen C, et al. Overexpression of the cardiac Na^+/Ca^{2+} exchanger increases susceptibility to ischemia/reperfusion injury in male, but not female, transgenic mice. Circ Res. 1998;83: 1215–23.

57. Sugishita M, Su Z, Li F, et al. Gender Influences $[Ca^{2+}]_i$ During Metabolic Inhibition in Myocytes Overexpressing the Na^+-Ca^{2+} Exchanger. Circulation. 2001;104:2101–6.

58. Hampton T, Wang J, DeAngelis J, et al. Enhanced gene expression of Na+/Ca2+ exchanger attenuates ischemic and hypoxic contractile dysfuction. Am J Physiol Heart Circ Physiol. 2000;279:H2846–54.

59. Ranu HK, Terracciano CM, Davia K, et al. Effects of Na^+/Ca^{2+}-exchanger overexpression on excitation-contraction coupling in adult rabbit ventricular myocytes. J Mol Cell Cardiol. 2002;34:389–400.

60. Zhang XQ, Song J, Rothblum LI, et al. Overexpression of Na^+/Ca^{2+} exchanger alters contractility and SR Ca^{2+} content in adult rat myocytes. Am J Physiol Heart Circ Physiol. 2001;281:H2079–88.

61. Fiset P, Soussi Gounni A. Antisense oligonucleotides: problems with use and solutions. Rev Biol Biotech. 2001;1:27–33.

62. Lipp P, Schwaller B, Niggli E. Specific inhibition of Na-Ca exchange function by antisense oligodeoxynucleotides. FEBS Lett. 1995;364:198–202.

63. Slodzinski MK, Juhaszova M, Blaustein MP. Antisense inhibition of Na+/Ca2+ exchange in primary cultured arterial myocytes. Am J Physiol Cell Physiol. 1995;269:C1340–5.

64. Slodzinski MK, Blaustein MP. Na^+/Ca^{2+} exchange in neonatal rat heart cells: antisense inhibition and protein half-life. Am J Physiol Cell Physiol. 1998;275: C459–67.

65. Takahashi K, Azuma M, Huschenbett J, et al. Effects of antisense oligonucleotides to the cardiac Na^+/Ca^{2+} exchanger on calcium dynamics in cultured cardiac myocytes. Biochem Biophys Res Commun. 1999;260:117–21.

66. Eigel BN, Hadley RW. Antisense inhibition of Na^+/Ca^{2+} exchange during anoxia/reoxygenation in

ventricular myocytes. Am J Physiol Heart Circ Physiol. 2001;281:H2184–90.

67. Reuter H, Henderson SA, Han T, et al. Cardiac excitation-contraction coupling in the absence of Na$^+$ - Ca^{2+} exchange. Cell Calcium. 2003;34:19–26.

68. Koushik SV, Bundy J, Conway SJ. Sodium-calcium exchanger is initially expressed in a heart-restricted pattern within the early mouse embryo. Mech Dev. 1999;88:119–22.

69. Cho CH, Lee SY, Shin HS, et al. Partial rescue of the Na$^+$-Ca^{2+} exchanger (NCX1) knock-out mouse by transgenic expression of NCX1. Exp Mol Med. 2003;35:125–35.

70. Henderson SA, Goldhaber JI, So JM, et al. Functional adult myocardium in the absence of Na$^+$-Ca^{2+} exchange: cardiac-specific knockout of NCX1. Circ Res. 2004;95:604–11.

71. O'Brien T, Lee K, Chien K. Positional specification of ventricular myosin light chain 2 expression in the primitive murine heart tube. Proc Natl Acad Sci USA. 1993;90:5157–61.

72. Fire A, Xu S, Montgomery MK, et al. Potent and specific genetic interference by double-stranded RNA in Caenorhabditis elegans. Nature. 1998;391:806–11.

73. Jorgensen R. Altered gene expression in plants due to trans interactions between homologous genes. Trends Biotechnol. 1990;8:340–4.

74. Romano N, Macino G. Quelling: transient inactivation of gene expression in *Neurospora crassa* by transformation with homologous sequences. Mol Microbiol. 1992;6:3343–53.

75. Fire A, Albertson D, Harrison S, et al. Production of antisense RNA leads to effective and specific inhibition of gene expression in C. elegans muscle. Development. 1991;113:503–14.

76. Pal-Bhadra M, Bhadra U, Birchler J. Cosuppression in *Drosophila*: gene silencing of *Alcohol dehydrogenase* by *white-Adh* transgenes is *Polycomb* dependent. Cell. 1997;90:479–90.

77. Lohmann J, Endl I, Bosch T. Silencing of developmental genes in Hydra. Dev Biol. 1999;214:211–14.

78. Ngo H, Tschudi C, Gull K, et al. Double-stranded RNA induces mRNA degradation in *Trypanosoma brucei*. Proc Natl Acad Sci USA. 1998;95:14687–92.

79. Denli A, Hannon G. RNAi: an ever-growing puzzle. Trends Biochem Sci. 2003;28:196–201.

80. Hannon GJ. RNA interference. Nature. 2002;418:244–51.

81. Elbashir SM, Harborth J, Lendeckel W, et al. Duplexes of 21-nucleotide RNAs mediate RNA interference in cultured mammalian cells. Nature. 2001;411:494–8.

82. Paddison PJ, Caudy AA, Bernstein E, et al. Short hairpin RNAs (shRNAs) induce sequence-specific silencing in mammalian cells. Genes Dev. 2002;16:948–58.

83. Ander BP, Hurtado C, Raposo CS, et al. Differential sensitivities of the NCX 1.1 and NCX 1.3 isoforms of the Na$^+$-Ca^{2+} exchanger to alpha-linolenic acid. Cardiovasc Res. 2007;73:395–403.

84. Hurtado C, Ander BP, Maddaford TG, et al. Adenovirally delivered shRNA strongly inhibits Na$^+$-Ca^{2+} exchanger

expression but does not prevent cardiac contraction. J Mol Cell Cardiol. 2005;38:647–54.

85. Hurtado C, Prociuk M, Maddaford TG, et al. Cells expressing unique sodium-calcium exchange (NCX1) splice variants exhibit different susceptibility to Ca^{2+} overload. Am J Physiol Heart Circ Physiol. 2006;290:H2155–62.

86. Hurtado C, Wigle JT, Dibrov E, et al. A comparison of adenovirally delivered molecular methods to inhibit Na$^+$/Ca^{2+} exchange. J Mol Cell Cardiol. 2007;43:49–53.

87. Pott C, Goldhaber JI, Philipson KD. Genetic manipulations of cardiac Na$^+$/Ca^{2+} exchanger protein expression. Biochem Biophys Res Commun. 2004;322:1336–40.

88. Imahashi K, Potts C, Goldhaber JI, et al. Cardiac specific ablation of the Na$^+$-Ca^{2+} exchanger confers protection against ischemia/reperfusion injury. Circ Res. 2005;97:916–21.

89. Komuro I, Ohtsuka M. Forefront of Na$^+$/Ca^{2+} exchanger studies: role of Na$^+$/Ca^{2+} exchanger – lessons learned from knock-out mice. J Pharmacol Sci. 2004;96:23–6.

90. Vetter R, Will H. Sarcolemmal Na-Ca exchange and sarcoplasmic reticulum calcium uptake in developing chick heart. J Mol Cell Cardiol. 1986;18:1267–75.

91. Vetter R, Kemsies C, Schulze W. Sarcolemmal Na$^+$/Ca^{2+} exchange and sarcoplasmic reticulum Ca2+ uptake in several cardiac preparations. Biomed Biochim Acta. 1987;46:S375–81.

92. Milerova M, Charvatova Z, Skarka L, et al. Neonatal cardiac mitochondria and ischemia/reperfusion injury. Mol Cell Biochem. 2010;335(1–2):147–53.

93. Eng S, Maddaford TG, Kardami E, et al. The effects of inhibition of two separate Na$^+$ entry pathways on myocardial ischemia/reperfusion injury. J Mol Cell Cardiol. 1998;30:829–35.

94. Hamming KS, Soliman D, Webster NJ, et al. Inhibition of beta-cell sodium-calcium exchange enhances glucose-dependent elevations in cytoplasmic calcium and insulin secretion. Diabetes. 2010;59(7):1686–93.

95. Blaustein MP, Zhang J, Chen L, et al. The pump, the exchanger, and endogenous ouabain: signaling mechanisms that link salt retention to hypertension. Hypertension. 2009;53(2):291–8.

96. Chandrasekaran S, Peterson RE, Mani SK, et al. Histone deacetylases facilitate sodium/calcium exchanger up-regulation in adult cardiomyocytes. FASEB J. 2009;23(11):3851–64.

97. Hilge M, Aelen J, Vuister GW. Ca^{2+} regulation in the Na$^+$/Ca^{2+} exchanger involves two markedly different Ca^{2+} sensors. Mol Cell. 2006;22:15–25.

98. Moyes CD, Tibbits GF. Gene structure evolution of the Na$^+$-Ca^{2+} exchanger (NCX) family. BMC Evol Biol. 2008;8:127.

99. Araujo IM, Carreira BP, Pereira T, et al. Changes in calcium dynamics following the reversal of the sodium-calcium exchanger have a key role in AMPA receptor-mediated neurodegeneration via calpain activation in hippocampal neurons. Cell Death Differ. 2007;14:1635–46.

100. Luo J, Wang Y, Chen X, et al. Increased tolerance to ischemic neuronal damage by knockdown of Na⁺-Ca²⁺ exchanger isoform 1. Ann NY Acad Sci. 2007;1099:292–305.

101. Bano D, Young KW, Guerin CJ, et al. Cleavage of the plasma membrane Na⁺/Ca²⁺ exchanger in excitotoxicity. Cell. 2005;120:275–85.

102. Li JP, Kajiya H, Okamoto F, et al. Three Na⁺/Ca²⁺ exchanger (NCX) variants are expressed in mouse osteoclasts and mediate calcium transport during bone resorption. Endocrinology. 2007;148: 2116–25.

103. Maddaford TG, Dibrov E, Hurtado C, et al. Reduced expression of the sodium-calcium exchanger in adult cardiomyocytes via adenovirally delivered shRNA results in resistance to simulated ischemic injury. Am J Physiol. 2010;298:H360–6.

104. Philipson KD, Nicoll DA. Sodium-calcium exchange: a molecular perspective. Annu Rev Physiol. 2000;62:111–33.

Scleraxis: A New Regulator of Extracellular Matrix Formation

Rushita A. Bagchi and Michael P. Czubryt

Abstract

Scleraxis is a transcription factor that appears to play a key role in both the development of extracellular matrix-rich tissues such as tendons, and in the synthesis of matrix itself by regulating matrix gene expression. Our understanding of how scleraxis works, how its activity and expression are regulated, and the specific role it plays in disease is largely incomplete. However, enough data have accumulated to date to identify scleraxis as a critical factor in tendon formation, and ongoing studies in our laboratory have implicated scleraxis as a previously unappreciated driver of cardiac fibrosis due to its role in regulating type I collagen formation. Scleraxis may in fact behave as a master regulator of fibrillar collagen formation in multiple tissues, and the development of therapies aimed at reducing scleraxis function may provide a novel means to control tissue fibrosis in multiple pathologies.

Keywords

Development • Extracellular matrix • Fibrosis • Gene expression • Heart • Heart valves • Tendons • Transcription factor

Introduction

By regulating the expression of a multitude of target genes, transcriptional regulators have the potential to play dramatic roles in cell, tissue, and organ physiology and pathophysiology. Understanding how these regulators function, and identifying their target genes, is thus critical for better understanding disease and developing new treatments. Scleraxis is a member of the basic-helix-loop-helix (bHLH) superfamily of transcription factors, and was originally considered to be a highly specific marker for progenitor cells destined to form tendons, ligaments, and bronchial cartilage [1–3]. Recent studies, however, suggest that scleraxis is expressed in a much wider variety of tissues, such as cardiac fibroblasts, and thus may have a broader range of activity than originally believed [4].

M.P. Czubryt (✉)
St. Boniface Research Centre and Department of Physiology, University of Manitoba, Winnipeg, Canada
e-mail: mczubryt@sbrc.ca

B. Ostadal et al. (eds.), *Genes and Cardiovascular Function*,
DOI 10.1007/978-1-4419-7207-1_6, © Springer Science+Business Media, LLC 2011

To date, the target genes regulated by scleraxis are largely unknown. Studies carried out over the past several years by our laboratory and others suggest that scleraxis regulates expression of a variety of connective tissue genes, including those encoding fibrillar collagens [4]. Our data indicate that scleraxis is involved in cardiac fibrosis, and the expression of scleraxis in other tissues suggests the intriguing possibility that it may play a regulatory role in other forms of organ fibrosis. Additional work is needed to further our understanding of the mechanisms by which scleraxis works, to identify its target genes, and to better understand how expression and activity of scleraxis itself is controlled. Indeed, despite the fact that it was cloned well over a decade ago, at the time of this writing there are fewer than 120 papers referencing scleraxis in the literature [3]. The need for additional research on this intriguing protein is thus significant.

Structure and Function

The various members of the bHLH transcription factor superfamily play critical roles in such varied processes as cell proliferation, differentiation, and regulation of oncogenesis [5–7]. Structurally, these proteins contain a bHLH moiety consisting of a short stretch of hydrophilic residues followed by a set of mainly hydrophobic residues located in two short helices separated by a non-conserved sequence of variable length which constitutes the loop [8, 9]. The basic domain of bHLH proteins constitutes the actual interface for DNA interaction. One helix is slightly smaller than the other to provide additional flexibility to facilitate dimerization by folding and packing against the other helix. Typically the larger helix contributes to the DNA interaction interface [10]. The bHLH proteins bind to signature motifs consisting of a core hexanucleotide sequence, CA*NN*TG (*N* represents any nucleotide), referred to as an E-box [3, 11, 12]. A transactivation domain, typically located in the C-terminal region, is responsible for the activity of these factors.

Small (~22 kDa), scleraxis is structurally very similar to other bHLH factors, including possession of an N-terminal bHLH motif and a C-terminal transactivation domain [3]. Scleraxis was first cloned in a yeast two-hybrid screen to identify interacting partners of E12 [3]. E12 is a ubiquitous Class A bHLH protein, also known as an E-protein [13]. Conversely, scleraxis is a Class B bHLH protein exhibiting a tissue-restricted expression pattern. Like other bHLH proteins, it binds specifically to E-boxes, and its ability to bind to oligonucleotides containing E-boxes from the muscle creatine kinase gene promoter is augmented by E12, suggesting that scleraxis heterodimerizes with E-proteins for full activity [3]. Using artificial promoter constructs, it has been shown that another E-protein, E47, also augments the ability of scleraxis to bind to E-boxes [14]. At present it is unclear how scleraxis "recognizes" specific E-boxes in target gene promoters. The identities of the two central nucleotides of the E-box hexamer are likely to be important, and it is possible that other nearby nucleotides also play a role in selectivity. Regardless of mechanism, it is clear that Class B E-box-binding bHLH proteins like scleraxis are not typically promiscuous. For example, while we noted that scleraxis strongly transactivated the human collagen Iα2 gene proximal promoter, which contains three E-boxes, the bHLH transcription factor MyoD had no effect on this promoter [4].

The Noda laboratory identified *aggrecan* as the first gene to be directly regulated by scleraxis, and noted that scleraxis was able to transactivate an aggrecan promoter reporter construct even without the addition of exogenous E-proteins E12 or E47 [15]. Deletion studies from our laboratory have shown that removal of the HLH domain, which mediates protein–protein interaction, resulted in an approximately 50% reduction in scleraxis activity [4]. This indicates that heterodimerization augments transactivation by scleraxis, but is not specifically required. This augmentation is likely to be context-specific, governed by the individual cell-type involved, the specific E-box sequence and the availability and identity of potential binding partners [15]. In contrast to the HLH domain, deletion of the basic DNA-binding domain completely attenuated transactivation by scleraxis, demonstrating an absolute requirement for DNA contact [4].

It is unclear whether scleraxis can interact with other proteins besides E12 and E47. However, specific experiments indicate that scleraxis does not appear to interact with the HLH inhibitory protein Id2 [14]. In our experiments, Id2 was able to inhibit scleraxis-mediated transactivation of the collagen Iα2 promoter, thus we hypothesized that Id2 may act by sequestering required scleraxis-binding partners [4]. Similarly, we have generated a mutant form of scleraxis lacking the basic DNA-binding domain and found that this mutant appears to act in a dominant negative fashion – also possibly by sequestration of binding partners. Nonetheless, it remains unclear whether these partners are E-proteins such as E12, or whether other critical partners exist. It is also unclear whether scleraxis is capable of forming homodimers to regulate gene expression. One novel binding partner for scleraxis is cAMP response element binding protein CREB2/ATF4, which represses scleraxis function in Sertoli cells [16].

Although the primary structure of scleraxis reveals a number of potential sites for posttranslational modification (e.g. phosphorylation), information is currently lacking as to whether such modifications may impact the transactivation activity, stability, or dimerization capabilities of scleraxis. It is thus difficult to theorize at this time exactly which intracellular signaling pathways may be important in mediating scleraxis function, although several such pathways have been demonstrated to be important. We have shown that scleraxis expression is up-regulated in response to TGF-β_1 signaling, but it is not yet known whether this effect is mediated by the canonical TGF-β-Smad pathway or some other mechanism [4]. Furthermore, it is unclear whether scleraxis-mediated transactivation of gene promoters is modulated by this pathway independently of its expression level, although a study in ROS17/2.8 osteoblastic osteosarcoma cells suggested that TGF-β stimulated the DNA-binding activity of scleraxis [17]. Scleraxis expression is also up-regulated by cAMP or follicle stimulating hormone in Sertoli cells, although the mechanism is unclear [18]. Smith et al. have reported that scleraxis expression is regulated by ERK1/2

signaling [19]. FGFs also appear to be important regulators of scleraxis expression. The transcription factors Pea3 and Erm, which function downstream of FGF signaling, regulate scleraxis somite expression, and FGF4 was sufficient to increase scleraxis expression in developing avian heart valves downstream of ERK and in chick limb tendons [20–22].

Gene Expression

The human scleraxis gene is currently identified in the NCBI sequence database as two variants *SCXA* and *SCXB*; however, these sequences represent a single gene located on chromosome 8 in the region of 8q24.3. The scleraxis protein itself is highly conserved, with nearly 100% identity between rats and mice, and approximately 90% identity between humans and lower mammals (see Fig. 1). This high degree of identity suggests that the biological function of scleraxis may be critical for proper development. Supporting this idea, knockout of scleraxis is associated with a significant decrease in the number of viable pups at birth, with greatly reduced survival at 2 months [23]. Scleraxis gene homologs have been identified in a variety of other organisms, including chicken, frog, cow, horse, and zebra fish.

During murine embryonic development, scleraxis is widely expressed at the time of gastrulation around embryonic day (E) 6.0, but its expression pattern becomes restricted soon thereafter [24]. Its expression can be detected as early as E9.5 in the sclerotome compartment of somites from which the ribs and vertebrae arise [3, 24]. Scleraxis is highly expressed in a number of pre-skeletal mesenchymal cells prior to chondrogenesis, but a decrease in its expression has been noted during ossification. There is abundant expression of scleraxis in progenitor cells destined to form ligaments, tendons, and bronchial cartilage [3]. High levels of this gene have also been noted throughout the pericardium [3]. It has been shown to be expressed during valvulogenesis in the developing *chordae tendinae* proximal to the papillary muscles of the embryonic chick heart as well as in semilunar valve precursor cells [25].

Fig. 1 Protein sequence alignment of scleraxis from mouse, rat, and human. NCBI protein sequences from mouse (accession NP_942588), rat (accession NP_001123980), and human (accession NP_001008272) were aligned using ClustalW2 (www.ebi.ac.uk). *Asterisks* denote amino acids conserved across all three species; *colons* denote conserved substitutions; *periods* denote semi-conserved substitutions. Inset: BLAST sequence alignment identity between mouse (*Mm*), rat (*Rr*), and human (*Hs*) scleraxis protein sequences

```
Mouse    MSFAMLRSAPPPGRYLYPEVSPLSEDEDRGSESSGSDEKPCRVHAARCGL  50
Rat      MSFAMLRSAPPPGRYLYPEVSPLSEDEDRGSESSGSDEKPCRVHAARCGL  50
Human    MSFATLRPAPP-GRYLYPEVSPLSEDEDRGSDSSGSDEKPCRVHAARCGL  49
         ****  **.*** ******************.*****************

Mouse    QGARRRAGGRRAAGSGPGPGGRPGREPRQRHTANARERDRTNSVNTAFTA  100
Rat      QGARRRAGGRRAAGSGPGPGGRPGREPRQRHTANARERDRTNSVNTAFTA  100
Human    QGARRRAGGRRAGGGGPG--GRPGREPRQRHTANARERDRTNSVNTAFTA  97
         ***********.*.***   ****************************

Mouse    LRTLIPTEPADRKLSKIETLRLASSYISHLGNVLLVGEACGDGQPCHSGP  150
Rat      LRTLIPTEPADRKLSKIETLRLASSYISHLGNVLLVGEACGDGQPCHSGP  150
Human    LRTLIPTEPADRKLSKIETLRLASSYISHLGNVLLAGEACGDGQPCHSGP  147
         ***********************************.*************

Mouse    AFFHSGRAGSPLPPPPPPP--PLARDGGENTQPKQICTFCLSNQRKLSKD  198
Rat      AFFHSGRAGSPLPPPPPPPPPLPLARDGGENTQPKQICTFCLSNQRKLSKD  200
Human    AFFHAARAGSPPPPPPPPPP----ARDG-ENTQPKQICTFCLSNQRKLSKD  192
         ****:.***** *******    ****  ********************

Mouse    RDRKTAIRS  207
Rat      RDRKTAIRS  209
Human    RDRKTAIRS  201
         *********
```

```
          Mm ⌐
89%       Rr  ⌐ 99%
          Hs ⌐ 88%
```

Scleraxis is highly expressed in the syndetome compartment of developing somites, a region that is spatially situated between future muscle- and bone-forming regions, and that is destined to generate tendons [2, 26]. This gene is highly expressed at the interface between muscles and skeletal primordial in E13.5 mouse embryos, but then becomes largely restricted to tendons by E15.5 [27]. One striking aspect of this expression pattern is that scleraxis tends to be expressed in precursors of tissues with significant extracellular matrix (ECM) composition.

Research to date has largely focused on the developmental expression pattern of scleraxis, and its expression in neonatal and adult tissues is only beginning to be explored. One of the barriers to this work has been the lack of an effective scleraxis antibody for use in tissue sections. An RT-PCR analysis of scleraxis expression in adult tissues showed expression in brain, heart, kidney, lung, muscle, spleen, and testis, but not in liver, prostate, or ovary [18]. Data from our laboratory show that scleraxis is expressed in adult rat

cardiac fibroblasts and myofibroblasts as well as in cardiomyocytes, i.e. it is expressed throughout the myocardium [4]. It remains unclear whether the various embryonic tissues that express scleraxis continue to do so in the adult, and whether new regions of scleraxis arise during maturation.

Physiological Role

Since scleraxis is expressed in a variety of tissues, its specific physiological role may vary according to tissue type. However, insight into its role may be obtained by identifying genes that are regulated by scleraxis, of which several have been identified to date. Collectively, these data suggest that scleraxis may be a general regulator of ECM formation, although the specific gene targets appear to vary by tissue type. Indeed, in some cases scleraxis appears to have opposing effects on gene expression depending on cell type.

In a number of studies, scleraxis expression has been associated with putative target gene expression, although a direct causal regulatory mechanism has not yet been demonstrated. For example, several lines of evidence suggest that scleraxis may regulate type II collagen production in a variety of cell types. Scleraxis overexpression in ROS17/2.8 cells resulted in increased expression of collagen II and the cartilage marker osteopontin, while at the same time leading to a decrease in expression of osteoblast markers collagen I and alkaline phosphatase [15, 28]. The coordinated up-regulation of scleraxis, collagen IIb, and aggrecan marks the differentiation of embryonic stem cells to a chondrocyte phenotype [29]. Scleraxis expression also correlates with expression of collagen II and tenascin during development of heart valves, and addition of FGF4 to developing avian heart valves resulted in increased expression of both scleraxis and tenascin [21, 25]. It was recently shown that scleraxis and E47 appear to work synergistically with Sox9 to regulate collagen $2\alpha 1$ gene expression, which is interesting since the expression patterns of scleraxis and Sox9 overlap in early tendon development [27, 30]. The expression of the tendon differentiation marker, tenomodulin, increases in cultured tendon-generating tenocytes in response to retroviral delivery of scleraxis, but whether scleraxis directly transactivates the tenomodulin gene or affects expression indirectly by acting on differentiation pathways is unknown. Both scleraxis and tenomodulin were concomitantly downregulated in myostatin-null mice, suggesting they are co-regulated [31].

Scleraxis has also been demonstrated to directly regulate a number of target genes. Aggrecan 1, a major proteoglycan component of cartilage, is directly up-regulated by scleraxis in ROS17/2.8 cells, due to interaction of scleraxis with the aggrecan 1 promoter [15, 32]. In Sertoli cells, scleraxis has been shown to up-regulate the expression of transferrin and androgen-binding protein, which may contribute to regulation of Sertoli cell function [18].

Recently, evidence from our laboratory and others has demonstrated that scleraxis directly regulates expression of type I collagen. Both scleraxis and collagen I genes were concomitantly expressed in pluripotent tendon-derived cell lines [33].

Type I collagen comprises two subunits, each expressed from its own gene – collagen $I\alpha 1$ and $I\alpha 2$. Scleraxis appears to directly regulate expression of both of these genes. Rossert's group recently demonstrated that the collagen $I\alpha 1$ gene is directly regulated by scleraxis via a short promoter element that was required for expression in rat tendon fibroblasts, in conjunction with NFATc [34]. Our laboratory has reported that scleraxis is expressed by fibroblasts and myofibroblasts, the primary collagen synthesizing cells of the heart, and that scleraxis expression increases more than fourfold during the phenoconversion of fibroblasts to myofibroblasts [4]. We found that scleraxis directly transactivates the human collagen $I\alpha 2$ gene promoter in both NIH 3T3 fibroblasts and primary rat cardiac fibroblasts. We also noted that cardiac fibroblast expression of scleraxis itself was strongly up-regulated by TGF-β_1, a potent pro-fibrotic factor implicated in fibrosis of multiple tissues including the heart, which was previously shown to up-regulate scleraxis expression in ROS17/2.8 cells [17]. It thus appears that a major role for scleraxis is as a master regulator of collagen synthesis. Experiments to examine how scleraxis interacts with the canonical collagen synthetic pathways, including Smad transcription factors, are under way in our laboratory. While there is this clear evidence that scleraxis regulates type I collagen gene expression, the finding that scleraxis over-expression in ROS17/2.8 cells leads to a down-regulation of type I collagen expression indicates that cell context is critical [15].

Additional insight into the role of scleraxis has come from mouse knockout studies. The initial study reporting the generation of scleraxis knockout animals suggested that it was essential for early embryonic development, since embryos homozygous for a targeted scleraxis knockout allele suffered mortality in the early stages of embryogenesis [24]. Recently however, Schweitzer's group produced a novel line of scleraxis-null animals, and found that the initial attempt had generated a hypomorph of an overlapping gene due to a neomycin-resistance selection cassette inserted into the scleraxis locus during generation of the mice. The scleraxis gene is located in the third intron of *Bop1*, a housekeeping gene essential for biogenesis of ribosomes; thus the presence of a Neo minigene may alter Bop1 splicing [35]. Schweitzer's laboratory performed elegant conditional recombination experiments in which they selectively excised the scleraxis coding region using a Cre/loxp approach, and excised the Neo cassette with Flp/frt [36]. Leaving the Neo cassette intact resulted in embryonic lethality similar to the previous knockout line but excision of the selection marker permitted the production of full-term pups.

Scleraxis knockout mice, though viable, had significant defects in load-bearing tendon formation [36]. These animals exhibited a dramatic disruption of tendon differentiation that was manifested in dorsal flexure of the forelimb paw, limited use of all paws, reduced functionality of the back muscles, and complete loss of ability to move the tail. Tendon defects were first noticed close to E13.5 in all tendons. Based on the phenotype observed in the scleraxis-null mice, it appears that scleraxis function is related to the incorporation of tendon progenitors into discrete tendons [36]. This is an important finding since there is little information on the molecular mechanisms that enable tenocytes to coordinate the secretion and organization of matrix structures during tendon genesis [37]. Scleraxis-null mice also showed alterations in their ability to produce tendon matrix, manifested in a dramatic decrease in the number of collagen fibres and their organization within the tendon matrix [36]. Significantly, there was a reduction or loss of collagen I expression in affected tendons, suggesting that scleraxis is required for normal collagen gene expression in agreement with our data in primary cardiac fibroblasts. However, since not all tendons were affected, and since type I collagen expression was relatively normal in some tissues, it is clear that scleraxis is not absolutely required for all such synthesis, and again suggests that cell context is likely to be critical. This study by Schweitzer's group presented the first demonstration of a tendon differentiation phenotype and provided significant insight into the role of scleraxis. Mice in which the myostatin gene has been knocked out appear with a milder phenotype of scleraxis-null mice: tendons are smaller and have reduced fibro-

blast density [31]. Furthermore, myostatin-null mice have reductions in tendon expression of type I collagen, scleraxis, and tenomodulin.

Recent work has also highlighted a potential role for scleraxis in periodontal ligament formation. Scleraxis is expressed in human periodontal ligament cells (hPDLC) and gingival fibroblasts (hGF), with highest expression in hPDLC and lowest in hGF [38, 39]. Indeed, scleraxis is frequently used as a marker for periodontal ligament cells or cell lines committed to a PDL fate [40–42]. Notably, there was a decrease in hPDLC scleraxis expression with increasing passage number in culture [38]. Another study investigated the role of scleraxis in modulating the effect of high glucose concentration on differentiation of hPDLC [43]. Scleraxis expression was up-regulated in hPDLC cultured in high glucose medium in vitro, concomitant with inhibition of osteogenetic differentiation in these cells [43]. These studies suggest that scleraxis expression persists in PDL cells, but is lost if these cells undergo osteogenetic differentiation. However, in contrast to these results it was recently reported that scleraxis expression in a PDL-derived cell line did not decrease with passage number, and appeared to only diminish minimally with osteogenetic induction [44]. The expression of tenomodulin decreased with passaging or osteogenesis induction, even though scleraxis did not appear to change. This is surprising, since an earlier study had identified scleraxis as a regulator of tenomodulin expression [28]. It should be noted, however, that most of these studies were performed in immortalized cultured cell lines derived from PDLs; thus the specific conditions employed may alter cell phenotype and make broad conclusions difficult. Further research into the potential role of scleraxis in inhibiting PDL differentiation is warranted.

Pathological Role

With such limited information to date on the normal roles and mechanism of function of scleraxis, it is perhaps not surprising that little is known about its role in disease and pathological processes. A number of diseases of connective tissue have been described, such as various classifications of Ehlers–Danlos syndrome in which various connective tissue components (particularly fibrillar collagens such as type III, V, and I) are mutated or otherwise incorrectly synthesized [45]. However, the possibility that scleraxis functionally affects initiation or progression of these diseases is completely unexplored to date. It was also previously reported that scleraxis expression is down-regulated in the brains of Down syndrome and Alzheimer disease patients, but this study reported only correlative data [46]. Nonetheless, potential roles for scleraxis in several pathologies are starting to be identified.

A recent study found concomitant increases in scleraxis and collagen $I\alpha1$ expression over several weeks in a mouse model of pathological patellar tendon injury [47]. Since scleraxis is expressed at much higher levels in cell cultures derived from patellar compared to Achilles tendons, it is possible that scleraxis plays a role specifically in the healing process of patellar tendons [48]. The possibility that scleraxis plays distinct roles in only a subset of tendons is further supported by the finding that scleraxis knockout largely affected only force-transmitting or intermuscular tendons [36].

The primary collagen constituent of the heart is type I fibrillar collagen, and this collagen is significantly up-regulated in cardiac fibrosis and in the formation of scar tissue following myocardial infarction [49]. We found a significant increase in scleraxis expression in the region of the infarct scar 4 weeks after surgically induced infarction in parallel with up-regulation of collagen $I\alpha2$ gene expression [4]. In contrast, these increases were not observed in distal non-infarcted myocardium or in sham-operated animals. We previously generated an acute heart failure model in transgenic mice by specifically expressing a constitutively active HDAC5 mutant in the heart [50]. Microarray analysis of these animals revealed a significant up-regulation of scleraxis expression several days prior to up-regulation of fibrillar collagens. Our data suggest that scleraxis may play a causal role in the induction of cardiac fibrosis. At this time, however, it is unclear whether scleraxis regulates type I collagen expression under basal conditions, in pathological conditions (e.g. post-infarct or during hypertension), or both.

Keloids are dermal thickenings or scars characterized by rampant over-expression of fibrillar type I or III collagen. Intriguingly, scleraxis expression is strongly induced in fibroblasts isolated from samples of dermal keloids [51]. In contrast, scleraxis is not expressed in normal dermal fibroblasts. Since our data indicate that scleraxis is sufficient to drive collagen $I\alpha2$ expression, it is intriguing to speculate that aberrant expression of scleraxis in dermal fibroblasts may contribute to the pathology of keloids. Since keloids represent a form of fibrosis, this finding in conjunction with our cardiac data suggests that scleraxis may be involved in the general induction of fibrosis, regardless of tissue type. If scleraxis is in fact a central player in multiple forms of fibrosis, then it may represent a convenient target for the development of novel anti-fibrotic therapies. The need for such therapies is significant, since pharmaceuticals specifically directed at reducing fibrosis are currently lacking [49].

Conclusions

The regulation of ECM formation plays a key role in mediating the function of many tissues. The association of scleraxis expression with that of a number of ECM genes suggests that it plays a central role in ECM synthesis, and thereby impacts ECM function through direct or indirect regulation of target genes. A clear role for scleraxis regulation of tendon development, structure, and function has been shown with the creation of scleraxis-null mice [36]. Data from our laboratory and others showing that scleraxis regulates type I collagen gene expression, that it is expressed in cardiac fibroblasts, and that its expression is associated with post-infarct cardiac remodeling indicate that scleraxis has other critical functions that are only beginning to be explored [4, 34]. Scleraxis may thus represent a candidate target for treatment of fibrosis in the heart and other tissues, but more work remains to be done before the promise of anti-fibrotic treatments based on interference with scleraxis function can be exploited.

References

1. Schweitzer R, Chyung JH, Murtaugh LC, et al. Analysis of the tendon cell fate using Scleraxis, a specific marker for tendons and ligaments. Development. 2001;128:3855–66.
2. Brent AE, Schweitzer R, Tabin CJ. A somitic compartment of tendon progenitors. Cell. 2003;113:235–48.
3. Cserjesi P, Brown D, Ligon KL, et al. Scleraxis: a basic helix-loop-helix protein that prefigures skeletal formation during mouse embryogenesis. Development. 1995;121:1099–110.
4. Espira L, Lamoureux L, Jones SC, et al. The basic helix-loop-helix transcription factor scleraxis regulates fibroblast collagen synthesis. J Mol Cell Cardiol. 2009;47:188–95.
5. Kadesch T. Consequences of heteromeric interactions among helix-loop-helix proteins. Cell Growth Differ. 1993;4:49–55.
6. Jan YN, Jan LY. Functional gene cassettes in development. Proc Natl Acad Sci USA. 1993;90:8305–7.
7. Olson EN, Klein WH. bHLH factors in muscle development: dead lines and commitments, what to leave in and what to leave out. Genes Dev. 1994;8:1–8.
8. Goldfarb AN, Lewandowska K. Nuclear redirection of a cytoplasmic helix-loop-helix protein via heterodimerization with a nuclear localizing partner. Exp Cell Res. 1994;214:481–5.
9. Littlewood TD, Evan GI. Helix-loop-helix transcription factors. 3rd ed. USA: Oxford University Press; 1998.
10. Chaudhary J, Skinner MK. Basic helix-loop-helix proteins can act at the E-box within the serum response element of the c-fos promoter to influence hormone-induced promoter activation in Sertoli cells. Mol Endocrinol. 1999;13:774–86.
11. Ephrussi A, Church GM, Tonegawa S, et al. B lineage–specific interactions of an immunoglobulin enhancer with cellular factors in vivo. Science. 1985;227:134–40.
12. Molkentin JD, Olson EN. Combinatorial control of muscle development by basic helix-loop-helix and MADS-box transcription factors. Proc Natl Acad Sci USA. 1996;93:9366–73.
13. Murre C, McCaw PS, Vaessin H, et al. Interactions between heterologous helix-loop-helix proteins generate complexes that bind specifically to a common DNA sequence. Cell. 1989;58:537–44.
14. Carlberg AL, Tuan RS, Hall DJ. Regulation of scleraxis function by interaction with the bHLH protein E47. Mol Cell Biol Res Commun. 2000;3:82–6.
15. Liu Y, Watanabe H, Nifuji A, et al. Overexpression of a single helix-loop-helix-type transcription factor, scleraxis, enhances aggrecan gene expression in osteoblastic osteosarcoma ROS17/2.8 cells. J Biol Chem. 1997;272:29880–5.
16. Muir T, Wilson-Rawls J, Stevens JD, et al. Integration of CREB and bHLH transcriptional signaling pathways through direct heterodimerization of the proteins: role in muscle and testis development. Mol Reprod Dev. 2008;75:1637–52.
17. Liu Y, Cserjesi P, Nifuji A, Olson EN, et al. Sclerotome-related helix-loop-helix type transcription factor (scleraxis) mRNA is expressed in osteoblasts and its level is enhanced by type-beta transforming growth factor. J Endocrinol. 1996;151:491–9.
18. Muir T, Sadler-Riggleman I, Skinner MK. Role of the basic helix-loop-helix transcription factor, scleraxis, in the regulation of Sertoli cell function and differentiation. Mol Endocrinol. 2005;19:2164–74.
19. Smith TG, Sweetman D, Patterson M, et al. Feedback interactions between MKP3 and ERK MAP kinase control scleraxis expression and the specification of rib progenitors in the developing chick somite. Development. 2005;132:1305–14.
20. Brent AE, Tabin CJ. FGF acts directly on the somitic tendon progenitors through the Ets transcription factors Pea3 and Erm to regulate scleraxis expression. Development. 2004;131:3885–96.
21. Zhao B, Etter L, Hinton Jr RB, et al. BMP and FGF regulatory pathways in semilunar valve precursor cells. Dev Dyn. 2007;236:971–80.
22. Edom-Vovard F, Schuler B, Bonnin MA, Teillet MA, Duprez D. Fgf4 positively regulates scleraxis and tenascin expression in chick limb tendons. Dev Biol. 2002;247:351–66.
23. Levay AK, Peacock JD, Lu Y, et al. Scleraxis is required for cell lineage differentiation and extracellular matrix remodeling during murine heart valve formation in vivo. Circ Res. 2008;103:948–56.
24. Brown D, Wagner D, Li X, Richardson JA, et al. Dual role of the basic helix-loop-helix transcription factor scleraxis in mesoderm formation and chondrogenesis during mouse embryogenesis. Development. 1999;126:4317–29.
25. Lincoln J, Alfieri CM, Yutzey KE. Development of heart valve leaflets and supporting apparatus in chicken and mouse embryos. Dev Dyn. 2004;230:239–50.
26. Dubrulle J, Pourquie O. Welcome to syndetome: a new somitic compartment. Dev Cell. 2003;4:611–12.
27. Asou Y, Nifuji A, Tsuji K, et al. Coordinated expression of scleraxis and Sox9 genes during embryonic development of tendons and cartilage. J Orthop Res. 2002;20:827–33.
28. Shukunami C, Takimoto A, Oro M, et al. Scleraxis positively regulates the expression of tenomodulin, a differentiation marker of tenocytes. Dev Biol. 2006;298:234–47.
29. zur Nieden NI, Kempka G, Rancourt DE, et al. Induction of chondro-, osteo- and adipogenesis in embryonic stem cells by bone morphogenetic protein-2: effect of cofactors on differentiating lineages. BMC Dev Biol. 2005;5:1.
30. Furumatsu T, Shukunami C, Amemiya-Kudo M, Shimano H, Ozaki T. Scleraxis and E47 cooperatively regulate the Sox9-dependent transcription. Int J Biochem Cell Biol. 2010;42:148–56.
31. Mendias CL, Bakhurin KI, Faulkner JA. Tendons of myostatin-deficient mice are small, brittle, and

hypocellular. Proc Natl Acad Sci USA. 2008; 105:388–93.

32. Watanabe H, Kimata K, Line S, et al. Mouse cartilage matrix deficiency (cmd) caused by a 7 bp deletion in the aggrecan gene. Nat Genet. 1994;7:154–7.

33. Salingcarnboriboon R, Yoshitake H, Tsuji K, et al. Establishment of tendon-derived cell lines exhibiting pluripotent mesenchymal stem cell-like property. Exp Cell Res. 2003;287:289–300.

34. Lejard V, Brideau G, Blais F, et al. Scleraxis and NFATc regulate the expression of the pro-alpha1(I) collagen gene in tendon fibroblasts. J Biol Chem. 2007;282:17665–75.

35. Strezoska Z, Pestov DG, Lau LF. Functional inactivation of the mouse nucleolar protein Bop1 inhibits multiple steps in pre-rRNA processing and blocks cell cycle progression. J Biol Chem. 2002;277:29617–25.

36. Murchison ND, Price BA, Conner DA, et al. Regulation of tendon differentiation by scleraxis distinguishes force-transmitting tendons from muscle-anchoring tendons. Development. 2007;134: 2697–708.

37. Kannus P. Structure of the tendon connective tissue. Scand J Med Sci Sports. 2000;10:312–20.

38. Liu Q, Xie H, Li WY, et al. Expression of Scleraxis in human periodontal ligament cells and gingival fibroblasts. Zhonghua Kou Qiang Yi Xue Za Zhi. 2006;41:556–8.

39. Shi S, Bartold PM, Miura M, et al. The efficacy of mesenchymal stem cells to regenerate and repair dental structures. Orthod Craniofac Res. 2005;8:191–9.

40. Tomokiyo A, Maeda H, Fujii S, et al. Development of a multipotent clonal human periodontal ligament cell line. Differentiation. 2008;76:337–47.

41. Yokoi T, Saito M, Kiyono T, et al. Establishment of immortalized dental follicle cells for generating periodontal ligament in vivo. Cell Tissue Res. 2007;327:301–11.

42. Fujii S, Maeda H, Wada N, et al. Investigating a clonal human periodontal ligament progenitor/stem cell line in vitro and in vivo. J Cell Physiol. 2008;215:743–9.

43. Yuan YD, Miao S, Xie H. Effect of high glucose on the expression of transcription factor Scleraxis in periodontal ligament cells in vitro. Zhonghua Kou Qiang Yi Xue Za Zhi. 2008;43:668–70.

44. Itaya T, Kagami H, Okada K, et al. Characteristic changes of periodontal ligament-derived cells during passage. J Periodontal Res. 2009;44:425–33.

45. Callewaert B, Malfait F, Loeys B, et al. Ehlers-Danlos syndromes and Marfan syndrome. Best Pract Res Clin Rheumatol. 2008;22:165–89.

46. Yeghiazaryan K, Turhani-Schatzmann D, Labudova O, et al. Downregulation of the transcription factor scleraxis in brain of patients with Down syndrome. J Neural Transm Suppl. 1999;57:305–14.

47. Scott A, Sampaio A, Abraham T, et al. Scleraxis expression is coordinately regulated in a murine model of patellar tendon injury. J Orthop Res. 2011;29:289–96.

48. Yeh LC, Tsai AD, Lee JC. Bone morphogenetic protein-7 regulates differentially the mRNA expression of bone morphogenetic proteins and their receptors in rat achilles and patellar tendon cell cultures. J Cell Biochem. 2008;104:2107–22.

49. Espira L, Czubryt MP. Emerging concepts in cardiac matrix biology. Can J Physiol Pharmacol. 2009;87:996–1008.

50. Czubryt MP, McAnally J, Fishman GI, et al. Regulation of peroxisome proliferator-activated receptor gamma coactivator 1 alpha (PGC-1 alpha) and mitochondrial function by MEF2 and HDAC5. Proc Natl Acad Sci USA. 2003;100:1711–16.

51. Naitoh M, Kubota H, Ikeda M, et al. Gene expression in human keloids is altered from dermal to chondrocytic and osteogenic lineage. Genes Cells. 2005;10: 1081–91.

Gender Impact on Pathophysiology of the Heart

Jane-Lise Samuel, Claude Delcayre,
and Bernard Swynghedauw

Abstract

Cardiovascular diseases are the leading cause of death in men and women in industrialized countries. The profound impact of biological sex on cardiovascular physiology of pathology has long been known, but the biological mechanisms responsible for sex-related differences have emerged more recently. Thus, this chapter is aimed at bringing a comprehensive review of the sex-based differences in cardiac structure and function in adults, during aging, and on the cardiac adaptability to pressure overload. The analysis of the major molecular mechanisms involved highlighted the impact of sex-based differences in pathophysiology of the heart. It emerged from the review that the sex-based difference is a variable that should be dealt with in both basic science and clinical research.

Keywords

Cardiac function • Cardiac hypertrophy • Coronary artery • Estrogens • Gender • Heart failure • Myocytes

Introduction

Cardiovascular diseases are the leading cause of death in men and women in industrialized countries, with aging, hypertension, and metabolic disorders being the major risk factors. The profound impact of biological sex on cardiovascular physiology or pathology has long been known, but the biological mechanisms responsible for sex-related differences have emerged more recently. This review aims to highlight the major differences in cardiac gene expression according to gender and/or female sex hormone in both basal conditions and in response to pathological situations such as severe pressure overload.

J.-L. Samuel (✉)
U942-INSERM, Hôpital Lariboisière Paris, France
e-mail: jane-lise.samuel@inserm.fr

B. Ostadal et al. (eds.), *Genes and Cardiovascular Function*,
DOI 10.1007/978-1-4419-7207-1_7, © Springer Science+Business Media, LLC 2011

Sex-Based Differences in Cardiac Structure and Function in Adults and During Aging

Before puberty there is no difference between men and women in terms of heart size and number and size of cardiomyocytes. However, after puberty the male myocardium is 15–30% larger than that of female, the size of cardiomyocytes is higher in males than in females, whereas the myocyte number is similar (review in [1]). This indicates a greater hypertrophic growth of the cardiomyocytes in men than in women during the adult life. With aging, sex-based differences are also reported. There is a preservation of cardiomyocyte number and sizes in elderly females whereas a significant loss of cardiomyocytes is described in age-matched men (review in [1]). In men, the number of cardiomyocytes significantly decreases (64 million are lost per year) through different processes including apoptosis and necrosis (review in [2]) (Table 1), whereas in the remaining cells, cardiomyocyte volume increases through a hypertrophic process [1, 3]. Women demonstrate a marked increase in the incidence of left ventricular (LV) hypertrophy after menopause, when the prevalence of arterial

Table 1 Biological parameters of female cardiomyocytes compared to male

Biological parameters	Female vs. male variation
Excitation-contraction coupling	
Ca^{2+} transients	Smaller
Amplitude of sparks	Lower
Gain of E-C coupling	Smaller
Time to peak	Smaller
Mitochondria	
Ca^{2+} uptake rates	Lower
Cardiac mitochondria content	Lower
Mitochondria efficiency	Better
H_2O_2 generation	Lower
β-Adrenergic system	
Density of β-adrenergic receptors	Lower
Inotropic response to β-adrenergic stimulation	Decreased

hypertension increases [4]. This cardiac hypertrophy can be significantly prevented by hormonal replacement therapy [1]. The occurrence of interstitial fibrosis, another classical feature of aging of the heart, is differentially regulated according to gender. Indeed, cardiac interstitial fibrosis is dramatically developed in males when compared to females (27% vs. 18% in the males and females septa, respectively) [5]. These histopathological findings are in-line with the sex-based differences observed through echocardiographic analysis. The diameter of the left ventricle (LV) increases with age only in men. Young women have a better diastolic function than men. With age, ventricular filling is impaired in both sexes, but the systolic function deteriorates only in men [6, 7]. Exercise reveals clearly sex-related differences in both healthy subjects and patients with asymptomatic aortic stenosis (AS) despite similar hemodynamic properties of the heart at rest [8–10] (Table 2). During exercise, the ejection fraction tends to increase more in men than in women whereas the cardiac output increases similarly in both. These data reflect the sex-based mechanisms involved in the adaptive responses of the heart to exercise. Women tend to increase their cardiac output primarily by increasing end-diastolic volume index without significantly increasing the ejection fraction whereas men primarily decrease the end-systolic volume index and raise the ejection fraction (reviews in [1, 10]) (Table 2).

Molecular Mechanisms of Sex-Specific Differences in Adult Heart and During Aging

The candidates to mediate sex-specific effects in the cardiovascular system are receptors for estrogens, progesterone, and androgens (ERs, PRs, and ARs, respectively). The two known ERs – ERα and ERβ – have been described in the human and rodent heart, (review in [11]). ERs, ARs, and PRs act by a number of genomic and non-genomic pathways. They are transcription factors able to initiate the transcription of hormone-sensitive

Table 2 Sex-based differences in cardiac function in humans

	Men	Women
Healthy subjects [10]		
LV stiffness constant β	0.011	0.012
Heart failure with normal ejection fraction [10]		
LV stiffness constant β	0.021	0.030*
Upright exercise of healthy subjects [8]		
Weight-adjusted peak O_2 consumption (mL/kg/min)	22.1	22.6
Ejection fraction at rest/during exercise (%)	62/77**	63/64
End-diastolic volume during exercise	+10%	+30%**
Increase in cardiac flow during exercise	+23%	+33%
Ratio of exercise to resting O_2 arteriovenous difference	+2.33	+2.34
Asymptomatic aortic stenosis [9]		
Ventricular mass (g/m²)	84	73*
End-diastolic volume (mL/m²)	50	39**
End-systolic volume (mL/m²)	18	13**
Increase in cardiac output during exercise (L/min)	8.0	5.4**

$*p < 0.05$; $**p \leq 0.01$

genes or to modulate the activity of other transcription factors. Upon binding of hormones, ER, AR, and PR might activate or interfere with multiple signaling pathways including phosphatidylinositol 3-kinase (PI3K).

In addition, many cardioprotective genes, such as HSP72 or HSP70, are up-regulated either directly or indirectly by estrogens (review in [1]). One of the major cellular targets for the sex-based differences in the cardiovascular system are the endothelial cells, mainly through the modulation of the endogenous vasodilator nitric oxide (NO). At baseline, the endothelial NO synthase NOS3 is present in both coronary vascular endothelium and cardiac endothelium. NOS3 is mainly targeted, through binding to caveolin-1 to plasmalemmal caveolae, microdomains that serve as sites for the sequestration of signaling molecules, review in [12]. Regarding the control of NOS3 activity in endothelial cells, the estrogens play a key role. Chambliss et al. [13] have shown in endothelial cells the non-genomic control of NOS3 via the estrogen receptor-α within the caveolae. Estrogen absence significantly affects the NOS3 activity [14, 15]. As reviewed by Fleming and Busse [15] chronic changes in estrogen status can differentially affect NOS3 and caveolin-1 protein levels in endothelial cells. In estrogen-depleted rat heart, a significant reduction in NOS3 activity

without change in the NOS3 expression but with enhanced NOS3–caveolin-1 interactions has been described [16]. Thus, the estrogen-dependent NOS3–caveolin interactions play an important role in the control of NOS3 activity and in turn in the endothelium-dependent vasodilation. In addition to the action on NO, the modulatory effects of estrogens on artery myogenic tone appear to involve regulation of calcium-activated potassium (BKCa) channels [17, 18]. In-line with these results, sex-based differences in coronary artery function have been observed in response to moderate increase in cardiac aldosterone production without alteration of cardiac function [19]. Indeed, a coronary dysfunction in aldosterone synthase-transgenic mice is observed only in males [20] and is demonstrated to be related to altered (1) calcium-activated potassium (BKCa) channels' expression in vascular smooth muscle and (2) coronary BKCa-dependent relaxation [21]. Recent results from our laboratory indicate that estrogens might counteract the effect of hyperaldosteronism on the BKCa-mediated coronary relaxation (Delcayre et al. unpublished data).

At the level of cardiomyocytes, there are sex differences in excitation-contraction (E-C) coupling in cardiac cells from adult rats; Ca^{2+} transients are smaller and the gain of E-C coupling is lower in female cardiomyocytes than in male cells and, in addition, aging-induced alterations of cardiac E-C coupling are more prominent in cardiomyocytes from males than in cells from females [3]. The difference in gain of E-C coupling between male and female cardiomyocytes reflects differences in the mean amplitude of sparks and the time to peak, which are smaller in female cells than in the male ones [22]. Other sex-based differences in intracellular calcium handling have been reported, such as phosphorylation state of phospholamban and L-type Ca^{2+} channel density. Revisiting gender-related differences in $K^{(+)}$ currents in mouse ventricle, it has been recently proposed that down-regulation of Kv4.3 and Kv1.5 transcripts by estrogens is one of the mechanisms defining gender-related differences in ventricular repolarization [23].

In addition, sex-based differences are found also in the uptake of Ca^{2+} by cardiac mitochondria – mitochondria from female rat heart having lower Ca^{2+} uptake rates; for a review see [24]. In addition, female rats exhibit lower cardiac mitochondria content; they are more efficient and generate less H_2O_2 than the males. Finally female myocytes have a lower density of β-adrenergic receptors and thus also a decreased inotropic response to β-adrenergic stimulation [24]. Of note, across the life span various biochemical characteristics (including telomerase activity and several components of the insulin-like growth factor system) vary differently in male and female cardiomyocytes [25].

In addition to the sex-based differences listed above, significant differences in the way male and female hearts respond to various challenges bring important insight into the mechanisms by which the female gender may influence favorably the remodeling and the adaptive response to myocardial insult.

Cardiac Adaptability to Pressure Overload and Impact of Sex-Based Differences

Hypertrophy per se is an independent risk factor for heart failure and sudden death (review in [2]). Mechanical pressure overload being secondary to either hypertension or to aortic stenosis, we will refer to both etiologies in this review. We have known for a long time the sex-specific ability of the myocardium to adapt to mechanical overload [26, 27]; sex differences in cardiovascular disease have been receiving increasing attention in both experimental and clinical research in the recent past [1, 7, 11, 16, 24, 28–31].

It is well assessed that premenopausal women have a better prognosis than do men in response to hypertension and aortic stenosis. Indeed, a clinical study of 29 women and 53 men with asymptomatic aortic stenosis has clearly demonstrated that men show an earlier and more severe systolic dysfunction than women [9]. Based on a clinical trial, the lines of evidence indicated that heart failure with normal ejection fraction (HFNEF) is much more common in women than in men [10]. This predominance has been demonstrated in a large American study, including 79% of women after adjusting the data for all available information. The study focuses on 19,710 patients (over 65 years) with heart failure, 35% of them having a normal ejection fraction. Of note, the diastolic function was not investigated in the cohort [32]. Similar results were found by Klapholz et al., [33] who conducted a prospective multicenter registry in a NY area to define the clinical characteristics, hospital course, treatment, and factors precipitating decompensation in patients hospitalized for HFNEF. A European study including 24 countries has led to similar conclusions, but again in the absence of left ventricular filling measures [34]. However, some authors have investigated the diastolic function by using echocardiography; review in [10]. Among them, "the Strong Heart Study" by Devereux et al. [35] deserves attention. This population-based study enrolled 3,184 patients aged between 47 and 81 years and was characterized by a high proportion of women (84%). It emerged that patients with HFNEF were old and overweight, in majority women, had renal dysfunction, impaired early diastolic LV relaxation, and concentric LV geometry. Conversely, patients with congestive heart failure and severe LV dysfunction were more often men, exhibiting a restrictive pattern of LV filling and eccentric LV hypertrophy. Other studies provide more nuanced

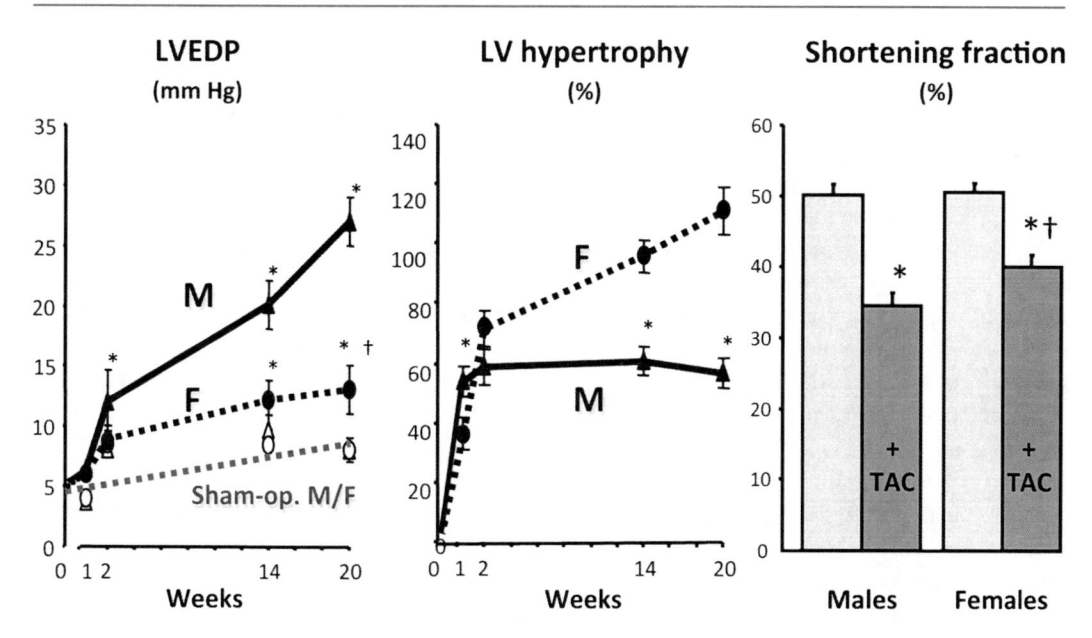

Fig. 1 Sex-related differences in responses to hemodynamic challenge. For a same level of aortic stenosis, LVEDP increases more and LV hypertrophy increases less in male rats than in females. In consequence, cardiac function is less depressed in females than in males (Redrawn from [30])

results, suggesting equal or greater prevalence of diastolic dysfunction in men (review in [10]). Thus, the greater rate of HFNEF in women might be related to sex-based differences in ventricular diastolic distensibility, in vascular stiffness and ventricular/vascular coupling, in skeletal muscle adaptation to HF, and in the perception of symptoms [10].

When focusing on patients with aortic stenosis (AS), [7, 36], women, and particularly elderly ones, develop a more concentric form of hypertrophy than men, with smaller ventricular diameters and less ventricular dilatation. In some, but not all studies, women had higher transvalvular gradients, greater relative wall thickness, and better systolic function. Furthermore, women with congestive heart failure have also been shown to survive better than men in some studies [7].

Interestingly enough, when analyzing hypertrophy regression after aortic valve replacement, LV hypertrophy reversed more frequently in women than in men [28].

Experimental data confirm and extend these sex-based differences in the development of cardiac hypertrophy to pressure overload. Different studies indicated that at the very early phase of a mechanical pressure overload, female rats develop more cardiac hypertrophy than male rats [27, 30] and that only males exhibit decreased signs of acute heart failure [30] (Fig. 1). However, in mice, the sex-based differences were observed only at later stages of cardiac hypertrophy (2 weeks after surgery) [37]. Thus, the differences in the adaptation of female and male hearts to pressure overload draw attention to the underlying mechanistic pathways.

Sex-Specific Differences in Gene Expression and Cardiac Adaptation to Pressure Overload

The sex-based differences in remodeling of the whole heart are mirrored by differences in intracellular signaling pathways and/or patterns of gene expression. One of the pioneer works on sex-based differences in cardiac response to severe pressure overload, such as thoracic aortic stenosis (TAC), demonstrated that ß-MyHC expression is greater in male than in female hypertrophic hearts, whereas the sarcoplasmic reticulum Ca^{2+}–ATPase mRNA levels are depressed in males only, and the Na^+–Ca^{2+} exchanger mRNA levels are increased independently of the gender, these transcriptional changes being associated with a preserved contractile reserve in female hypertrophic hearts [38]. In contrast, mRNA microarray analysis using the transverse aortic constriction (TAC) model in mice does not show differences in the selection of hypertrophy markers such as α-actin, ANP, and BNP [37, 39]. However, several genes controlling mitochondrial functions including PGC-1 had a lower expression in males [37]. A whole female/male gene network analysis reveals that female-specific genes are mainly related to mitochondria and metabolism and male-specific ones to extracellular matrix and biosynthesis [37]. Of note, the number of differentially regulated genes in response to acute pressure overload is greater (greater than twofold) in males than in females, whereas the response to chronic pressure overload is similar in males and females [39].

Marked sex-based differences in the development of fibrosis associated with cardiovascular disease, and particularly with pressure overload, have been observed both in human [40] and in experimental models [37, 41]. In this microarray analysis [37, 41], genes associated with extracellular matrix remodeling exhibited a lower expression in female hearts (collagen 3, MMP 2, TIMP2, and TGF-β2) after TAC in mice. Although the molecular mechanisms underlying gender dimorphism are complex and are still not well understood, it emerged that steroid sex hormones (estrogens, progesterone, and testosterone) and their respective receptors play a key role (review in [31]). It is established that estrogens reduce the turnover of the extracellular matrix, especially the collagen network. Estrogens inhibit fibroblast proliferation and collagen synthesis of type 1, but activate the expression of genes encoding metalloproteinase [42, 43]. It is worthy of note the recent insights into the sex-specific regulation of fibrosis-related genes using genetic models and in vitro approaches. Indeed, ß-estradiol significantly increased collagen-I and -III gene expressions in male fibroblasts and had opposite effects in female

cells [28]. Using the genetic model ER-beta(−/−), it is demonstrated that sex-based difference in cardiac fibrosis after TAC was abolished in ER-beta (−/−) mice [41]. The sex-based differences observed in the regulation of genes encoding ECM proteins and metalloproteinase and, in turn, in the development of fibrosis in response to pressure overload might represent (1) one of the major mechanisms slowing the progression to heart failure in females and (2) a positive element allowing more rapid hypertrophy regression following surgery for aortic valve replacement.

Other lines of evidence of estrogen-induced cardioprotection were provided by studies devoted to NO bioavailability and/or endothelial dysfunction. It has been demonstrated that NO had direct systolic as well as diastolic myocardial effects (review in [12]). The reduction in the bioavailability of NO is a key feature of endothelial dysfunction, classically described during heart failure. This decreased dilatation in small arteries is mainly secondary to the chronic decrease in blood flow [44], which is probably involved in the decrease in the expression and/or the activity of NOS3 in the failing myocardium in human [45] and experimental [46–48] models. Besides, a role of the protein–protein interactions, or posttranslational modification controlling NOS3 activity, such as caveolin-1 binding, NOS3 phosphorylation has been proposed [49, 50] to modulate NOS3 activity. At least, the NO reduction could be due to the increased peroxynitrites or to NOS3 decoupling (review in [12]). During the development of cardiac hypertrophy, the NOS3 expression varies according to the hypertrophic stimuli. The development of physiological cardiac hypertrophy during gestation is associated with a transient increase of cardiac NOS3 expression (up to 14 days pc) that is paralleled by an increase of cGMP [51]. In response to a severe pressure overload secondary to a thoracic aorta coarctation (TAC), gender differences in changes in NOS3 activity are observed [30]. In female rats, the NOS3 activity in the hypertrophied heart remained constant, although the enzyme expression increased before appearance of HF signs [16]. After TAC, the absence of estrogen prevents the increase in

NOS3 expression and worsens the cardiac dysfunction without affecting the development of cardiac hypertrophy. These data highlight the role of NOS3 through estrogen in the cardiac adaptation to new load conditions [16]. One novel pathway to mediate the protective effects through NOS activity on the vasculature and heart may be the increase of protein S-nitrosylation in the vascular endothelium by estrogen and mainly ß-estradiol [52].

Besides the putative role of NOS3-derived NO, the implication of NOS1-derived NO has been demonstrated during the development of cardiac hypertrophy and failure [53–55]. In addition, it was shown that male mice lacking both NOS isoforms NOS1/3(−/−) have a twofold higher mortality compared to females whereas gender does not affect survival when only one NOS gene was knocked out. Notably, the development of cardiomyocyte hypertrophy and interstitial fibrosis with age in NOS1/3(−/−) mice is independent of the gender [56].

Conversely to failing heart, in rats as well as in humans, in which NOS1 activity increased together with a redistribution of the enzyme at the sarcolemmal level through binding with caveolin-3 [53, 54], the subcellular relocalization of NOS1, particularly the translocation toward the sarcolemma, is not observed in hypertrophic hearts following TAC. Furthermore, the NOS1 activity is shown to depend upon enzyme expression level without influence of molecular partners such as caveolin-3 [16]. Sex-based differences have been observed: NOS1/caveolin-3 association is significantly higher in females versus males in response to cardiac injury in mice [57] or following pressure overload in rats [30]. In these models, ß-estradiol per se modulates neither NOS1 expression nor activity, whatever the hypertrophy status [16]. Thus according to Murphy et al. [58], the increase in NOS1 near caveolin-3 in females under stress conditions (I/R) associated with increased calcium (which activates NOS) results in increased S-nitrosylation of the L-type calcium channel, lower calcium entry, and therefore less calcium loading, constituting a cardioprotective mechanism as previously discussed [52].

Lines of evidence indicated that mechanosensitive pathways trigger NOS1 expression and activity in muscle cells including cardiomyocytes (review in [12]). During the early phase after TAC, the higher parietal stress in males than in females [27] has been proposed to be one of the triggers for the early NOS1 induction in rat hearts after TAC [30]. In addition, it was demonstrated that NOS1 expression in cardiac muscle following TAC was independent of estrogen level [16]. Thus according to the pressure overload and estrogen status, there is a differential regulation of NOS expression and activity, the mechanotransduction pathway being mainly involved in the induction of NOS1, while the ER pathway regulated NOS3 activity and, in turn, cardiac function. This differential response in NOS expression and activity during development of cardiac hypertrophy and according to gender might affect the molecular mechanisms by which NO influences myocardial function, particularly cGMP-activated pathways [59]. In addition to NO, ANP is known to modulate cGMP levels in cardiomyocytes [60], and to alter their function.

The association of natriuretic peptides (NPs), such as BNP and ANP, with gender was examined in several studies; despite disparity, some studies report a higher BNP concentration in females compared to males. Indeed in normal patients, NT-proBNP, like BNP, tends to be higher in female patients and older individuals, through mechanisms involving either the clearance receptor for BNP or increase in expression [61, 62]. On the other hand, a population-based study indicated that in women, LV mass and NP concentrations increase to a lesser extent and only with severe LV dysfunction when compared to men [63]. In the same way, experimental models indicate that ANP mRNA level is greater in male than in female TAC-induced hypertrophy rat hearts [38]. Regarding women, hormone replacement therapy has been associated with higher BNP levels, suggesting that BNP expression may be sensitive to estrogen regulation in humans [62]. The role of estrogens in the control of ANP expression during the development of cardiac hypertrophy has been evidenced in experimental models [64]. In-line with these findings, it has been shown that in vitro estrogens exert antihypertrophic effects on cardiomyocytes, by transactivation of the ANP gene [65, 66]. Estrogen-induced ANP accumulation in the ventricular cardiomyocytes most likely results in ANP receptor activation in an autocrine/paracrine manner which, in turn, evokes cytoplasmic cGMP signaling downstream [65]. Furthermore, the increase in cGMP mediated by ANP, but not by NO, prevents cardiomyocyte hypertrophy [66]. Interestingly, during the development of pregnancy-induced cardiac hypertrophy, the down-regulation of cardiac NPs as BNP and receptors in LV during may be physiologically required to allow the development of physiological LV hypertrophy. Of note is the expression of NPs increasing postpartum, when the development of cardiac hypertrophy has to be stopped [51]. Taken together it emerged that the tight regulation of NP expression is of importance for the sex-based differences in the development of cardiac hypertrophy.

Conclusions

In summary, the differences in cardiac gene expression according to gender and/or female sex hormone described here would help to stress that gender is a variable that should be dealt with in both basic science and clinical research. It is clear that the response of humans and animals to various disease states can be profoundly affected by sex.

References

1. Bhupathy P, Haines CD, Leinwand LA. Influence of sex hormones and phytoestrogens on heart disease in men and women. Womens Health (Lond Engl). 2010;6:77–95.
2. Swynghedauw B. Molecular mechanisms of myocardial remodeling. Physiol Rev. 1999;79:215–62.
3. Howlett SE. Age-associated changes in excitation-contraction coupling are more prominent in ventricular myocytes from male rats than in myocytes from female rats. Am J Physiol Heart Circ Physiol. 2010;298:H659–70.
4. Lopez-Ruiz A, Sartori-Valinotti J, Yanes LL, et al. Sex differences in control of blood pressure: role of oxidative stress in hypertension in females. Am J Physiol Heart Circ Physiol. 2008;295:H466–74.
5. Forman DE, Cittadini A, Azhar G, et al. Cardiac morphology and function in senescent rats: gender-related differences. J Am Coll Cardiol. 1997;30: 1872–7.
6. Swynghedauw B, Besse S, Assayag P. Biology of cardiac and vascular senescence. Bull Acad Natl Méd. 2006;190:783–92.
7. Luczak ED, Leinwand LA. Sex-based cardiac physiology. Annu Rev Physiol. 2009;71:1–18.
8. Higginbotham MB, Morris KG, Coleman RE, Cobb FR. Sex-related differences in the normal cardiac response to upright exercise. Circulation. 1984;70:357–66.
9. Legget ME, Kuusisto J, Healy NL, et al. Gender differences in left ventricular function at rest and with exercise in asymptomatic aortic stenosis. Am Heart J. 1996;131:94–100.
10. Regitz-Zagrosek V, Brokat S, Tschope C. Role of gender in heart failure with normal left ventricular ejection fraction. Prog Cardiovasc Dis. 2007;49:241–51.
11. Regitz-Zagrosek V. Therapeutic implications of the gender-specific aspects of cardiovascular disease. Nat Rev Drug Discov. 2006;5:425–38.
12. Loyer X, Heymes C, Samuel JL. Constitutive nitric oxide synthases in the heart from hypertrophy to failure. Clin Exp Pharmacol Physiol. 2008;35:483–8.
13. Chambliss KL, Shaul PW. Rapid activation of endothelial NO synthase by estrogen: evidence for a steroid receptor fast-action complex (SRFC) in caveolae. Steroids. 2002;67:413–9.
14. Mendelsohn ME, Karas RH. The protective effects of estrogen on the cardiovascular system. N Engl J Med. 1999;340:1801–11.
15. Fleming I, Busse R. Molecular mechanisms involved in the regulation of the endothelial nitric oxide synthase. Am J Physiol Regul Integr Comp Physiol. 2003;284:R1–12.
16. Loyer X, Damy T, Chvojkova Z, et al. 17beta-estradiol regulates constitutive nitric oxide synthase expression differentially in the myocardium in response to pressure overload. Endocrinology. 2007;148:4579–84.
17. Geary GG, Krause DN, Duckles SP. Estrogen reduces myogenic tone through a nitric oxide-dependent mechanism in rat cerebral arteries. Am J Physiol Heart Circ Physiol. 1998;275:H292–300.
18. Rosenfeld CR, White RE, Roy T, et al. Calcium-activated potassium channels and nitric oxide coregulate estrogen-induced vasodilation. Am J Physiol Heart Circ Physiol. 2000;279:H319–28.
19. Benard L, Milliez P, Ambroisine ML, et al. Effects of aldosterone on coronary function. Pharmacol Rep. 2009;61:58–66.
20. Garnier A, Bendall JK, Fuchs S, et al. Cardiac specific increase in aldosterone production induces coronary dysfunction in aldosterone synthase-transgenic mice. Circulation. 2004;110:1819–25.
21. Ambroisine ML, Favre J, Oliviero P, et al. Aldosterone-induced coronary dysfunction in transgenic mice

involves the calcium-activated potassium (BKCa) channels of vascular smooth muscle cells. Circulation. 2007;116:2435–43.

22. Farrell SR, Ross JL, Howlett SE. Sex differences in mechanisms of cardiac excitation-contraction coupling in rat ventricular myocytes. Am J Physiol Heart Circ Physiol. 2010;299:H36–45.

23. Saito T, Ciobotaru A, Bopassa JC, et al. Estrogen contributes to gender differences in mouse ventricular repolarization. Circ Res. 2009;105:343–52.

24. Ostadal B, Netuka I, Maly J, et al. Gender differences in cardiac ischemic injury and protection–experimental aspects. Exp Biol Med (Maywood). 2009;234: 1011–9.

25. Deschepper CF, Llamas B. Hypertensive cardiac remodeling in males and females: from the bench to the bedside. Hypertension. 2007;49:401–7.

26. Douglas PS, Otto CM, Mickel MC, et al. Gender differences in left ventricle geometry and function in patients undergoing balloon dilatation of the aortic valve for isolated aortic stenosis. NHLBI Balloon Valvuloplasty Registry. Br Heart J. 1995;73:548–54.

27. Douglas PS, Katz SE, Weinberg EO, et al. Hypertrophic remodeling: gender differences in the early response to left ventricular pressure overload. J Am Coll Cardiol. 1998;32:1118–25.

28. Petrov G, Regitz-Zagrosek V, Lehmkuhl E, et al. Regression of myocardial hypertrophy after aortic valve replacement: faster in women? Circulation. 2010;122:S23–8.

29. Konhilas JP, Leinwand LA. The effects of biological sex and diet on the development of heart failure. Circulation. 2007;116:2747–59.

30. Loyer X, Oliviero P, Damy T, et al. Effects of sex differences on constitutive nitric oxide synthase expression and activity in response to pressure overload in rats. Am J Physiol Heart Circ Physiol. 2007;293: H2650–8.

31. Bernardo BC, Weeks KL, Pretorius L, et al. Molecular distinction between physiological and pathological cardiac hypertrophy: experimental findings and therapeutic strategies. Pharmacol Ther. 2010;128: 191–227.

32. Masoudi FA, Havranek EP, Smith G, et al. Gender, age, and heart failure with preserved left ventricular systolic function. J Am Coll Cardiol. 2003;41:217–23.

33. Klapholz M, Maurer M, Lowe AM, et al. Hospitalization for heart failure in the presence of a normal left ventricular ejection fraction: results of the New York Heart Failure Registry. J Am Coll Cardiol. 2004;43:1432–8.

34. Cleland JG, Swedberg K, Follath F, et al. The EuroHeart Failure survey programme – a survey on the quality of care among patients with heart failure in Europe. Part 1: patient characteristics and diagnosis. Eur Heart J. 2003;24:442–63.

35. Devereux RB, Roman MJ, Liu JE, et al. Congestive heart failure despite normal left ventricular systolic function in a population-based sample: the Strong Heart Study. Am J Cardiol. 2000;86:1090–6.

36. Regitz-Zagrosek V, Oertelt-Prigione S, Seeland U, et al. Sex and gender differences in myocardial hypertrophy and heart failure. Circ J. 2010;74:1265–73.

37. Witt H, Schubert C, Jaekel J, et al. Sex-specific pathways in early cardiac response to pressure overload in mice. J Mol Med. 2008;86:1013–24.

38. Weinberg EO, Thienelt CD, Katz SE, et al. Gender differences in molecular remodeling in pressure overload hypertrophy. J Am Coll Cardiol. 1999;34:264–73.

39. Weinberg EO, Mirotsou M, Gannon J, et al. Sex dependence and temporal dependence of the left ventricular genomic response to pressure overload. Physiol Genomics. 2003;12:113–27.

40. Villari B, Campbell SE, Schneider J, et al. Sex-dependent differences in left ventricular function and structure in chronic pressure overload. Eur Heart J. 1995;16:1410–9.

41. Fliegner D, Schubert C, Penkalla A, et al. Female sex and estrogen receptor-beta attenuate cardiac remodeling and apoptosis in pressure overload. Am J Physiol Regul Integr Comp Physiol. 2010;298:R1597–606.

42. Xu Y, Arenas IA, Armstrong SJ, et al. Estrogen modulation of left ventricular remodeling in the aged heart. Cardiovasc Res. 2003;57:388–94.

43. Mahmoodzadeh S, Dworatzek E, Fritschka S, Pham TH, Regitz-Zagrosek V. 17beta-estradiol inhibits matrix metalloproteinase-2 transcription via MAP kinase in fibroblasts. Cardiovasc Res. 2010;85:719–28.

44. Devaux C, Iglarz M, Richard V, et al. Chronic decrease in flow contributes to heart failure-induced endothelial dysfunction in rats. Clin Exp Pharmacol Physiol. 2004;31:302–5.

45. Drexler H, Kastner S, Strobel A, et al. Expression, activity and functional significance of inducible nitric oxide synthase in the failing human heart. J Am Coll Cardiol. 1998;32:955–63.

46. Crabos M, Coste P, Paccalin M, et al. Reduced basal NO-mediated dilation and decreased endothelial NO-synthase expression in coronary vessels of spontaneously hypertensive rats. J Mol Cell Cardiol. 1997;29:55–65.

47. Wiemer G, Linz W, Hatrik S, et al. Angiotensin-converting enzyme inhibition alters nitric oxide and superoxide release in normotensive and hypertensive rats. Hypertension. 1997;30:1183–90.

48. Bauersachs J, Bouloumie A, Mulsch A, et al. Vasodilator dysfunction in aged spontaneously hypertensive rats: changes in NO synthase III and soluble guanylyl cyclase expression, and in superoxide anion production. Cardiovasc Res. 1998;37:772–9.

49. Drab M, Verkade P, Elger M, et al. Loss of caveolae, vascular dysfunction, and pulmonary defects in caveolin-1 gene-disrupted mice. Science. 2001;293: 2449–52.

50. Ratajczak P, Damy T, Heymes C, et al. Caveolin-1 and -3 dissociations from caveolae to cytosol in the heart during aging and after myocardial infarction in rat. Cardiovasc Res. 2003;57:358–69.

51. Jankowski M, Wang D, Mukaddam-Daher S, et al. Pregnancy alters nitric oxide synthase and natriuretic

peptide systems in the rat left ventricle. J Endocrinol. 2005;184:209–17.

52. Chakrabarti S, Lekontseva O, Peters A, et al. 17beta-estradiol induces protein S-nitrosylation in the endothelium. Cardiovasc Res. 2010;85:796–805.

53. Damy T, Ratajczak P, Shah AM, et al. Increased neuronal nitric oxide synthase-derived NO production in the failing human heart. Lancet. 2004;363:1365–7.

54. Bendall JK, Damy T, Ratajczak P, et al. Role of myocardial neuronal nitric oxide synthase-derived nitric oxide in beta-adrenergic hyporesponsiveness after myocardial infarction-induced heart failure in rat. Circulation. 2004;110:2368–75.

55. Loyer X, Gomez AM, Milliez P, et al. Cardiomyocyte overexpression of neuronal nitric oxide synthase delays transition toward heart failure in response to pressure overload by preserving calcium cycling. Circulation. 2008;117:3187–98.

56. Barouch LA, Cappola TP, Harrison RW, et al. Combined loss of neuronal and endothelial nitric oxide synthase causes premature mortality and age-related hypertrophic cardiac remodeling in mice. J Mol Cell Cardiol. 2003;35:637–44.

57. Sun J, Picht E, Ginsburg KS, et al. Hypercontractile female hearts exhibit increased S-nitrosylation of the L-type Ca^{2+} channel alpha1 subunit and reduced ischemia/reperfusion injury. Circ Res. 2006;98:403–11.

58. Murphy E, Steenbergen C. Gender-based differences in mechanisms of protection in myocardial ischemia-reperfusion injury. Cardiovasc Res. 2007;75:478–86.

59. Balligand JL, Cannon PJ. Nitric oxide synthases and cardiac muscle. Autocrine and paracrine influences. Arterioscler Thromb Vasc Biol. 1997;17:1846–58.

60. Francis SH. The role of cGMP-dependent protein kinase in controlling cardiomyocyte cGMP. Circ Res. 2010;107:1164–6.

61. Costello-Boerrigter LC, Boerrigter G, Redfield MM, et al. Amino-terminal pro-B-type natriuretic peptide and B-type natriuretic peptide in the general community: determinants and detection of left ventricular dysfunction. J Am Coll Cardiol. 2006;47:345–53.

62. Redfield MM, Rodeheffer RJ, Jacobsen SJ, et al. Plasma brain natriuretic peptide concentration: impact of age and gender. J Am Coll Cardiol. 2002;40:976–82.

63. Luchner A, Brockel U, Muscholl M, et al. Gender-specific differences of cardiac remodeling in subjects with left ventricular dysfunction: a population-based study. Cardiovasc Res. 2002;53:720–7.

64. van Eickels M, Grohe C, Cleutjens JP, et al. 17beta-estradiol attenuates the development of pressure-overload hypertrophy. Circulation. 2001;104:1419–23.

65. Babiker FA, De Windt LJ, van Eickels M, et al. 17beta-estradiol antagonizes cardiomyocyte hypertrophy by autocrine/paracrine stimulation of a guanylyl cyclase A receptor-cyclic guanosine monophosphate-dependent protein kinase pathway. Circulation. 2004;109:269–76.

66. Horio T, Nishikimi T, Yoshihara F, et al. Inhibitory regulation of hypertrophy by endogenous atrial natriuretic peptide in cultured cardiac myocytes. Hypertension. 2000;35:19–24.

Part III

Mitochondrial Diseases

Mitochondrial DNA and Heart Disease

Chihiro Shikata, Masami Nemoto,
Takanori Ebisawa, Akihiro Nishiyama,
and Nobuakira Takeda

Abstract

The relationship between abnormalities of myocardial mitochondrial DNA and heart disease is reviewed. Myocardial mitochondrial DNA abnormalities can induce both hypertrophic and dilated cardiomyopathies. In mitochondrial encephalomyopathy, abnormalities of myocardial mitochondrial DNA can also induce cardiac involvement, for example, heart failure and arrhythmia. The influence of acquired mitochondrial DNA mutations is also discussed.

Keywords

Arrhythmia • Cardiomyopathy • Heart failure • Kearns–Sayre syndrome • MELAS • MERRF • Mitochondrial DNA • Mitochondrial encephalomyopathy

Introduction

Mitochondria have their own DNA besides nuclear DNA. Abnormalities of mitochondrial DNA decrease cellular energy production and induce impairment of organ function.

Mitochondria possess an energy-producing system composed of NADH dehydrogenase, cytochrome, and cytochrome oxidase, which are encoded and regulated by mitochondrial DNA as well as nuclear DNA. Human mitochondrial DNA is double stranded and circular, consisting of 16,569 base pairs and containing 11 structural genes for the subunits of respiratory enzyme complexes and two genes for two subunits of F0- ATPase, as well as for 22 tRNA molecules and two rRNA molecules [1]. Each cardiac myocyte contains 2,000–3,000 mitochondria, each of which possesses two or three DNAs.

Mitochondrial DNA mutations are inherited from the mother [2, 3]. This DNA is easily damaged because it is continually exposed to free radicals and contains neither histones nor introns, and the mitochondrial DNA repair system is relatively primitive. Oxygen-derived free radicals generated by the mitochondrial inner membrane convert deoxyguanosine (dG) in mitochondrial DNA to 8-hydroxy-dG, which is misread as another base during duplication. An increase of 8-hydroxy-dG

N. Takeda (✉)
Department of Internal Medicine, Aoto Hospital,
Jikei University, Tokyo, Japan
e-mail: ntakeda@jikei.ac.jp

is consequently synonymous with the accumulation of point mutations in mitochondrial DNA.

Ozawa and colleagues have succeeded in determining the entire mitochondrial DNA sequence using direct sequencing [4, 5]. Mitochondrial DNA mutation may lead to impairment of mitochondrial function, for example, deficiency of mitochondrial respiratory chain enzymes or ATPase related to the subunits encoded by mitochondrial DNA. The term "mitochondrial cardiomyopathy" has been coined to describe cardiomyopathy induced by mitochondrial DNA mutations [6].

Cardiomyopathy

Cardiomyopathy can have several forms, including hypertrophic, dilated, and restrictive cardiomyopathies, and arrhythmogenic right ventricular dysplasia. The etiologies of these conditions are still unknown, but recent developments in molecular biology have provided suggestive evidence, such as the detection of mutations of the genes encoding myocardial contractile proteins such as myosin, actin, tropomyosin, and troponin. Myocardial mitochondrial DNA mutations have also been detected by Ozawa et al. in cardiomyopathic patients [7–9], and a number of other reports have documented similar mutations and their potential role in cardiomyopathy [10–22].

A point mutation that alters adenine (A) to guanine (G) within the mitochondrial tRNALeu(UUR) gene is common in patients with the syndrome of mitochondrial myopathy, encephalopathy, lactic acidosis, and stroke-like episodes (MELAS) [9]. PCR and Southern blot analysis have revealed multiple mitochondrial DNA deletions in a pedigree of inherited dilated cardiomyopathy [23], but the extent to which these mitochondrial DNA mutations are involved in the etiology of idiopathic cardiomyopathy remains to be elucidated.

All humans appear to have the potential to develop cardiomyopathy because the myocardium degenerates with age due to the accumulation of free radical-induced damage to the mitochondrial DNA. Abnormal acceleration of

mitochondrial DNA mutations, especially those related to mitochondrial protein synthesis, can induce premature aging and severe mitochondrial cardiomyopathy [24]. An A-to-G point mutation at position 3,260 of the mitochondrial tRNALeu(UUR) gene has been found in a maternally inherited disorder that was manifested as a combination of adult-onset myopathy and cardiomyopathy [10]. An A-to-G substitution has also been found at position 4,269 in the tRNAIle gene of a patient with fatal cardiomyopathy [12], and an A-to-G mutation at position 15,923 of the mitochondrial tRNAThr gene is associated with neonatal cardiomyopathy [25].

Other patients with fatal infantile cardiomyopathy have also been reported [26, 27], as has the development of severe mitochondrial cardiomyopathy in young people with an A-to-G transition at position 827 of the mitochondrial 12S rRNA gene [28]. It has also been suggested that a G-to-A point mutation at 12,192 in the tRNAHis gene may be an evolutionary risk factor for cardiomyopathy [29]. Therefore, the detection of mitochondrial DNA deletions has been proposed as a new method for investigating sudden cardiac death in which ischemic damage is the primary cause [30].

No clear correlation has been found between the severity of clinical manifestations and the mutations detected by conventional analysis of limited regions of the entire mitochondrial DNA. In contrast, comprehensive analysis of mitochondrial DNA by the direct base sequencing technique has revealed a close correlation between the mitochondrial DNA genotype and clinical phenotype [5, 28]. Each cardiac myocyte contains 2,000–3,000 mitochondria, each of which possesses two or three circular mitochondrial DNAs. Thus, cells can contain normal and mutant mitochondrial DNA in varying proportions (heteroplasmy). This may result in marked differences of energy production among myocardial cells, which may induce arrhythmias.

If the mitochondrial DNA mutation is extensive, oxidative phosphorylation will be depressed, leading to a decrease of energy production and the development of heart failure. Mutations in nuclear DNA encoding the mitochondrial respiratory enzyme complex subunits can also affect energy production. Furthermore, it has been suggested that mitochondrial DNA mutations might activate the mitochondrial apoptosis pathway, thus causing dilated cardiomyopathy [31]. The investigation of mitochondrial DNA mutations may therefore yield various clues to the etiology of arrhythmias and cardiac dysfunction.

Some characteristic phenomena have been observed in patients with mitochondrial cardiomyopathy: the level of lactic acid in serum or spinal fluid is over 1.5 times the normal upper limit; there is a defect of mitochondrial enzymes involved in the electron transport system, glycolysis, and lipid metabolism; and changes in mitochondrial morphology have been revealed in skeletal and cardiac muscles using Gomori trichrome staining, that is, the presence of ragged-red fibers. The diagnosis of mitochondrial cardiomyopathy can be confirmed by detection of mitochondrial DNA mutations in myocardial biopsy samples. Electron microscopy can show changes in the size or number of mitochondria. Mitochondrial DNA mutations are observed in hypertrophic and dilated cardiomyopathies. In fact, it has been reported that about 3% of dilated cardiomyopathies are induced by mitochondrial DNA mutations.

Encephalomyopathy

In patients with mitochondrial encephalomyopathy, abnormalities occur in the skeletal muscles and the central nervous system, and cardiac abnormalities are also sometimes present [32–38)

1. Kerns–Sayre syndrome (KSS)
   Kerns–Sayre syndrome is characterized by chronic progressive external ophthalmoplegia, heart block, and pigmented retinopathy. The main cause is thought to be mitochondrial DNA deletions [39–44], although mitochondrial dysfunction induced by abnormal nuclear DNA may also be involved [45]. The cardiac manifestations of this disease are arrhythmias, such as atrioventricular block, premature ventricular contractions, supraventricular or ventricular

tachycardia, sinus dysrhythmia, ST segment and T-wave changes, and cardiac dilatation and failure [46–52]. In many patients, implantation of a pacemaker is required to prevent sudden death, and some patients may acquire the need for a pacemaker at an advanced age.

2. Mitochondrial myopathy, encephalopathy, lactic acidosis, and stoke-like episode (MELAS)
   MELAS usually occurs at a young age and is characterized by headache, vomiting, and stroke-like episodes such as hemiplegia [53]. This disease is induced by point mutations of the mitochondrial tRNALeu(UUR) gene, from A to G at position 3,243 [54, 55] or from thymine (T) to cytosine (C) at position 3,271 [56]. Cardiac involvement results in the onset of cardiomyopathy [57, 58].

3. Myoclonic epilepsy with ragged-red fibers (MERRF)
   Myoclonic epilepsy is the cardinal symptom of patients with MERRF, which is induced by an A-to-G point mutation at position 8,344 of the mitochondrial tRNALys gene [59]. Cardiac involvement results in onset of cardiomyopathy.

Pathogenic mechanisms of mtDNA mutations were described in literatures [60–62].

Acquired Mutations

Mitochondrial DNA mutations can occur after birth. An age-dependent increase of deletions in mitochondrial DNA has been observed in the myocardium of both humans and rats [63–68]; mitochondrial DNA deletions have been found in myocardial autopsy specimens from patients with diabetes or myocardial infarction [69, 70], and patients who have been treated with doxorubicin [70]. Autopsy and biopsy specimens of ischemic hearts are reported to show a higher degree of mitochondrial DNA damage than normal hearts [71]. In addition, myocardial mitochondrial DNA damage and deletions induced by doxorubicin have been demonstrated in experimental animals [72, 73]. Therefore, free radicals may play a role in inducing mitochondrial DNA mutations related to the pathological conditions described earlier.

Treatment

Some reports and review articles have indicated the possibility of L-carnitine and coenzyme Q10 therapy for patients with impairment of cardiac function due to mitochondrial DNA mutations, as well as the use of gene therapy [74–82].

References

1. Anderson S, Bankier AT, Barrel BG, et al. Sequence and organization of the human mitochondrial genome. Nature. 1981;290:457–65.
2. Giles RE, Blanc H, Cann HM, et al. Maternal inheritance of human mitochondrial DNA. Proc Natl Acad Sci USA. 1980;77:6715–9.
3. Ozawa T, Yoneda M, Tanaka M, et al. Maternal inheritance of deleted mitochondrial DNA in a family with mitochondrial myopathy. Biochem Biophys Res Commun. 1988;154:1240–7.
4. Tanaka M, Sato W, Ohno K, et al. Direct sequencing of deleted mitochondrial DNA in myopathic patients. Biochem Biophys Res Commun. 1989;164:156–63.
5. Ozawa T, Katsumata M, Hayakawa M, et al. Mitochondrial DNA mutations and survival rate. Lancet. 1995;345:189.
6. Ozawa T. Mitochondrial cardiomypathy. Herz. 1994;19:105–18.
7. Ozawa T, Tanaka M, Sugiyama S, et al. Multiple mitochondrial DNA deletions exist in cardiomyocytes of patients with hypertrophic or dilated cardiomyopathy. Biochem Biophys Res Commun. 1990;170:830–6.
8. Hattori K, Ogawa T, Kondo T, et al. Cardiomyopathy with mitochondrial DNA mutations. Am Heart J. 1991;122:866–9.
9. Obayashi T, Hattori K, Sugiyama S, et al. Point mutations in mitochondrial DNA in patients with hypertrophic cardiomyopathy. Am Heart J. 1992;124:1263–9.
10. Zeviani M, Gellera C, Antozzi C, et al. Maternally inherited myopathy and cardiomyopathy: association with mutation in mitochondrial DNA tRNA(Leu) (UUR). Lancet. 1991;338:143–7.
11. Ozawa T, Sugiyama S, Tanaka M, et al. Mitochondrial DNA mutations and disturbances of energy metabolism in myocardium. Jpn Circ J. 1991;55:1158–64.
12. Taniike M, Fukushima H, Yanagihara I, et al. Mitochondrial tRNA(Ile) mutation in fatal cardiomyopathy. Biochem Biophys Res Commun. 1992;186:47–53.
13. Mariotti C, Tiranti V, Carrara F, et al. Defective respiratory capacity and mitochondrial protein synthesis in transformant cybrids harboring the tRNA(Leu)(UUR) mutation associated with maternally inherited myopathy and cardiomyopathy. J Clin Invest. 1994;93:1102–7.
14. Hayashi J, Ohta S, Kagawa Y, et al. Functional and morphological abnormalities of mitochondria in human cells containing mitochondrial DNA with pathogenic point mutations in tRNA genes. J Biol Chem. 1994;269:19060–6.
15. Tanaka M, Obayashi T, Yoneda M, et al. Mitochondrial DNA mutations in cardiomyopathy; combination of replacements yielding cysteine residues and tRNA mutations. Muscle Nerve. 1995;3:S165–74.
16. Zeviani M, Mariotti C, Antozzi C, et al. OXPHOS defects and mitochondrial DNA mutations in cardiomyopathy. Muscle Nerve. 1995;3:S170–4.
17. Takei Y, Ikeda S, Yanagisawa N, et al. Multiple mitochondrial DNA deletions in a patient with mitochondrial myopathy and cardiomyopathy but not ophthalmoplegia. Muscle Nerve. 1995;18:1321–5.
18. Ozawa T, Mitochondrial DNA. mutations in myocardial diseases. Eur Heart J. 1995;16(Suppl):10–4.
19. Turner LF, Kaddoura S, Harrington D, et al. Mitochondrial DNA in idiopathic cardiomyopathy. Eur Heart J. 1998;19:1725–9.
20. Khogali SS, Mayosi BM, Beattie JM, et al. A common mitochondrial DNA variant associated with susceptibility to dilated cardiomyopathy in two different populations. Lancet. 2001;357:1265–7.
21. Li YY, Chen D, Watkins SC, et al. Mitochondrial abnormalities in tumor necrosis factor-alpha-induced heart failure are associated with impaired DNA repair activity. Circulation. 2001;104:2492–7.
22. Taylor RW, Giordano C, Davidson MM, et al. A homoplasmic mitochondrial transfer ribonucleic acid mutation as a cause of maternally inherited hypertrophic cardiomyopathy. J Am Coll Cardiol. 2003;42:1786–96.
23. Suomalainen A, Paetau A, Leinonen H, et al. Inherited idiopathic dilated cardiomyopathy with multiple deletions of mitochondrial DNA. Lancet. 1992;340:1319–20.
24. Katsumata K, Hayakawa M, Tanaka M, et al. Fragmentation of human heart mitochondrial DNA associated with premature aging. Biochem Biophys Res Commun. 1994;202:1012–110.
25. Yoon KL, Ernst SG, Rasmussen C, et al. Mitochondrial disorder associated with newborn cardiopulmonary arrest. Pediatr Res. 1993;33:433–40.
26. Papadopoulou LC, Sue CM, Davidson MM, et al. Fatal infantile cardioencephalomyopathy with COX deficiency and mutations in SCO2, a COX assembly gene. Nat Genet. 1999;23:333–7.
27. Akita Y, Koga Y, Iwanaga R, et al. Fatal hypertrophic cardiomyopathy associated with an A8296G mutation in the mitochondrial tRNA(Lys) gene. Hum Mutat. 2000;15:382.
28. Ozawa T, Katsumata K, Hayakawa M, et al. Genotype and phenotype of severe mitochondrial cardiomyopathy; a recipient of heart transplantation and the genetic control. Biochem Biophys Res Commun. 1995;207:613–20.
29. Shin WS, Tanaka M, Suzuki J, et al. Novel homoplasmic mutation in mtDNA with a single evolutionary origin as a risk factor for cardiomyopathy. Am J Hum Genet. 2000;67:1617–20.
30. Fouret PJ, Nicolas G, Lecomte D. Detection of the 4977 base pair mitochondrial DNA deletion in

paraffin-embedded heart tissue using the polymerase chain reaction – a new method to probe sudden cardiac death molecular mechanism? Forensic Sci. 1994; 39:693–8.

31. Zhang D, Mott JL, Farrar P, et al. Mitochondrial DNA mutations activate the mitochondrial apoptotic pathway and cause dilated cardiomyopathy. Cardiovasc Res. 2003;57:147–57.

32. Vydt TC, de Coo RF, Soliman OI, et al. Cardiac involvement in adults with m.3243A>G MELAS gene mutation. Am J Cardiol. 2007;99:264–9.

33. Ruiter EM, Siers MH, van den Elzen C, et al. The mitochondrial 13513 G>A mutation is most frequent in Leigh syndrome combined with reduced complex I activity, optic atrophy and/or Wolff-Parkinson-White. Eur J Hum Genet. 2007;15:155–61.

34. Wortmann SB, Rodenburg RJ, Backx AP, Schmitt E, Smeitink JA, Morava E. Early cardiac involvement in children carrying the A3243G mtDNA mutation. Acta Paediatr. 2007;96:450–1.

35. Sproule DM, Kaufmann P, Engelstad K, et al. Wolff-Parkinson-White syndrome in patients with MELAS. Arch Neurol. 2007;64:1625–7.

36. Wang SB, Weng WC, Lee NC, et al. Mutation of mitochondrial DNA G13513A presenting with Leigh syndrome, Wolff-Parkinson-White syndrome and cardiomyopathy. Pediatr neonatol. 2008;49:145–9.

37. Wahbi K, Larue S, Jardel C, et al. Cardiac involvement is frequent in patients with the m.8344A>G mutation of mitochondrial DNA. Neurology. 2010;74:674–7.

38. Limongelli G, Tome-Esteban M, Dejthevaporn C, et al. Prevalence and natural history of heart disease in adults with primary mitochondrial respiratory chain disease. Eur J Heart Fail. 2010;12:114–21.

39. Holt IJ, Cooper JM, Morgan-Hughes JA, et al. Deletions of muscle mitochondrial DNA. Lancet. 1988;1:1462.

40. Zeviani M, Moraes CT, DiMauro S, et al. Deletions of mitochondrial DNA in Kearns-Sayre syndrome. Neurology. 1988;38:1339–46.

41. Moraes CT, DiMauro S, Zeviani M, et al. Mitochondrial DNA deletions in progressive external ophthalmoplegia and Kearns-Sayre syndrome. N Engl J Med. 1989;320:1293–9.

42. Obermaier-Kusser B, Mueller-Hoecker J, Nelson I, et al. Different copy numbers of apparently identically deleted mitochondrial DNA in tissues from a patient with Kearns-Sayre syndrome detected by PCR. Biochem Biophys Res Commun. 1990;169:1007–15.

43. Ponzetto C, Bresolin N, Bordoni A, et al. Kearns-Sayre syndrome: different amounts of deleted mitochondrial DNA are present in several autoptic tissues. J Neurol Sci. 1990;96:207–10.

44. Bosbach S, Kornblum C, Schroeder R, et al. Executive and visuospatial deficits in patients with chronic progressive external ophthalmoplegia and Kearns-Sayre syndrome. Brain. 2003;126:1231–40.

45. Soumalainen A, Majander A, Haltia M, et al. Multiple deletions of mitochondrial DNA in several tissues of a patient with severe retarded depression and familial

46. Gerbitz KD, Obermaier-Kusser B, Zierz S, et al. Mitochondrial myopathies: divergences of genetic deletions, biochemical defects and the clinical syndromes. J Neurol. 1990;237:5–10.

47. Melacini P, Angelini C, Buja G, et al. Evolution of cardiac involvement in progressive ophthalmoplegia with deleted mitochondrial DNA. Jpn Heart J. 1990;31:115–20.

48. Kenny D, Wetherbee J. Kearne-Sayre syndrome in the elderly: mitochondrial myopathy with advanced heart block. Am Heart J. 1990;120:440–3.

49. Bordarier C, Duyckaerts C, Robain O, et al. Kearns-Sayre syndrome. Two clinicopathological cases. Neuropediatrics. 1990;21:106–9.

50. Tranchant C, Mousson B, Mohr M, et al. Cardiac transplantation in an incomplete Kearns-Sayre syndrome with mitochondrial DNA deletion. Neuromuscul Disord. 1993;3:561–6.

51. Sato W, Tanaka M, Sugiyama S, et al. Deletion of mitochondrial DNA in a patient with conduction block. Am Heart J. 1993;125:550–2.

52. Ulicny KS, Detterbeck FC, Hall CD. Sinus dysrhythmia in Kearns-Sayre syndrome. PACE. 1994;17:991–4.

53. Montagna P, Gallassi R, Medori R, et al. MELAS syndrome: characteristic migrainous and epileptic features and maternal transmission. Neurology. 1988;38:751–4.

54. Goto Y, Nonaka I, Horai A. A mutation in the tRNA[Leu(UUR)] gene associated with MELAS subgroup of mitochondrial encephalomyopathies. Nature. 1990; 348:651–3.

55. Tanaka M, Ino H, Ohno K, et al. Mitochondrial DNA mutations in mitochondrial myopathy, lactic acidosis, and stoke-like episodes (MELAS). Biochem Byophys Res Commun. 1991;174:861–8.

56. Goto Y, Nonaka I, Horai S. A new mtDNA mutation associated with mitochondrial myopathy, encephalopathy, lactic acidosis and stroke-like episodes (MELAS). Biochim Biophys Acta. 1991;1097:238–40.

57. Matthews PM, Hopkin J, Brown RM, et al. Comparison of the relative levels of the 3243(A G) mtDNA mutation in heteroplasmic adult and fatal tissues. J Med Genet. 1994;31:41–4.

58. Sato W, Tanaka M, Sugiyama S, et al. Cardiomyopathy and angiopathy in patients with mitochondrial myopathy, encephalopathy, lactic acidosis, and stroke-like episodes. Am Heart J. 1994;128:733–41.

59. Shoffner JM, Lott MT, Lezza AM, et al. Myoclonic epilepsy and ragged-red fiber disease (MERRF) is associated with a mitochondrial DNA tRNA[Lys] mutation. Cell. 1990;61:931–7.

60. Carelli V, Giordano C, d'Amati G. Pathogenic expression of homoplasmic mtDNA mutations needs a complex nuclear-mitochondrial interaction. Trends Genet. 2003;19:257–62.

61. Hess JF, Parisi MA, Bennett JL, et al. Impairment of mitochondrial transcription termination by a point mutation associated with the MELAS subgroup of

mitochondrial encephalomyopathies. Nature. 1991; 351:236–9.

62. Schon EA, Koga Y, Davidson M, et al. The mitochondrial tRNA$^{Leu(UUR)}$ mutation in MELAS: a model for pathogenesis. Biochim Biophys Acta. 1992;1101:206–10.

63. Cortopassi GA, Arnheim N. Detection of a specific mitochondrial DNA deletion in tissues of older humans. Nucleic Acids Res. 1990;18:6927–93.

64. Sugiyama S, Hattori K, Hayakawa M, et al. Quantitative analysis of age-associated accumulation of mitochondrial DNA with deletion in human hearts. Biochem Biophys Res Commun. 1991;180:894–9.

65. Hattori K, Tanaka M, Sugiyama S, et al. Age-dependent increase in deleted mitochondrial DNA in the human ear: possible contributory factor to presbycardia. Am Heart J. 1991;121:1735–42.

66. Hayakawa M, Hattori K, Sugiyama S, et al. Age-associated oxygen damage and mutations in mitochondrial DNA in human heart. Biochem Biophys Res Commun. 1992;189:979–85.

67. Hayakawa M, Sugiyama S, Hattori K, et al. Age-associated damage in mitochondrial DNA in human hearts. Mol Cell Biochem. 1993;119:95–103.

68. Baumer A, Zhang C, Linnane AW, et al. Age-related human mtDNA deletions: a heterogeneous set of deletions arising at a single pair of directly repeated sequences. Am J Hum Genet. 1994;54:618–30.

69. Takeda N, Tanamura A, Iwai T. Mitochondrial DNA deletion in human myocardium. Mol Cell Biochem. 1993;119:105–8.

70. Takeda N, Tanamura A, Iwai T, et al. Mutations of myocardial DNA in diabetic patients. In: Dhalla NS, Pierce GN, Panagia V, Beamish RE, editors. Heart Hypertrophy and Failure. Boston: Kluwer Academic Publishers; 1995. p. 59–66.

71. Corral-Debrinski M, Stepien G, Shoffner JM, et al. Hypoxemia is associated with mitochondrial DNA damage and gene induction. JAMA. 1991;266:1812–6.

72. Elles CN, Ellis MB, Blakemore WS. Effect of adriamycin on heart mitochondrial DNA. Biochem J. 1987;245:309–12.

73. Adachi K, Fujiura Y, Mayumi A, et al. A deletion of mitochondrial DNA in murine doxorubicin-induced cardiotoxicity. Biocem Biophys Res Commune. 1993; 195:945–51.

74. Suzuki S, Hinokio Y, Ohtomo M, et al. The effects of coenzyme Q10 treatment on maternally inherited diabetes mellitus and deafness, and mitochondrial DNA 3243 (A to G) mutation. Diabetologia. 1998;41:584–8.

75. Fosslien E. Review: Mitochondrial medicine-cardiomyopathy caused by defective oxidative phosphorylation. Ann Clin Lab Sci. 2003;33:371–95.

76. Dimauro S, Mancusu M, Naini A. Mitochondrial encephalomyopathies: therapeutic approach. Ann NY Acad Sci. 2004;1011:232–45.

77. Salles JE, Moises VA, Almeida DR, et al. Myocardial dysfunction in mitochondrial diabetes treated with coenzyme Q10. Diab Res Clin Pract. 2006;72:100–3.

78. DiMauro S, Mancuso M. Mitochondrial diseases: therapeutic approaches. Biosci Rep. 2007;27:125–37.

79. Kyriakouli DS, Boesch P, Taylor RW, et al. Progress and prospects: gene therapy for mitochondrial DNA disease. Gene Ther. 2008;15:1017–23.

80. Sproule DM, Kaufmann P. Mitochondrial encephalopathy, lactic acidosis, and stroke-like episodes: basic concepts, clinical phenotype, and therapeutic management of MELAS syndrome. Ann NY Acad Sci. 2008;1142:133–58.

81. Komaki H, Nishigaki Y, Fuku N, et al. Pyruvate therapy for Leigh syndrome due to cytochrome c oxidase deficiency. Biochim Biophys Acta. 2010;1800:313–15.

82. Azevedo O, Vilarinho L, Almeida F, et al. Cardiomyopathy and kidney disease in a patient with maternally inherited diabetes and deafness caused by the 3243A>G mutation of mitochondrial DNA. Cardiology. 2010;115:71–4.

A Novel Algorithm from Personal Genome to the Pathogenic Mutant Causing Mitochondrial Cardiomyopathy

Teruhiko Toyo-oka, Toshihiro Tanaka, Licht Toyo-oka, and Katsushi Tokunaga

Abstract

Amazing progresses in both human genome analysis and bioinformatics *in silico* have made it possible to reach whole genome profiling in a short period with a reasonable cost and time. In this review, we have introduced the next step after reading the full genome sequence of both nuclear and mitochondrial genomes to identify the pathogenic site(s) in several cardiomyopathies. Considering ~3 million sites of single nucleotide polymorphism (SNP) per person, it is difficult to reach not a personal variant but a pathogenic site. The current algorithm might be promising for the identification of responsible gene, even in the case of polygenic nature.

Keywords

Electron microscopy • Genome • Heteroplasmy • Magnetic resonance spectroscopy • Mitochondrial cardiomyopathy • Mitochondriosis • Open reading frame (ORF) • Oxidative phosphorylation • Pathogenic mutant • Revised Cambridge resequencing system (rCRS) • Risk factor • transgene

Introduction

Human whole genome was reported just 10 years ago and the aim of coming decades is addressed to the clinical translation of personal genetic

T. Toyo-oka (✉)
Department of Cardiovascular Medicine, Postgraduate School of Medicine, University of Tokyo, Tokyo, Japan

Department of Molecular Cardiology, Tohoku University Bioengineering Research, Sendai, Japan

Department of Cardioangiology, Postgraduate School of Medicine, Kitasato University, Sagamihara, Japan
e-mail: toyooka_2im@hotmail.com

background of each patient, searching for the precise mechanism of pathogenicity, gene counseling, and/or tailored medicine to provide most suitable option for treatment [1]. For the assessment of genetic origin of heart failure and/or dilated cardiomyopathy (DCM), the mitochondrial (mt) genome represents one of the most informative and cost-effective researches, because of (1) the abundant rate of exons over introns, not like a nuclear genome, (2) short genome size to determine the whole DNA sequence [2] to profile the progression of various diseases [3], (3) repeating the beating throughout life with consuming and producing huge amount of adenosine triphosphate (ATP) in

Table 1 Homology of mt-DNA sequence (8551–9300) to NUMT (Mitochondrial DNA-like sequences in the nucleus) of human genome. Also, note an accurate criticism raised by Yao et al. [39]

Sequences producing significant alignments			
Accession	Description	E value	Max ident
NC 001807.4	Homo sapiens mitochondrion, complete genome	0	99%
NT 004350.19	Home sapiens chromosome 1 genomic contig, GRCh37 reference primary assembly	0	98%
NT 034772.6	Home sapiens chromosome 5 genomic contig, GRCh37 reference primary assembly	0	88%
NW 001838563.2	Homo sapiens chromosome 1 genomic contig, alternate assembly (based on HuRef), whole genome shotgun sequence	0	98%
NT 022184.15	Homo sapiens chromosome 2 genomic contig, GRCh37 reference primary assembly	4.00E–91	96%
NT 167187.1	Homo sapiens chromosome 8 genomic contig, GRCh37 reference primary assembly	2.00E–55	85%
NW 001839126.2	Homo sapiens chromosome 8 genomic contig, alternate assembly (based on HuRef), whole genome shotgun sequence	2.00E–55	85%
NW 923907.1	Homo sapiens chromosome 8 genomic contig, alternate assembly (based on Celera), whole genome shotgun sequence	2.00E–55	85%
NT 032977.9	Homo sapiens chromosome 1 genomic contig, GRCh37 reference primary assembly	2.00E–29	100%
NW 001838577.2	Homo sapiens chromosome 1 genomic contig, alternate assembly (based on HuRef), whole genome shotgun sequence	2.00E–29	100%
NW 921351.1	Homo sapiens chromosome 1 genomic contig, alternate assembly (based on Celera), whole genome shotgun sequence	2.00E–29	100%
NT 007299.13	Homo sapiens chromosome 6 genomic contig, GRCh37 reference primary assembly	2.00E–24	86%
NW 001838987.1	Homo sapiens chromosome 6 genomic contig, alternate assembly (based on HuRef), whole genome shotgun sequence	2.00E–24	86%
NW 923184.1	Homo sapiens chromosome 6 genomic contig, alternate assembly (based on Celera), whole genome shotgun sequence	2.00E–24	86%

their own cells, and (4) continuous exposure to reactive oxygen species (ROS) produced in the oxidative phosphorylation with much fewer protective actions than nuclear genome.

The mt-genome includes abundant variants not related to the pathogenicity but reflecting the haplogroup or phylogeny to adopt extracellular environment [1]. Accordingly, mt-genome study is so meaningful and fascinating but it includes widespread problems, as follows: (1) ethical conflicts originated in a disclosure of patient's privacy [2], (2) methodological arguments to sample considerable amount of living human cardiomyocytes to evaluate the mutant's phenotype, (3) changes in the hetroplasmy rate during tissue culture, as is convenient for the analysis and the amplification [3], (4) environmental difference of cardiomyocytes in situ under mechanical and/or chemical stress(es) from cultured cells in vitro, and the resultant modification of the phenotype, (5) the case with no identical variant in rodent to prepare transgenic models [4], and (6) intrinsic problems to patents and licensing [5]. In this short review, we present a new scheme to overcome these dilemmas and to clarify the pathogenic mechanism of various mt-diseases, based on abundant sources of bioinformatics *in silico*. The homology of mt-DNA sequence with that of nuclear-DNA is shown in Table 1.

An Algorithm to Reach the Pathogenic Mutant in mtCM

Necessity for Full Sequencing of the mt-Genome

In the outpatient section of the Tokyo University Hospital, we have followed ~80 cases with hypertrophic cardiomyopathy (HCM) and DCM, of which diagnosis was based on clinical and laboratory data including morphological, physiological, biochemical, serological, and, most importantly, pathological characteristics of endomyocardial biopsy samples [6]. For the conventional measurement of gene survey, we have employed gene polymorphism using PCR (polymerase chain reaction)-amplified SSCP (single-stranded conformation polymorphism) or RFLP (restriction-fragment-length polymorphism, Fig. 1) for ~15 years. In the recent 5 years, we have shifted to more time-saving and accurate modality, sequence-specific primer cycle elongation-fluorescence correlation spectroscopy (SSPCE-FCS), as described previously [7]. As candidate genes, we have selected several variants popular in Japan [8] and detected three pedigrees with identical mutations [9].

The classical methods to utilize PCR-based gene amplification often cause misreading of not the responsible, but the pseudogene(s) located in the other site. Particularly, nuclear genes preserve an incredible amount of pseudogenes with the same sequence as the ancient mtDNA [NUMT, Ref. 10] in part, even when the original mtDNA has already altered adapting to a new environment (Fig. 2). Consequently, whole mt-genome sequencing is preferable over the classical methods and would be essential in future to avoid misdiagnosis.

New Modality to Read the Whole mt-DNA Sequence

The whole mt-DNA sequences of all three probands and 10 Japanese volunteer patients without CM or heart failure as an internal standard were determined with GeneChip® Human Mitochondrial Resequencing Array 2.0 [11, Toyo-oka et al., submitted]. The DNA sequences different from the

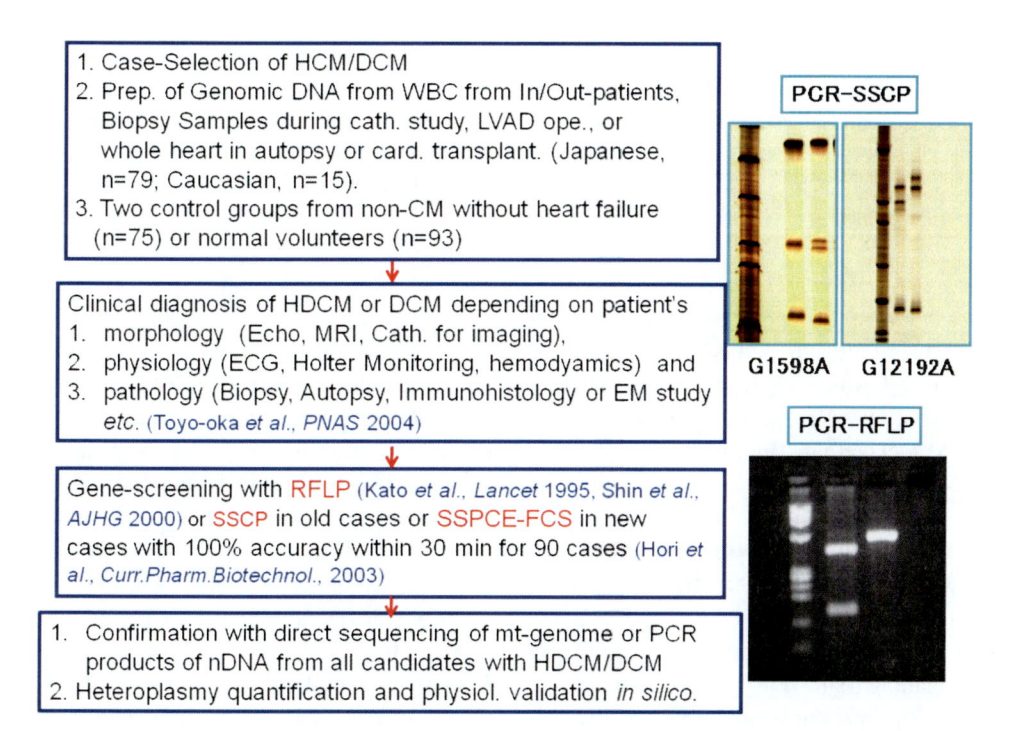

Fig. 1 Classical screening steps of wide variety of DCM/HCM in nuclear and mitochondrial genomes

a

tRNAT	species	5888 95	97	15901 7	10	11	16 23 28 32	37	40	46 53
Primates	Homo sapiens	GTCCTTG TA	GTAT	AAACTA ATAC	A	CCAGT	CTTGTAA ACCGG AGAT GAAAA	CCT	TTTTC	CAAGGACA
	Gorilla gorilla	GCCCTTG TA	GTAC	AGACCA ATAC	A	CCAGT	CTTGTAA ACCGG AAAC GAAGA	CCT	CCTTC	CAAGGGCA
	Pan troglodytes	GCCCTTG TA	GTAT	AAACTA ATAC	A	CCGGT	CTTGTAA ACCGG AAAC GAAAA	CTT	TCTTC	CAAGGACA
	Hylobates lar	GCCCTTG TA	GTAT	AAGCCA ATAC	A	CCGGT	CTTGTAA GCCGG AACT GAAAT	CTT	CCTTC	CAAGGACA
	Pongo pygmaeus	GCCCCTGTA	GTAC	AAATAA GTAC	G	CCAGC	CTTGTAA CCTGA AAAT GAAGC	CCC	CCTTC	CACGGGCA
	Papio hamadryas	GCCCTTG TA	GTAC	AAACTA ATAC	A	CTGGT	CTTGTAA ACCAG AAAT GGAGC	A	CCTCC	CCAGGGTA
	Bos taurus	GTCTTTG TA	GTAC	ATCTA ATAT	A	CTGGT	CTTGTAA ACCAG AGAA GGAGA	ACAACTAA	CCTCC	CTAAGACT
	Cebus albifrons	GTCCTTG TA	GTAT	ATCCAA TTAC	C	CCGGC	CTTGTAA ACCGG AAAA GGAGG	CACGCTA	ACTCC	CCAGGACA
	Lemur catta	GCCCTTG TA	GTAT	AACTTA ATAC	C	CTGGT	CTTGTAA ACCAG ACAT GGAGA	ACCCCCT	CCTCC	CAAGGACA
	Macaca mulatta	GCCCTCGTA	GTAT	AAATTA GTAC	A	CTGGC	CTTGTAA ACCAG AAAT GAACA	C	TCTTC	CTAGGGCA
	Tarsius bancanus	GTCCTCG TA	GTAT	AACCA TTAC	C	TTGGT	CTTGTAA ACCAA AAAT GAAGG	AACCCAA	CCTCC	CTAGGACC
Dermoptera	Cynocephalus variegatus	GTCCCTG TA	GTAT	AATAA TTAC	T	CTAGT	CTTGTAA ACCAG AAAT GGAGG	GAGCAC	CCTCC	CCAGGACA
Oryctero-podidae	Orycteropus afer	GTCCTTG TA	GTAT	AAACTA TTAC	C	ATGGT	CTTGTAA ACCAT AAAT GGATC	TAAC	CCTCC	CCAGGACA
Cetartio-dactyla	Balaenoptera acutorostrata	GTCTTTG TA	GTAT	AACTAA TTAC	C	CCGGT	CTTGTAA ACCGG AAAA GGAGA	GCGAACCACACCTCC		CTAAGACT

b

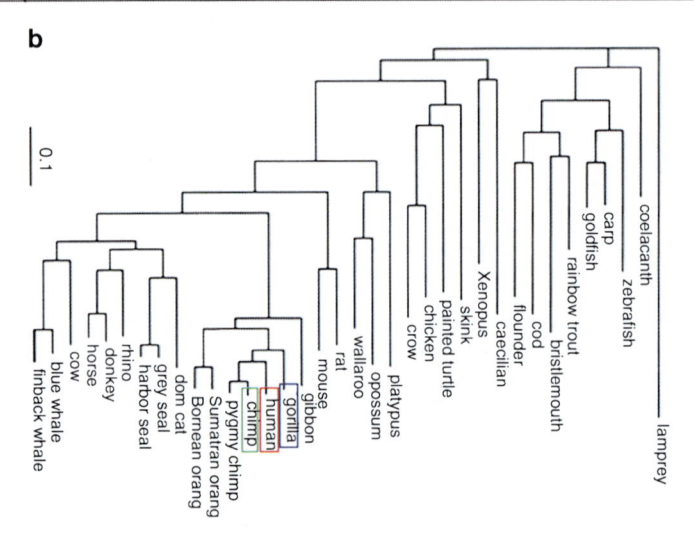

Fig. 2 (**a**) The maximum likelihood estimate of tRNA^Thr in vertebrate phylogeny, focusing on primates. Red-, green-, and blue-colored nucleotides indicate a modifier gene of the current HDCM or DCM, several neurodegenerative disease, and modulator gene of LHON (Leber's hereditary optic neuropathy), respectively. (**b**) The estimation of mtDNA in vertebrate phylogeny (Cited from, Broughton et al. [40])

world-standard rCRS were confirmed with the classical dye-terminator method (Sanger sequencing) equipped with size separation in capillary using mitoSEQ™ Resequencing System for the Human Mitochondrial Genome.

Identification of Pathogenic Mutant in the ORF of the mt-Genome

For the evaluation of physiological significance of open reading frame (ORF), it would be reasonable to assume that the synonymous mutation has no or less meaning in the pathogenesis, except the modification of codon usage in nuclear or mitochondrial genome [12–14]. The mutation within ORF would directly cause the conformational change in the encoded protein (transgene) and accordingly result in the functional modification, if any. For the integration of all 13 polypeptides coded by the mt-gene into the inner membrane, most of mt-proteins abundantly include hydrophobic domains and are buried in the phospholipid bilayer. Among the mt-proteins, ATPase 6 is the most hydrophobic peptide and mutation of the current case from alanine to threonine occurred in the midst of the hydrophobic rigid structure (Toyo-oka et al., submitted). Thus, it would be conceivable to assume that the present mutation causes a serious alteration in oxidative phosphorylation at the final step to synthesize ATP. Another mutation to cause NARP (neuropathy, ataxia, and retinitis pigmentosa) confirmed the scheme described above in the same *ATP6* gene [15].

The other mutations in ORF constitute the main source of the mitochondrial gene-related diseases and the predicted structure of the transgene, that is, LHON in *ND1*, *ND4*, or *ND6* [16–19] or KSS with the large 5 kb deletion spanning from *ATP8* to *ND5* of [20, 21] a wait a more fine analysis like an ionic charge of the constituent amino acids, modulation of helical structure, and intragenic suppressor action in LHON *ND1* gene [22]. For the functional prediction, the higher-ordered structure of the ND6 gene [23] or gene interference between nuclear and mt-genomes might be much more informative to estimate the mutant function (Toyo-oka et al., submitted).

Pathogenic Mutation in tRNA of the mt-Genome

The tRNA is another large source of mt-gene mutations, because tRNA is situated at the critical step of protein synthesis and the defect will cause a serious problem in the production rate of each component protein in mitochondria. Several mutations have been reported on MELAS 3,243 in tRNA[Leu(UUR)] [24, 25] and MERRF 8,344 in tRNA[Lys] [26, 27] or dilated cardiomyopathy (DCM) in tRNA[Thr] (Toyo-oka et al., submitted). McFarland et al. raised five criteria [28]:

1. ~Three-fourths of mutation sites in stem regions of the secondary structure
2. Pathogenic hot spots in both the acceptor and anticodon stems
3. Disruption of Watson–Crick base pairs
4. More common pathogenicity in C-G base pairing than A-T pairing secondary to the lower thermodynamic energy
5. Preferential pathogenicity in loop structure with unusual number of nucleotides that may

affect the tertial structure. To these criteria, we add here the following three items more for pathogenicity:

6. Medical records describing the identical mutation in other mitochondrion-related diseases, especially in energy-consuming tissues, like neurodegenerative diseases in brain, inner ear, or retina; skeletal or cardiac muscles, like myopathy, HCM, or DCM; and endocrine organs, like diabetes mellitus with or without angiopathy
7. Conservation of the wild-type sequence in nonhuman primates, suggesting the biological significance
8. Pathological features of mitochondriosis in the electron microscopy of biopsy samples

When each criterion is precisely inspected, each item is not independent, but some overlap among these stratifications. Furthermore, each item may require scoring for the more exact prediction in future. Particularly, the morphological observation using fresh sample to avoid the postmortem degeneration is critical to proceed to an advanced step of an accurate diagnosis for the genetic diseases.

The endomyocardial biopsy samples provide several characteristic findings in mitochondria, involving accumulation of a huge number of bizarre-formed mitochondria, that is, mitochondriosis (Toyo-oka et al., submitted), concentric cristae [24], hypertrophic mitochondria within myocytes, and vessel walls with or without paracrystalline mitochondrial inclusions [25, 26].

Other Comments on Gene Analysis

The DNA sequence in rRNA is meaningful for exact and efficient protein synthesis but the clinical significance of the mutant is still obscure, except the rare case of A1555G mutation in 12S-rRNA with sensory hearing loss or DEAF gene [29, 30].

As the initial step of assignment of the pathogenic mutations coding a mitochondrial gene, the nuclear gene should be separately or independently examined not to be mixed with each other. Then the combination of two analyses would yield unexpected results that show double or sometimes triple mutation, and pathogenesis

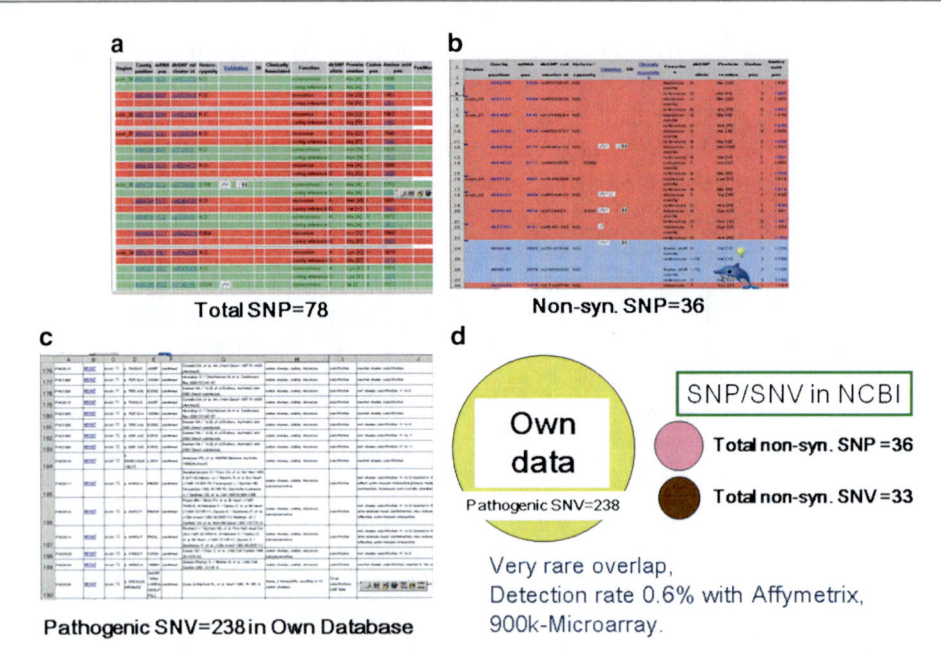

Fig. 3 Less agreement of the microarray commercially available now, comparing NIH SNP/SNV data to our handmade database of *MYH7* gene. Note that the overlap was very rare among these databases and that the detection rate between the two databases was 0.6% with Affymetrix, 900k-Microarray

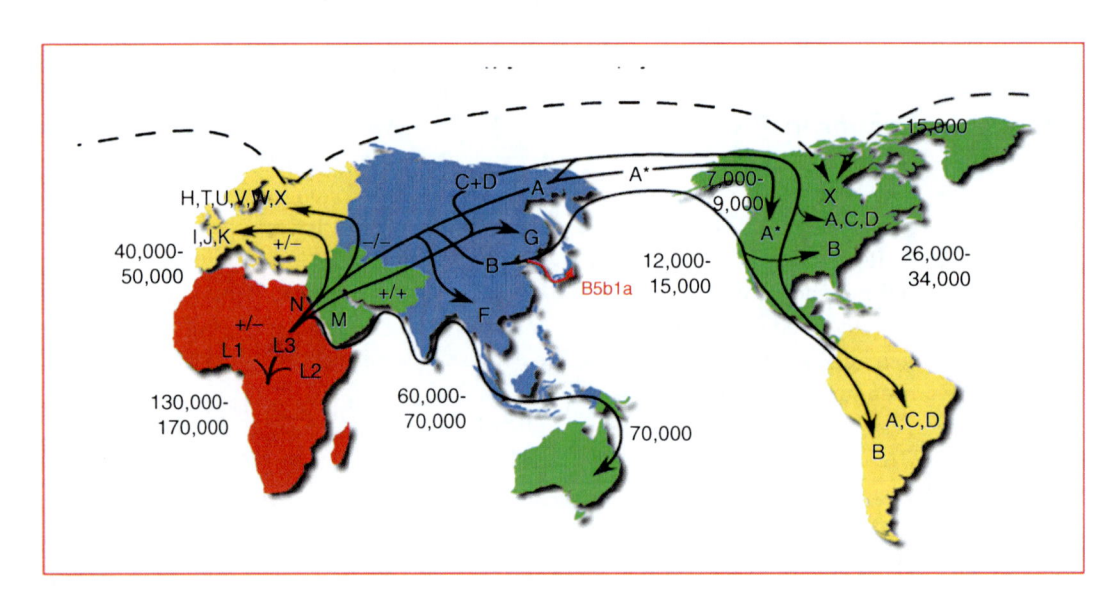

Fig. 4 Human mtDNA migrations (cited from MITOMAP: A human mitochondrial genome database. http://www. mitomap.org, 2009)

of the complex familial disease is clarified or the classical "penetrance" is explained by the multiple gene defect with the different time course (Toyo-oka et al., submitted). The SNP microarray commercially available now is still at the primitive stage to cover pathogenic mutants or variants near the responsible locus, even when a 900 k gene chip is used for the analysis (Fig. 3).

In addition, magnetic resonance spectroscopy (MRS), together with ^{1}H-magnetic resonance imaging (^{1}H-MRI), will be promising for the elucidation of an actual effect of mutant(s) on cardiac function, especially to detect the energy metabolism with ^{31}P-MRS in the case with mtCM [31, 32], though both bore size and magnetic intensity of superconducting coils are insufficient for precise measurement of human hearts in vivo within a limited measuring time.

It is very meaningful to determine the belonging haplogroup as a risk factor. From the worldwide survey [32–37], we identified that the present mutation belonged to the B5b1a subhaplogroup (Toyo-oka et al., submitted). The same G15927A mutation in *tRNA^{Thr}* has been reported to modify the pathogenesis of other neurological diseases [38]. In addition, the current sequence was restricted to the Japanese and no similarity to Chinese or Koreans has been reported [9], which may imply that the new haplogroup has branched from East Asians after their ancestors left the Eurasian continent (Fig. 4).

Conclusions

The sequence of both nuclear and mitochondrial genomes has been identified in different cardiomyopathies. The full resequencing together with comprehensive gene analysis would clarify the controversial results obtained from PCR analysis using a partial amplification in mitochondrial gene mutation.

Acknowledgments This study was financially supported by the Research Fund from the Ministry of Education, Culture, Science and Sports; the Ministry of Health, Welfare and Labor; and the Motor Vehicle Foundation Japan.

References

1. Walalce DC. Colloquium paper: bioenergetics, the origins of complexity, and the ascent of man. Proc Natl Acad Sci USA. 2010;107(Suppl 2):8947–53.
2. Hodgkinson K, Dicks E, Connors S, et al. Translation of research discoveries to clinical care in arrhythmogenic right ventricular cardiomyopathy in Newfoundland and Labrador: lessons for health policy in genetic disease. Genet Med. 2009;11:859–65.
3. Suen DF, Narendra DP, Tanaka A, et al. Parkin overexpression selects against a deleterious mtDNA mutation in heteroplasmic cybrid cells. Proc Natl Acad Sci USA. 2010;107:11835–40.
4. Smithies O, Maeda N. Gene targeting approaches to complex genetic diseases: atherosclerosis and essential hypertension. Proc Natl Acad Sci USA. 1995; 92:5266–72.
5. Angrist M, Chandrasekharan S, Heaney C, et al. Impact of gene patents and licensing practices on access to genetic testing for long QT syndrome. Genet Med. 2010;12(4 Suppl):S111–54.
6. Toyo-oka T, Kawada T, Nakata J, et al. Translocation and cleavage of myocardial dystrophin as a common pathway to advanced heart failure. Proc Natl Acad Sci USA. 2004;101:7381–5.
7. Hori K, Shin WS, Hemmi C, et al. High fidelity SNP genotyping using sequence-specific primer elongation and fluorescence correlation spectroscopy. Curr Pharm Biotec. 2003;4:477–84.
8. Kato M, Takazawa K, Kimura A, et al. Altered actin binding with myosin mutation in hypertrophic cardiomyopathy and sudden death. Lancet. 1995;345:1247.
9. Shin WS, Tanaka M, Suzuki J, et al. A novel homoplasmic mutation in mtDNA with a single evolutionary origin as a risk factor for cardiomyopathy. Am J Hum Genet. 2000;67:1617–20.
10. Mishmar D, Ruiz-Pesini E, Brandon M, et al. Mitochondrial DNA-like sequences in the nucleus (NUMTs): insights into our African origins and the mechanism of foreign DNA integration. Hum Mut. 2004;23:125–33.
11. Warrington JA, Shah NA, Chen X, et al. New developments in high throughput resequencing and variation detection using high-density microarrays. Hum Mutat. 2002;19:402–9.
12. Tuller T, Carmi A, Vestsigian K, et al. An evolutionarily conserved mechanism for controlling the efficiency of protein translation. Cell. 2010;141: 344–54.
13. Cannarozzi G, Schraudolph NN, Faty M, et al. A role for codon order in translation dynamics. Cell. 2010; 141:355–67.
14. Jia W, Higgs PG. Codon usage in mitochondrial genomes: distinguishing context- dependent mutation from translational selection. Mol Biol Evol. 2008;25: 339–51.
15. Pastores GM, Santorelli FM, Shanske S. Leigh syndrome and hypertrophic cardiomyopathy in an infant with a mitochondrial DNA point mutation (T8993G). Am J Med Genet. 1994;50:265–71.
16. Howell N, Kubacka I, Xu M, et al. Leber hereditary optic neuropathy: involvement of the mitochondrial ND I gene and evidence for an intragenic suppressor mutation. Am J Hum Genet. 1991;148:935–42.
17. Qu J, Li R, Tong Y, et al. Only male matrilineal relatives with Leber's hereditary optic neuropathy in a large Chinese family carrying the mitochondrial DNA G11778A mutation. Biochem Biophys Res Commun. 2005;328:1139–45.
18. Ji Y, Zhang AM, Jia X, et al. Mitochondrial DNA haplogroups M7b1'2 and M8a affect clinical expression of Leber hereditary optic neuropathy in Chinese families with the m.11778G-->a mutation. Am J Hum Genet. 2008;83:760–8.

19. Qu J, Zhou X, Zhang J, et al. Extremely low penetrance of Leber's hereditary optic neuropathy in 8 Han Chinese families carrying the ND4 G11778A mutation. Ophthalmology. 2009;116:558–564 e3.

20. Kearns TP, Sayre GP. Retinitis pigmentosa, external ophthalmoplegia, and complete heart block: Unusual syndrome with histological study in one of two cases. AMA Arch Ophthalmol. 1958;60:280–9.

21. Shoffner JM, Lott MT, Voljavec AS, et al. Spontaneous Kearns-Sayre/chronic external ophthalmoplegia plus syndrome associated with a mitochondrial DNA deletion: a slip- replication model and metabolic therapy. Proc Natl Acad Sci USA. 1989;86:7952–6.

22. Pello R, Martín MA, Carelli V, et al. Mitochondrial DNA background modulates the assembly kinetics of OXPHOS complexes in a cellular model of mitochondrial disease. Hum Mol Genet. 2008;17:4001–11.

23. Keeney PM, Xie J, Capaldi RA, et al. Parkinson's disease brain mitochondrial complex I has oxidatively damaged subunits and is functionally impaired and misassembled. J Neurosci. 2006;26:5256–64.

24. Gilchrist JM, Sikirica M, Stopa E, et al. Adult-onset MELAS. Evidence for involvement of neurons as well as cerebral vasculature in stroke like episodes. Stroke. 1996;27:1420–3.

25. Prayson RA, Wang N. Mitochondrial myopathy, encephalopathy, lactic acidosis, and stroke like episodes (MELAS) syndrome: an autopsy report. Arch Pathol Lab Med. 1998;122:978–81.

26. Shoffner JM, Lott MT, Lezza AM, et al. Myoclonic epilepsy and ragged-red fiber disease (MERRF) is associated with a mitochondrial DNA tRNA(Lys) mutation. Cell. 1990;61:931–7.

27. Yoneda M, Tanno Y, Horai S, et al. A common mitochondrial DNA mutation in the t-RNA^{Lys} of patients with myoclonus epilepsy associated with ragged-red fibers. Biochem Int. 1990;21:789–96.

28. McFarland R, Elson JL, Taylor RW, et al. Assigning pathogenicity to mitochondrial tRNA mutations. Trends Genet. 2004;20:591–6.

29. Prezant TR, Agapian JV, Bohlman MC, et al. Mitochondrial ribosomal RNA mutation associated with both antibiotic-induced and non-syndromic deafness. Nat Genet. 1993;4:289–2949.

30. Fischel-Ghodsian N, Prezant TR, Bu X, et al. Mitochondrial ribosomal RNA gene mutation in a patient with sporadic aminoglycoside ototoxicity. Am J Otolaryngol. 1993;14:399–403.

31. Toyo-oka T, Nagayama K, Suzuki J, et al. Noninvasive assessment of cardiomyopathy development with simultaneous measurement of topical ^{1}H- and ^{31}P-magnetic resonance spectroscopy. Circulation. 1992;86:295–301.

32. Harris KM, Spirito P, Maron MS, et al. Ventricular remodeling in the end-stage phase of hypertrophic cardiomyopathy. Circulation. 2006;114:216–25.

33. Finnila S, Lehtonen MS, Majamaa K. Phylogenetic network for European mtDNA. Am J Hum Genet. 2001;68:1475–84.

34. Herrnstadt C, Elson JL, Fahy E, et al. Reduced-median-network analysis of complete mitochondrial DNA coding-region sequences for the major African, Asian, and European haplogroups. Am J Hum Genet. 2002;70:1152–71.

35. Starikovskaya EB, Sukernik RI, Derbeneva OA, et al. Mitochondrial DNA diversity in indigenous populations of the southern belt of Siberia and its implications for the origins and evolution of Native American haplogroups. Ann Hum Genet. 2005;69(Pt 1):67–89.

36. Kong QP, Bandelt HJ, Sun C, et al. Updating the East Asian mtDNA phylogeny: a prerequisite for the identification of pathogenic mutations. Hum Mol Genet. 2006;15:2076–86.

37. Tanaka M, Cabrera VM, Gonzalez AM, et al. Mitochondrial genome variation in eastern Asia and the peopling of Japan. Genome Res. 2004;14(10A):1832–50.

38. Wang X, Lu J, Zhu Y, et al. Mitochondrial tRNAThr G15927A mutation may modulate the phenotypic manifestation of ototoxic 12S rRNA A1555G mutation in four Chinese families. Pharmacogenet Genom. 2008;18:1059–70.

39. Yao YG, Macauley V, Kivisild T, et al. To trust or not to trust an idiosyncratic mitochondrial data set. Am J Hum Genet. 2003;72:1341–6.

40. Broughton RE, Milam JE, Roe BA. The complete sequence of the zebra fish (Danio rerio) mitochondrial genome and evolutionary patterns in vertebrate mitochondrial DNA. Genome Res. 2001;11:1958–67.

MELAS Syndrome: Mediated by Impaired Taurinomethyluridine Synthesis

Stephen W. Schaffer and Chian Ju Jong

Abstract

Taurine (2-aminoethanesulfonate) is a ubiquitous β-amino acid found in a very high concentration in excitable tissue. One of its most important functions is its conjugation with uridine located in the wobble position of tRNA$^{\text{Leu(UUR)}}$. Because the wobble modification stabilizes the UG base pairing, it facilitates the decoding of UUG codons. Consequently, taurine deficiency, which reduces the wobble modification, decreases the synthesis of proteins whose mRNA has a high UUG codon content. The synthesis of one such protein, ND6, plunges 60% after a 50% decline in taurine content. Because ND6 is a subunit of respiratory chain complex I, taurine depletion also leads to a decline in the activity of the electron transport chain. A similar sequence of events occurs in the mitochondrial disease, MELAS (mitochondrial myopathy, encephalopathy, lactic acidosis, and stroke-like episodes). The initial event in most MELAS patients is the appearance of one mutation in tRNA$^{\text{Leu(UUR)}}$, which in turn blocks the taurinomethyl modification of the wobble nucleotide. As a result, the synthesis of ND6 and other UUG-dependent proteins falls. As respiratory function declines, the generation of ATP is compromised and in some cases the mitochondria begin to produce oxidants. Because mutations in tRNA$^{\text{Leu(UUR)}}$ trigger multiple events, the identification of which event causes mitochondrial dysfunction has been challenging. The taurine-deficient model has aided in the identification of at least one pathological pathway that contributes to the development of the MELAS disorder.

S.W. Schaffer (✉)
Department of Pharmacology, College of Medicine,
University of South Alabama,
Mobile, AB, USA
e-mail: sschaffe@jaguar1.usouthal.edu

B. Ostadal et al. (eds.), *Genes and Cardiovascular Function*,
DOI 10.1007/978-1-4419-7207-1_10, © Springer Science+Business Media, LLC 2011

Keywords

β-Alanine • Cardiomyopathy • MELAS syndrome • Mitochondria-encoded proteins • Mitochondrial disease • ND6 • Posttranscriptional modification • Respiratory chain activity • Taurine • Taurinomethyluridine • tRNA aminoacylation • tRNA$^{Leu(UUR)}$ • Wobble nucleotide

Introduction

Characteristics of Mitochondrial Diseases

Mitochondrial diseases are a heterogeneous group of disorders that arise from mutations in either mitochondrial or nuclear genomes and produce deficiencies in the mitochondrial respiratory chain [1]. Mutations in the nuclear genome can cause mitochondrial diseases by affecting the synthesis of mitochondria-encoded proteins, the encoding of respiratory chain subunits, the alteration of energy metabolism and the delivery of reducing equivalents to the respiratory chain, and the generation of proteins that regulate the integrity of the respiratory chain. On the other hand, mitochondrial mutations trigger mitochondrial diseases largely by affecting the synthesis of mitochondria-encoded proteins, which combine with other subunits to produce the respiratory chain complexes. While some mitochondrial mutations are localized to genes of individual mitochondria-encoded proteins and ribosomal RNA [1–3], most of the mitochondrial mutations occur in genes encoding mitochondrial tRNAs. Amazingly, 21 of the 22 mitochondrial DNA genes for tRNAs can harbor mutations [2, 3], with the gene for tRNA$^{Leu(UUR)}$ experiencing the largest number of potential mutations (18 in 17 different positions). These mutations differ in origin and frequency. While point mutations of the mitochondrial genome are largely maternally inherited and relatively frequent, large-scale rearrangements (deletions and insertions) are fairly uncommon and often arise spontaneously.

Disorders attributed to mitochondrial DNA mutations are usually manifested as pathological lesions in the nervous system and skeletal muscle but can involve either a single organ (such as the eye in Leber hereditary optic neuropathy) or multiple organ systems. Because of the importance of electron transport chain flux and adenosine triphosphate (ATP) generation in the maintenance of myocardial contractile function, mitochondrial DNA mutations often lead to the development of myocardial remodeling and failure [4–6]. However, some mitochondrial mutations lead to catastrophic biochemical alterations that are incompatible with life and result in fatal infantile cardiomyopathies [6]. Because cells contain a mixture of normal and abnormal DNA, the severity of a given mitochondrial disorder depends upon the ratio of normal to mutant DNA.

Mutations in mitochondrial tRNA genes usually result in multisystem disorders, with the MELAS (mitochondrial myopathy, encephalopathy, lactic acidosis, and stroke-like episodes) syndrome being one of the most characterized multisystem disorders. The primary symptoms of the MELAS syndrome include lactic acidosis, episodic vomiting, seizures, hearing loss, migraine-like headaches, short stature, and recurrent cerebral insults that resemble a stroke. However, patients with the MELAS syndrome are also prone to the development of a cardiomyopathy [7, 8]. The primary lesions associated with the development of the MELAS syndrome are mutations A3243G and T3271C of the mitochondrial tRNA$^{Leu(UUR)}$ gene. Nonetheless, other mutations in the tRNA$^{Leu(UUR)}$ gene (G3244A, T3258C, T3291C) also trigger the development of the MELAS syndrome [9–12]. The syndrome can also arise from mitochondrial point mutations of respiratory chain components and from large-scale mitochondrial deletions [11]. Because cardiomyocytes of MELAS patients harbor both normal and mutant mitochondrial DNA, a threshold percentage of mutant DNA must be present to initiate defects in respiration and the appearance of clinical symptoms.

Cybrid lines and tissue containing mutated tRNA$^{Leu(UUR)}$ genes generally exhibit decreased rates of mitochondrial protein synthesis, respiratory chain deficiency, reduced mitochondrial electrochemical potential, and diminished rates of respiration [13–16]. The onset of these events is initiated by malfunction of the mutated tRNAs. Three theories have been advanced to explain the effect of tRNA mutations on mitochondrial protein synthesis and respiratory chain activity. One theory attributes the decline in mitochondrial protein synthesis to impaired aminoacylation of the tRNA. The second theory attributes impaired mitochondrial function to reduced rates of transcription [17]. The other major theory implicates tRNA wobble modification deficiency in the development of mitochondrial dysfunction.

Role of Reduced Aminoacylation and Impaired Transcription in MELAS-Associated Mutations

The structure and function of cytosolic and mitochondrial tRNAs depend upon posttranscriptional modification of key nucleotides. Approximately 10% of the nucleotides in cytosolic tRNAs and 6–12% in mitochondrial tRNAs undergo posttranscriptional modification [18]. Figure 1 shows the clover-leaf structure and sequence of human mitochondrial tRNA$^{Leu(UUR)}$. Among the notable posttranscriptional modifications of tRNA$^{Leu(UUR)}$ are base methylation (m^{1}U,m^{5}C,etc.) and conversion of unmodified base to a ribothymidine moiety (T), a 5-taurinomethyluridine moiety (U*), a pseudouridine moiety (Ψ), and a dihydrouridine moiety (D). Helm et al. [18] found that the A3243G MELAS mutation is associated with undermethylation of base G3239 (m^{2}G). While the undermethylation of m^{2}G might decrease the stability of the mutated tRNA, a more important consequence of the A3243G mutation is decreased aminoacylation [2, 19]. According to Hao et al. [20] a wide range of mutations, including those

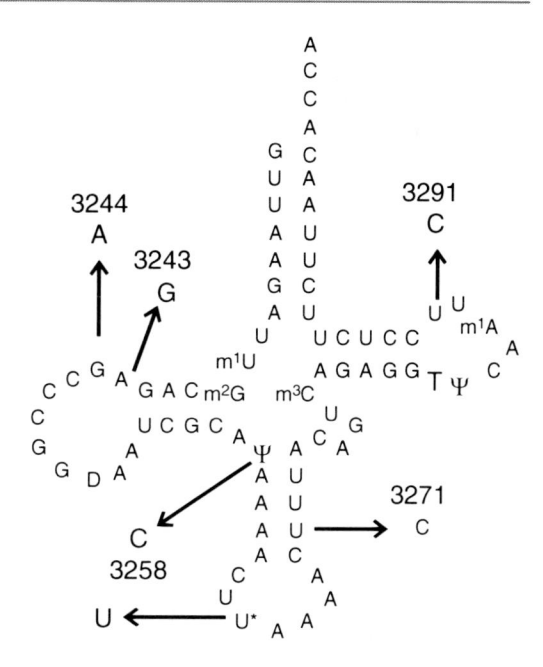

Fig. 1 Secondary structure of human tRNA$^{Leu(UUR)}$. Human tRNA$^{Leu(UUR)}$ contains nine nucleotides that undergo post-transcriptional modification [methylation – m^{1}U, m^{2}G, etc.; dihydrouridine (D), pseudouridine (Ψ), taurinomethyluridine (U*), ribothymidine (T)]. The tRNA assumes a clover-leaf configuration with several distinct regions. Shown are five MELAS mutations (A3243G, G3244A, T3258C, T3271C, and T3291C) that cause a wobble modification defect (failure to convert U to U*)

in the D-loop, the anticodon stem, and the TΨC loop of tRNA$^{Leu(UUR)}$, decrease the leucylation of the mutated tRNA. This decline in leucyl-tRNA content invariably leads to reduced rates of mitochondrial protein synthesis [21]. Among the mitochondrial proteins exhibiting marked declines in protein synthesis as a result of reduced leucyl tRNA content is the NADH dehydrogenase subunit, ND6. However, the impairment in ND6 synthesis and that of other mitochondria-encoded proteins cannot be attributed to abnormal elongation, as the synthesis of the mitochondria-encoded proteins is not directly related to the number of UUR codons per leucine residue found in the mitochondrial protein [2]. Moreover, the reduction in protein synthesis cannot be attributed to mis-incorporation of leucine into proteins during translation, as the tRNA$^{Leu(UUR)}$ mutant is amino-acylated only with leucine [22]. Nonetheless, over-expression of mitochondrial leucyl-tRNA

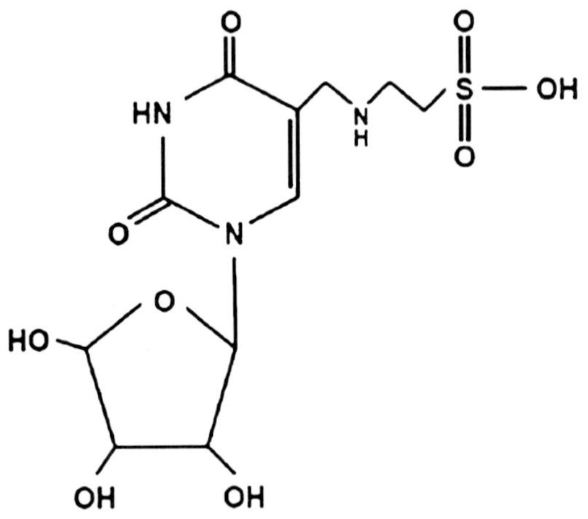

Fig. 2 Structure of taurinomethyluridine

synthetase increases both the percentage of aminoacylated $tRNA^{Leu\ (UUR)}$ and the steady-state levels of $tRNA^{Leu(UUR)}$ in cybrid cells harboring the A3243G mutation [14]. Despite the improvement in aminoacylation efficiency, oxygen consumption is only modestly improved in cells containing elevated levels of leucyl tRNA synthetase, suggesting that factors other than reduced aminoacylation and impaired rates of transcription contribute to mitochondrial dysfunction in cells carrying the A3243G mutant.

Wobble Modification Defect in the MELAS Syndrome

One of the most important posttranscriptional modifications of $tRNA^{Leu(UUR)}$ involves the taurinomethylation of a uridine base situated in the wobble position of the anticodon (Figs. 1 and 2). Using an *E. coli* cell-free translation system, Takai et al. [23] found that the modification of the wobble base of $tRNA^{Ser}$ leads to enhanced wobbling, implying that the posttranscriptional modification of the wobble position affects the reading of the codon. This occurs because the posttranscriptional modification of uridine located in the wobble position affects the unusual base-pairing at the wobble position, allowing expansion of the decoding capability of the tRNA [24]. In the case of $tRNA^{Leu(UUR)}$, taurinomethylation of uridine in the

wobble position permits equal decoding of UUA and UUG, while $tRNA^{Leu(UUR)}$ lacking the taurinomethylation modification preferentially decodes UUA [25]. Interestingly, the posttranscriptional taurinomethyl modification of the wobble base is dramatically reduced in cybrid cells containing $tRNA^{Leu(UUR)}$, harboring one of five mutations associated with the MELAS syndrome (A3243G, G3244A, T3258C, T3271C, and T3291C) [12, 26]. This effect is important because mutated $tRNA^{Leu(UUR)}$ lacking the wobble modification shows weak binding of the anticodon to the UUG codon but not to the UUA codon.

The formation of a stable and geometrically favorable codon–anticodon interaction allows translation to proceed. However, mismatches in the interaction alter the codon–anticodon minihelical structure, which slows the process of translation and can actually terminate it. Nonetheless, the ribosome accommodates most modifications in the wobble position. While the first two positions of the anticodon are restricted by Watson–Crick canonical base-pair interactions, the wobble position allows considerable flexibility. As a result, the synthesis of mitochondria-encoded proteins, whose mRNA is rich in UUG codons, proceeds uninterrupted in normal tissue. However, $tRNA^{Leu(UUR)}$ mutations that restrict the wobble modification, such as those often seen in the MELAS syndrome, exhibit reduced rates in the synthesis of UUG-dependent mitochondria-encoded proteins. The respiratory chain complex I subunit, ND6, is unique among the mitochondria-encoded proteins because its mRNA is rich in UUG codons and its synthesis is highly dependent on the wobble modification. Thus, it is not surprising that Hayashi et al. [27] found that cybrid cells containing $tRNA^{Leu(UUR)}$ harboring the MELAS 3271 mutation exhibit depressed respiratory chain complex I activity and impaired synthesis of ND6. It is noteworthy that overall protein synthesis is not appreciably altered by the T3271C $tRNA^{Leu(UUR)}$ mutation, suggesting that the T3271C mutation only causes distinct changes in mitochondrial function triggered by defects in the wobble modification and the synthesis of proteins whose mRNA harbors a high UUG content [27]. These data support the view that $tRNA^{Leu(UUR)}$

mutations initiate a sequence of events that begin with a reduction in taurinomethylation of the wobble base and proceed to the reduction in UUG-dependent protein synthesis, slowing in electron transport and the development of clinical symptoms of the MELAS syndrome [12].

Taurine Deficiency Triggers a MELAS-Like Condition

Taurine is a β-amino acid found in very high concentration in excitable tissues [28]. The reaction that links taurine to the MELAS syndrome is the taurinomethylation of uridine located in the wobble position of tRNA$^{Leu(UUR)}$. The posttranscriptional modification of the wobble base stabilizes the UG base pairing of the codon–anticodon complex, thereby facilitating the decoding of UUG codons. Although the conjugation enzyme responsible for the taurinomethylation reaction has not been identified, it is reasonable to assume that the formation of taurinomethyluridine depends upon the ability of the conjugation enzyme to recognize taurine and tRNA$^{Leu(UUR)}$ as substrates and the availability of taurine to bind to the active site of the enzyme. Taurine depletion presumably reduces the levels of taurine below the Km of the conjugation enzyme, thereby diminishing the wobble modification. Like MELAS mutations, reductions in taurinomethyluridine content as a result of taurine depletion reduce UUG decoding and produce a MELAS-like syndrome. However, taurine depletion is unlikely to promote other complications of the MELAS syndrome, such as defects in aminoacylation and in other posttranscriptional modifications that alter the structure and stability of the tRNA.

Three models have been developed to examine the effects of cellular taurine depletion: a nutritional model of taurine depletion in certain species, a model produced by knocking out the taurine transporter, and a model dependent on the inhibition of the taurine transporter by taurine analogues. All three models lead to the development of a cardiomyopathy [29–31]. However, mitochondrial function has only been evaluated in the latter

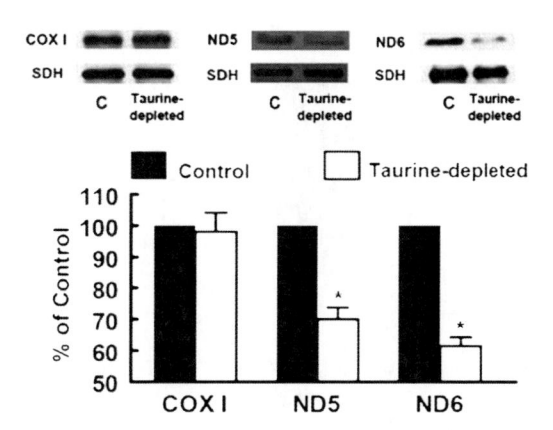

Fig. 3 Effect of taurine depletion on mitochondrial levels of respiratory chain subunits. Upper panel reveals representative gels of untreated (control) and β-alanine treated (taurine-deficient) cardiomyocytes. In all gels, succinate dehydrogenase content (SDH) serves as a loading control. Lower panel shows changes in the protein levels of cytochrome c oxidase I (COX I), ND5, and ND6 in cells treated with β-alanine to reduce cellular taurine levels. Data represent means ± S.E.M. of six to eight different cellular preparations. Asterisks denote significant differences between untreated (solid bars) and taurine-deficient (open bars) cells. The mitochondrial protein experiencing the greatest decline in response to taurine loss is ND6, whose mRNA contains a high content [6] of UUG codons. On the other hand, cytochrome c oxidase 1 (COX1), whose mRNA lacks the UUG codon, is unaffected by taurine deficiency. ND5, whose mRNA contains 2 UUG codons, exhibits an intermediate decline in proteins levels upon taurine depletion

model. In that model, 50% of cellular taurine levels are lost upon treatment of isolated cardiomyocytes with medium containing the taurine analogue, β-alanine (5 mM) [32]. The decline in taurine content is associated with a decrease in the levels of specific mitochondria-encoded proteins, with ND6 suffering the greatest decline in cellular content (Fig. 3). However, there is a poor correlation between the number of UUG codons in a protein's mRNA and the cellular level of that protein. While the number of UUG codons in rat ND6, ND5, and COI (cytochrome c oxidase I) is 6, 2, and 0, respectively, the decline in the levels of the three proteins in response to taurine depletion in rat cardiomyocytes is 40%, 30% and 0%, respectively [26]. Thus, like the MELAS syndrome, taurine depletion appears to reduce the synthesis of mitochondria-encoded proteins with a high UUG

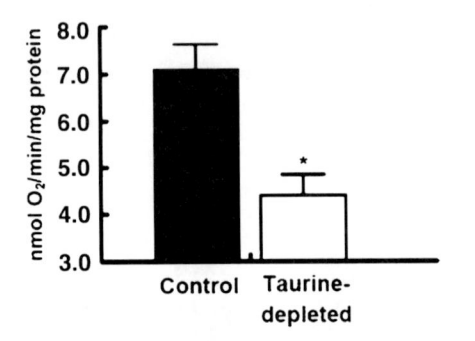

Fig. 4 Effect of taurine depletion on the rate of oxygen consumption. Isolated cardiomyocytes were incubated for 3 days with medium containing (taurine-depleted) or lacking (control) the taurine transport inhibitor, β-alanine. Oxygen consumption was measured using a Clark oxygen electrode. Data are normalized relative to protein content. Values shown represent means ± S.E.M. of five different cell preparations. Asterisks denote significant difference between control and taurine-deficient cells ($p < 0.05$)

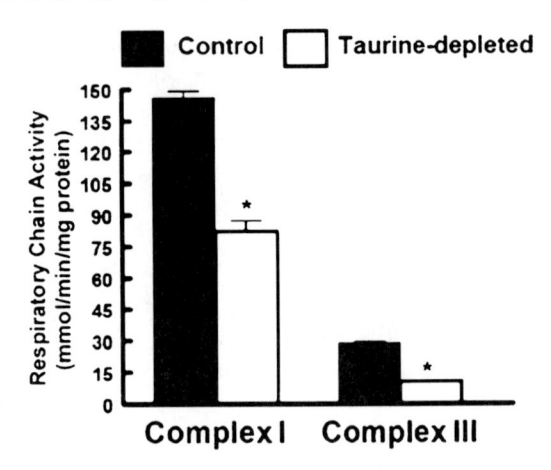

Fig. 5 Effect of taurine depletion on respiratory chain complex activities. Cells were treated with β-alanine as described in Fig. 4. After isolation of mitochondria, the activity of respiratory chain complexes I and III was determined. Data represent means ± S.E.M. of three to five cell preparations. Asterisks denote significant difference between control and taurine-deficient cells ($p < 0.05$)

codon/UUR codon ratio, but the relationship between the protein synthetic rate and UUG codon content is not linear [2, 33]. One interesting feature of the taurine depletion models is that they serve as models of the MELAS syndrome because they mimic the defects arising from a wobble modification deficiency. However, taurine deficiency does not mimic the features of the MELAS syndrome caused by changes in the status of other posttranscriptional modifications or in aminoacylation defects. Although MELAS patients are prone to the development of a cardiomyopathy, the importance of the mitochondrial defects toward the development of the taurine-deficient cardiomyopathy remains to be established.

It is widely recognized that the rate of mitochondria-encoded protein synthesis is a determinant of respiratory chain activity [34]. Thus, it is not surprising that taurine depletion is associated with a 30% decrease in respiration, a 50% decline in complex I activity, and a 65% reduction in complex III activity (Figs. 4 and 5). It is significant to note that like taurine depletion, the A3243G tRNA[Leu(UUR)] MELAS mutation also leads to reductions in complex I activity and oxygen consumption [14, 33].

Although the mechanism underlying the development of the MELAS disorder and other mitochondrial diseases has not been definitively established, it is known that impaired electron transport chain function causes both a loss in ATP generation and enhanced production of reactive oxygen species [34]. Indeed, some mitochondrial mutations also lead to enhanced oxidative stress [35].

Conclusions

The MELAS disorder is associated with a complex web of interacting factors that contribute to the pathological and biochemical alterations of the mitochondrial disease. With so many events affecting respiratory function, it is not surprising that the identity of the distinct events that initiate the onset of the mitochondrial disorder remain to be established. Clearly, the use of a simplified model, such as the taurine deficiency model, helps in uncovering the identity of distinct pathophysiological pathways initiated by MELAS mutations.

Acknowledgments The present study was supported with a grant from the American Heart Association.

References

1. Kleist-Retzow JC, Schauseil-Zipf J, Michalk DV, et al. Mitochondrial diseases: an expanding spectrum of disorders and affected genes. Exp Physiol. 2003;88:155–66.
2. Chomyn A, Enriquez JA, Micol V, et al. The mitochondrial myopathy, encephalopathy, lactic acidosis, and stroke-like syndrome-associated human mitochondrial tRNA$^{Leu (UUR)}$ mutation causes aminoacylation deficiency and concomitant reduced association of mRNA with ribosomes. J Biol Chem. 2000;275:19198–209.
3. Sohm B, Sissler M, Park H, et al. Recognition of human mitochondrial tRNA$^{Leu(UUR)}$ by its cognate leucyl-tRNA synthetase. J Mol Biol. 2004;339:17–29.
4. Tsutsui H, Kinugawa S, Matsushima S. Mitochondrial oxidative stress and dysfunction in myocardial remodeling. Cardiovasc Res. 2009;81:449–56.
5. Anan R, Nakagawa M, Higuchi I, et al. Cardiac involvement in mitochondrial diseases: A study on 17 patients with documented mitochondrial DNA defects. Circulation. 1995;91:955–61.
6. Casademont J, Miro O. Electron transport chain defects in heart failure. Heart Fail Rev. 2002;7:131–9.
7. Limongelli G, Tome-Esteban M, Dejthevaporn C, et al. Prevalence and natural history of heart disease in adults with primary mitochondrial respiratory chain disease. Eur J Heart Fail. 2010;12:114–21.
8. Vydt TCG, de Coo RFM, Soliman OII, et al. Cardiac involvement in adults with m.3243A>G MELAS gene mutation. Am J Cardiol. 2007;99:264–9.
9. Goto YI, Nonaka I, Horai S. A mutation in the tRNA$^{Leu (UUR)}$ gene associated with the MELAS subgroup of mitochondrial encephalomyopathies. Nature. 1990;348:651–3.
10. Goto YI, Nonaka I, Horai S. A new mtDNA mutation associated with mitochondrial myopathy, encephalopathy, lactic acidosis and stroke-like episodes (MELAS). Biochim Biophys Acta. 1991;1097:238–40.
11. Finsterer J. Mitochondriopathies. Eur J Neurol. 2004;11:163–86.
12. Kirino Y, Goto YI, Campos Y, et al. Specific correlation between the wobble modification deficiency in mutant tRNAs and the clinical features of a human mitochondrial disease. Proc Natl Acad Sci USA. 2005;102:7127–32.
13. King MP, Koga Y, Davidson M, et al. Defects in mitochondrial protein synthesis and respiratory chain activity segregate with the tRNA$^{Leu (UUR)}$ mutation associated with mitochondrial myopathy, encephalopathy, lactic acidosis and stroke-like syndrome. Mol Cell Biol. 1992;12:480–90.
14. Li R, Guan MX. Human mitochondrial leucyl-tRNA synthetase corrects mitochondrial dysfunction due to the tRNA$^{Leu (UUR)}$ A3243G mutation, associated with mitochondrial encephalomyopathy, lactic acidosis, and stroke-like symptoms and diabetes. Mol Cell Biol. 2010;30:2147–54.
15. Mariotti C, Tiranti V, Carrara F, et al. Defective respiratory capacity and mitochondrial protein synthesis in transformant cybrids harbor the tRNA$^{Leu (UUR)}$ mutation associated with maternally inherited myopathy and cardiomyopathy. J Clin Invest. 1994;93:1102–7.
16. Ikawa M, Kawai Y, Arakawa K, et al. Evaluation of respiratory chain failure in mitochondrial cardiomyopathy by assessments of ^{99m}Tc-MIBI washout and ^{123}I-BMIPP/^{99m}Tc-MIBI mismatch. Mitochondrion. 2007;7:164–70.
17. Hess JF, Parisi MA, Bennett JL, et al. Impairment of mitochondrial transcription termination by a point mutation associated with the MELAS subgroup of mitochondrial encephalomyopathies. Nature. 1991; 351:236–9.
18. Helm M, Florentz C, Chomyn A, et al. Search for differences in post-transcriptional modification patterns of mitochondrial DNA-encoded wild-type and mutant human tRNA^{Lys} and tRNA$^{Leu (UUR)}$. Nucleic Acid Res. 1999;27:756–63.
19. Park H, Davidson E, King MP. The pathogenic A3243G mutation in human mitochondrial tRNA$^{Leu (UUR)}$ decreases the efficiency of aminoacylation. Biochemistry. 2003;42:958–64.
20. Hao R, Yao YN, Zheng YG, et al. Reduction of mitochondrial tRNA$^{Leu (UUR)}$ aminoacylation by some MELAS-associated mutations. FEBS Lett. 2004;578: 135–9.
21. Lofgren DJ, Thompson LH. Relationship between histidyl-tRNA level and protein synthesis rate in wild-type and mutant Chinese hamster ovary cells. J Cell Physiol. 1979;99:303–12.
22. Yasukawa T, Suzuki T, Ueda T, et al. Modification defect at anticodon Wobble nucleotide of mitochondrial tRNA$^{Leu(UUR)}$ pathogenic mutations of mitochondrial myopathy, encephalopathy, lactic acidosis, and stroke-like episodes. J Biol Chem. 2000;275:4251–7.
23. Takai K, Okumura S, Hosono K, et al. A single uridine modification at the wobble position of an artificial tRNA enhances wobbling in an Escherichia coli cell-free translation system. FEBS Lett. 1999;447:1–4.
24. Weixlbaumer A, Murphy IV FV, Dziergowska A, et al. Mechanism for expanding the decoding capacity of transfer RNAs by modification of uridines. Nat Struct Mol Biol. 2007;14:498–502.
25. Kurata S, Weixlbaumer A, Ohtsuki T, et al. Modified uridines with C$_5$-methylene substituents at the first position of the tRNA anticodon stabilize U-G wobble pairing during decoding. J Biol Chem. 2008;283: 18801–11.
26. Kirino Y, Yasukawa T, Oha S, et al. Codon-specific translation defect caused by wobble modification deficiency in mutant tRNA from a human mitochondrial disease. Proc Natl Acad Sci USA. 2004;101:15070–5.
27. Hayashi J, Ohta S, Takai D, et al. Accumulation of mtDNA with a mutation at position 3271 in tRNA$^{Leu(UUR)}$ gene introduced from a MELAS patient to HeLa cells lacking mtDNA results in progressive inhibition of mitochondrial respiratory function. Biochem Biophys Res Commun. 1993;197:1049–55.
28. Huxtable RJ. Physiological actions of taurine. Physiol Rev. 1992;72:101–63.

29. Pion PD, Kittleson MD, Rogers QR, et al. Myocardial failure in cats associated with low plasma taurine: a reversible cardiomyopathy. Science. 1987;237:764–8.

30. Eley DW, Lake N, ter Keurs HEDJ. Taurine depletion and excitation-contraction coupling in rat myocardium. Circ Res. 1994;74:11210–19.

31. Ito T, Kimura Y, Uozumi Y, et al. Taurine depletion caused by knocking out the taurine transporter gene leads to a cardiomyopathy and cardiac atrophy. J Mol Cell Cardiol. 2008;44:927–37.

32. Pastukh V, Ricci C, Solodushko V, et al. Contribution of PI 3-kinase/Akt survival pathway toward osmotic preconditioning. Mol Cell Biochem. 2005;269:59–67.

33. Sasarman F, Antonicka H, Shoubridge EA. The A3243G tRNA$^{Leu\ (UUR)}$ mutation causes amino acid misincorporation and a combined respiratory chain assembly defect partially suppressed by overexpression of EFTu and EFG2. Hum Mol Genet. 2008;17:3697–707.

34. Ricci C, Pastukh V, Leonard J, et al. Mitochondrial DNA damage triggers mitochondrial superoxide generation and apoptosis. Am J Physiol. 2008;294: C413–22.

35. Lenaz G, Baracca A, Carelli V, et al. Bioenergetics of mitochondrial diseases associated with mtDNA mutations. Biochim Biophys Acta. 2004;1658:89–94.

Part IV

Ischemic Heart Disease

Genetics of Myocardial Infarction

Rudolf Poledne and Jaroslav A. Hubacek

Abstract

Numerous teams are trying to find a genetic determination of individuals with high risk of myocardial infarction. Originally more attention was paid to candidate genes of atherosclerosis risk factors – hypercholesterolemia and hypertension. Out of several hundreds of potential genes involved, only effect of polymorphism of apolipoprotein E was reproduced in different settings and populations. Attention was focused to genes involved in monocyte behavior, arterial wall metabolism, and thromboembolic process more recently. Still the significant effect of few genes is low (OR 1.2–1.7), and in addition reproducibility is very low. Genome-wide scan has been used recently and most discriminative part was identified in chromosome 9 (but without any known protein function). Low reproducibility in different projects is probably related to low number of cases and controls. On the other hand, project with several thousands of individuals in compared groups suffered from inadequate characteristics of individuals, and gene environment interaction might also have substantial effect in reproducibility. Participation of high number of candidate genes with very small or negligible effect is supposed.

Keywords

Acute coronary syndrome • Candidate genes • Gene–environment interaction • Genetics • Myocardial infarction • Wide genome scan

Introduction

Myocardial infarction (MI) is the most common cause of death in almost all industrialized countries, and it is becoming the leading reason of death also in most developing countries. It is not only that this event is most prevalent but it is fatal usually for almost one-third of individuals when

R. Poledne (✉)
Institute for Clinical and Experimental Medicine and Centre for Cardiovascular Research, Prague, Czech Republic
e-mail: rupo@ikem.cz

B. Ostadal et al. (eds.), *Genes and Cardiovascular Function*,
DOI 10.1007/978-1-4419-7207-1_11, © Springer Science+Business Media, LLC 2011

it is first diagnosed. It is a complex clinical complication as a consequence of long-lasting development of atherosclerosis combined with an acute thrombosis. MI occurs when thrombosis is precipitated by ruptured atherosclerotic plaque leading to obstruction of an artery and consequently ischemia followed by necrosis of a part myocardium. Similar to other pathologies, these atherothrombotic events have a part in environmental effects but also a genetic background. Genetic predisposition has been known for almost a century as a positive family history of cardiovascular disease is one of the important risk factors of MI. It is well known that in addition to atherosclerosis, risk factors like dyslipoproteinemia, hypertension, insulin resistance, smoking and age, and family history of parental MI play very important role of MI risk even after adjustment for other risk factors. The importance of genetic compartment of MI was proved also in large twin study [1, 2].

Fast development of methods of molecular genetics resulted in enormous scientific activities searching for genes responsible for a genetic predisposition of MI. Several monogenic disorders have been identified with high relative risk of MI but they are very rare and represent a very small proportion of all MI. The most common form of MI are examples of multifactorial disease resulting as a combination of variants within many genes but each of them with a relatively small effect sometimes difficult to detect. Two main approaches have been used to identify genes involved in the genetic risk of MI – gene association studies and more recently genome-wide linkage.

Genetic Component of MI Due to Genetic Determination of One of the Risk Factors

Dyslipoproteinemia and Hypertension

Three main risk factors for premature MI (dyslipoproteinemia, hypertension, and insulin resistance) have been known for almost half a century.

Their genetic predisposition is of course in relation to all other effects. As increased concentration of atherogenic low-density lipoprotein (LDL) particles is one of the main and most frequently studied risks of MI, it is not surprising that its genetic determination attracts interest of geneticists. Familial hypercholesterolemia discovered in the sixties of the last century is the best example of substantial increased risk of MI. Individuals with familial cholesterolemia displaying high cholesterol concentration practically independently of diet and defects in LDL receptors are playing a dominant role in the appearance of high-risk phenotype. Homozygotes with this genetic defect displaying total cholesterol concentration of more than 20 mmol/L die at children age (without any other risk factors with the exception of high LDL) and they are the best example of genetic risk of MI. Fortunately the frequency of this metabolic defect is very small (1:1,000,000). But also heterozygotes of this disease (frequency 1:500) are at high risk of premature MI. Identification of families with a defect of the function of LDL receptor in the majority of industrially developed countries is successful, and its treatment starting in childhood and pharmacotherapy with very potent statins is one of the most important successes of application of genetics in practical medicine. Unfortunately, the majority of genetically predisposed high sensitivity to diet-increasing LDL cholesterol concentration is polygenic. Most frequently studied candidate genes for high intravasal LDL cholesterol concentration (apoB, apoE, HMgCoR, LDLr, PCSK9, ABCA1, LPL) were proved to be involved not only in the risk of hypercholesterolemia but also in the risk of MI [3]. Although numerous genes were identified to influence high-density lipoprotein (HDL) cholesterol concentrations, their effect on risk of MI has not been found with the exception of Copenhagen City Heart Study. In this large prospective study, a small but significant effect of polymorphisms in the ABCA receptor gene family (participating in HDL and reverse cholesterol transport) on MI risk was found [4].

Also genetic factors or other risk factors of atherosclerosis and MI have been studied for almost three decades. Understandably, increased blood pressure is a complicated network of numerous pathophysiological defects involving numerous genes participating in this pathology. High number of candidate genes has been identified also for diabetes and insulin insufficiency [5], but similar to hypercholesterolemia and hypertension only few of the candidate genes were confirmed in different population studies.

Genetics of hypertension is the most frequent pathology in older age and represents a very import risk of MI. More detailed description of genetic background of dyslipoproteinemia and hypertension is presented in another chapter of this book.

Obesity and Insulin Resistance

The importance of visceral obesity and metabolic syndrome in acceleration of atherogenesis and risk of MI has increased during the last three decades. Cardiometabolic risk was defined as a combination of central obesity, high blood pressure, increased concentration of triacylglycerols and decreased HDL cholesterol concentration, and a decrease of insulin sensitivity [6]. It has been shown recently as a very strong individual risk for MI with hazard ratio of 2.40 for men and even 3.84 for women compared to individuals who do not have this phenotype [7]. We were able to document a shift from the dominating risk of LDL cholesterol concentration to substantial effect of low HDL and central obesity in the Czech population during last three decades. Numerous candidate genes have been found participating in the central obesity phenotype and high triacylglycerol and low HDL concentrations. For example, polymorphism in antipoietic-like protein is independent of lipid concentration, and a large prospective study demonstrated an increase of the risk ratio of MI to 1.48 [8]. FTO gene is one of the most documented genes participating in the increase of body mass index (BMI). Gene variants in this locus are also increasing risk in MI development but, in addition, it also increases total mortality independent of fatness [9].

Genetics of Proinflammatory Status

Presence of a proinflammatory status (and its genetic part) has been determined very frequently during the last decade after C-reactive protein (CRP) concentration was proved as an independent risk factor for MI. Although CRP (as a marker of proinflammation) concentration is related to numerous environmental and metabolic effects, namely obesity and visceral fat volume, it is also under genetic control and several genes might be involved. Central obesity is influencing a risk of MI not only due to insulin-resistance-related dyslipoproteinemia, but it can also influence a risk of MI more directly due to an increase of the proinflammatory status. The effect of proinflammatory status risk measured as high sensitivity determination of CRP (hsCRP) has been documented more than 10 years ago but its genetic component has not been discovered yet although its heritability is known.

We have documented that proinflammatory status is significantly increased in siblings (both sons and daughters) of young patients with coronary atherosclerosis (compared to age-matched controls) [10]. Analyzing polymorphisms in seven candidate genes related to cholesterol metabolism and proinflammatory status (including IL-6, TNF, IL-20, HMGcoR, and apoE) [11], Licastro identified individuals with low and high risk using a statistical model. Proinflammatory gene variants taken together determine an individual risk for MI, especially in young age. It is not due to a similar environmental effect in the family as patient's wife did not differ in CRP concentration from age-matched controls. We were also able to prove participation of two genes determining proinflammatory status and influencing CRP concentration. Both genes were related to lipoprotein metabolism (genes for apoCI and apoE) [10]. Participation of three other genes related directly to the CRP gene was described in two large studies. With application of rather complicated statistical model, the other group of authors was able to prove the effect of participation of few other genes related to diabetes and proinflammation status (IL-6, IL-10, and TNF). Although no marker of proinflammatory status was included in this study, the author concludes participation of these genes related to inflammation.

Because CRP concentration is influenced by BMI, it is not surprising that genes related to BMI play a role in MI risk [10]. Recently fatness-associated FTO gene variants were shown to increase mortality independently of fatness [9]. We have recently also documented that this gene polymorphism increases the risk of MI and this significant effect was also unrelated to BMI [13].

Looking for the Candidate Gene of MI

For more than 10 years, numerous research groups have searched for MI candidate gene using gene-association method [14]. On the other hand, low consistency and reproducibility of already published association of individual candidate gene alleles leads to a certain doubt if genetic epidemiology is able to bring additional information to family history in the identification of individuals with increased risk of premature MI.

An exponential increase in the number of MI candidate gene studies over this period would expect a substantial increase in the understanding of genetic predisposition of MI. The original idea of genetic epidemiology was to construct a substantial tool of clinical value of identifying individuals with higher risk of this disease. Now it is evident that there is only a relatively small effect of association of any single genotype with premature MI, ranging usually between 1.1 and 1.7 (OR, odds ratio) [14, 15]. It is understandable partly due to the multifactorial effect of coronary artery disease development combined with different methodological approach to its clinical complication. Genes related to different risk factors of atherosclerosis as well as genes related to thrombosis and arterial wall metabolism might be involved.

A list of most frequently studied candidate genes is in Table 1. This list of genes might document also a distribution of interest in different parts of atherothrombosis disease: its risk factors, reactivity of arterial wall, monocyte characteristic, and later thrombotic events. A dominant portion of candidate genes studied is related to lipoprotein

metabolism (15%) and inflammation (16%), followed by genes determining arterial wall behavior after atherogenic stimuli (12%) and then to blood pressure regulation, monocyte activity, oxidation, and coagulation (6–8%). Whereas in the late nineties attention was focused on lipoprotein metabolism [1, 15] and blood pressure regulation, more attention has been paid to inflammation and atherothrombosis-regulating genes [11, 16].

Our experiences are similar to other groups applying epidemiology genetics to study a genetic background of MI. We compared 1,399 patients with transmural and non-transmural premature MI (under 65 years in men and 75 years in women) with quite complete clinical, biochemical, anthropometric, and socioeconomic data, and we compare them with sex and age-matched individuals selected from a large representative sample of the same (Czech) population. Data obtained from patients and the control group are identical and their collection is based on the WHO MONICA Study. (More than 20 populations over the world were followed for development of cardiovascular risk factors using the same methodology.) Out of numerous polymorphisms analyzed till now, significant influence of only two genes – apolipoprotein E and FTO (related to obesity) – were proved to participate in the individual risk in this case-control study [13, 17].

Fast development of molecular genetics finally drives attention to constructing genetic chips that allow to analyze hundreds or thousands of variants within genes in one study. Although this method is rather expensive, an engagement of private companies already helps to solve this disadvantage. Recent analysis of possible participation of more than 17,000 SNPs in MI was published by a group of Cardiovascular Research Institute, UCSF [18]. They used analysis of pooled DNA samples in three independent case-control studies and identified 5 SNPs in four genes associated with MI. One is related to thrombus formation which is critical to this clinical complication, and two others related to mitochondrial oxidation, and the last one with high Lp(a) concentration or probably to "more deleterious" form of Lp(a). Unfortunately, none of these genes was confirmed by the first whole gene scan [19]

Table 1 List of the most frequently analyzed candidate genes for premature myocardial infarction

Gene symbol	Gene name : gene function
ABCA1	ATP-binding cassette A1 participating in HDL metabolism
ACE	Angiotensin I converting enzyme (peptidyl-dipeptidase A) 1 : vasodilatator
ADD1	Adducin 1 (α) : binds calciomodulin
AGT	Angiotensinogen : cofactor
AGTR1	Angiotensin II receptor, type 1
ALOX5AP	Arachidonate 5-lipoxygenase-activating protein
ANGPT L 40 K	Angiogenic-related protein participating in fatty acid metabolism
APOA1	Apolipoprotein A-I : participates in reverse cholesterol transport
APOA5	Apolipoprotein A5 participating in triglyceride-rich lipoproteins
APOE	Apolipoprotein E : ligand for apoB/E receptor
CCL11	Chemokine (C-C motif) ligand 11 : inflammatory reaction
CCR2	Chemokine (C-C motif) receptor 2 : chemikinese receptor
CCR5	Chemokine (C-C motif) receptor 5 : immune response
CD14	CD14 molecule: LPS receptor on monocyte membrane
CETP	Cholesteryl ester transfer protein : LPS exchange in plasma compartment
COMT	Catechol-O-methyltransferase : inactivation of catacholamine hormones
CX3CR1	Chemokine (C-X3-C motif) receptor 1 : mediates adhesive and migratory function
CYP11B2	Cytochrome P450 : corticosterone metabolism
CYP2C9	Cytochrome P450 : monooxygenase
ENPP1	Ectonucleotide pyrophosphatase/phosphodiesterase 1 : soft tissue calcification
ESR1	Estrogen receptor 1 : cellular proliferation
F12	Coagulation factor XII : blood coagulation, fibrinolysis
F13A1	Coagulation factor XIII : stabilazing fibrin clod
F2	Coagulation factor II (thrombin) : blood homeostasis, inflammation
F5	Coagulation factor V : activation of prothrombin
FGB	Fibrinogen β-chain : cofactor of platelet aggregation
FTO	Fatness-associated gene
GJA4	Gap junction protein : alfa connexon
GP1BA	Glycoprotein Ib (platelet) : formation of platelet plaques
GRL (NR3C1)	Nuclear receptor subfamily 3 : inflammatory response
GSTT1	Glutathione transferase participating in lipoprotein oxidation
HFE	Hemochromatosis : binding to transferrin receptor
HSL	Hormone-sensitive lipase regulating fatty acid release from adipocytes
HNF1	Hepatic nuclear factor, inflammation, influence on CRP gene
HTR2A	5-Hydroxytryptamine (serotonin) receptor 2A : involved in contraction
ICAM1	Intercellular adhesion molecule 1 : adhesion molecule for monocytes
IL1B	Interleukin 1, β : inflammatory response
IL6	Interleukin 6 (interferon, β 2) : monocyte differentiation and inflammation
IL18	Interleukin 18, immune response
ITGA2	Integrin, α 2 : adhesion of platelets to collagen
ITGB3	Integrin, β 3 : binding of metaloproteinase
KIF6	Kinesin-like protein 6 involved in cytokinesis and microtubule transport
LDL R	LDL receptor, cell-surface receptor binding apoB/E
LIPC	Hepatic lipase : important for HDL metabolism
LPL	Lipoprotein lipase : involved in triglyceride-rich lipoproteins
LRP1	Low-density lipoprotein-related protein 1 : clearence of lipoprotein remnants
MGP	Matrix Gla protein : associates with organic matrix of bone

(continued)

Table 1 (continued)

Gene symbol	Gene name : gene function
MMP3	Matrix metallopeptidase (stromelysin1) : degradation of collagen and proteoglycans
MTHFR	5,10-Methylenetetrahydrofolate reductase : homocysteine metabolism
MTP	Microsomal triglyceride transfer protein : regulation of apoB containing LP in liver
MTR	5-Methyltetrahydrofolate-homocysteine methyltransferase : homocysteine metabolism
OLR1	Oxidized low-density lipoprotein receptor 1 : internalization of ox-LDL
p22-PHOX (CYBA)	Cytochrome b-245, α polypeptide : generates superoxide
PAI1 (SERPINE1)	Serpin peptidase inhibitor, plasminogen activator inhibitor : regulation of fibrinolysis
PECAM	Platelet/endothelial cell adhesion molecule : transendothelial migration of monocytes
PON 1 + 2	Paraoxonase 1 and 2 : prevents LDL oxidation
PPARG	Peroxisome proliferator-activatation glucose homeostasis, adipocyte differentiation
PTGS2	Prostaglandin-endoperoxide synthase 2 : mediator of inflammation
RECQL2 (WRN)	Werner syndrome : cell junction
SELE	Selectin E : immunoadhesion
SELP	Selectin P : inflammation, monocyte reaction
TFPI	Tissue factor pathway inhibitor (lipoprotein-associated coagulation inhibitor)
THBD	Thrombomodulin : endothelial cell receptor, cell-to-cell interaction
THPO	Thrombopoietin : regulator of circulating platelet reaction
TLR4	Toll-like receptor 4 : immune response to lipopolysaccharides
TNF	Tumor necrosis factor : inflammation factor secreted by macrophages
TNFRSF1A	Tumor necrosis factor : signal function in inflammation reaction
UCP-2	Uncoupling protein 2 participating in lipoprotein oxidation

as none of them was genotyped. It is a similar situation to participation of gene for apoE [19, 20] as this most frequently proved candidate gene for MI was not included in the chip for the whole gene scan in any study published yet.

A new approach to analyze the genetic background of MI was presented recently. These authors stated that SNPs in some biomarkers provide new tools for investigating a causal relationship with the disease [21]. Analyzing almost a thousand of SNPs, they found in addition to the effect of already proved lipid relation genes (apoB, LDL-R, CETP, apoAV, and PCSK9) an association with several gene polymorphisms related to a biomarker of inflammation and for CRP concentration.

Gene Score

An alternative approach is to construct a set of selected candidate genes with a well documented effect and to calculate certain gene score to increase the informative value of molecular genetics for clinical practice. The best example was published by the group of University College London [21]. Humphries and his coworkers selected genes repeatedly proved to participate in the risk of MI. This set of candidate genes makes it possible to calculate a score which is as useful in analyzing individual risk as the complete set of traditional risk factors (LDL-C, HDL-C, BP, sex).

Steve Humphries and coworkers from London followed more than 2,000 men in the prospective Northwick Park Heart Study II for 10 years. In stepwise multivariate risk analysis, they included 12 genes previously associated with MI risk [21]. Four of them remain in the model at the end – uncoupling protein 2, apolipoproteins A4 and E, and lipoprotein lipase. The combined discriminative effect of all these four genes was almost identical compared to the effect of most important traditional risk factors (age, triacylglycerols, and cholesterol concentration and blood pressure). Combining the effect of candidate risk factors with genotype improved significantly dissociation of cases and controls ($p = 0.001$). This approach seems to be potentially possible for application in practical medicine.

The Whole Genome Scan

As attempts of identifying genetic variants that affect the risk of MI have been hampered by poor reproducibility of identified candidate genes in one population, an alternative approach was completed during the last years [19, 22, 23]. Technological advances have led to the development of relatively inexpensive genotyping arrays that contain thousands of variants covering the majority of the genome.

Genome-wide scan has been used to study several pathologies recently and this approach has reached a really exponential gradient. While there were only two GWS published in 2000, 1,252 papers were published till now. More than 50% of these papers studied genetic predisposition of risks factors related to cardiovascular disease, but only 10% were related to atherosclerosis and its clinical complications. Only a few of them tried to analyze the individual risk of MI as it is understandable that this problem of multifactorial disease is much more complicated to elucidate.

Well-powered genome-wide scan has now identified several novel putative loci that increase the risk of MI. In 2007 two independent genome-wide scan completed in two populations presented strong association of a common variation in the position of chromosome 9p21[21–23] with MI. Another scan of whole genome in two European studies identified 7 chromosome loci with statistically significant association with coronary artery disease displaying a certain association with classical risk factors of MI (e.g., locus on chromosome 1 is strongly associated with LDL cholesterol concentration). The most significant effect was identified on chromosome 9 and this result is in agreement with earlier published studies. This association in chromosome 9 has not demonstrated any relation to hypercholesterolemia, hypertension, and diabetes. Recently two large genome-wide scans analyzing individual risk of MI were published [19, 21]. They identified four positions highly significantly different from the control group. The first one is in position 9p21.3 with OR 1.20 (CI 1.16–1.25). The other one with similar OR displays a signal in positions 1p13.3, 1q41, and 10q11.21.

Reproducibility of Results

The most important problem of case-control association studies is their rather low reproducibility. Very often a significant difference in genotype frequencies of MI survivors group and controls published is not reproduced in other studies [14]. What might be the reason for this low reproducibility? One possible reason (applied mainly to earlier studies) is in the very small size of groups compared. A significant difference after comparison of a low number of cases with the same size of "healthy controls" might be only a product of small number of genotypes in each of the compared groups. Recently, the majority of case-control studies comprise around several hundreds of individuals, so the probability of random positive effect is much smaller [18]. On the other hand, large studies of several thousands of MI survivors and controls are negatively influenced by inadequate quality and non-homogeneity of data of individuals included that might be another source of false results. This type of studies is usually based on a collection of different projects analyzed in the same laboratory. Also, construction of a control group might influence the results of case-control gene-association studies. So called "healthy control" selected from different databases need not be the real control group. Probably a better way is to select age- and sex-matched control from a large representative population sample of the same population as cases-MI survivors. Large prospective studies in homogeneous populations represent probably the best methodological approach if the number of cases ranges in several hundreds and controls are matched from the same project.

Gene–Environment Interaction

Gene–environment interaction has been intensively studied during the last decade [24–26]. Numerous interactions at different gene locuses have been documented leading to a new era of nutrigenomics and pharmacogenomics.

It is understandable that different lifestyle conditions in different populations might also influence a lower reproducibility of different candidate genes participating in early onset of MI. For example, low saturated fatty acid intake in Japanese population together with high intake of protective n3 fatty acids and high vegetable intake are potentially able to cover differences in candidate genes related to lipoprotein metabolism. On the other hand, a large prevalence of smoking in this population might influence the comparison to the results of population with lower smoking prevalence but high LDL concentration and less healthy diet.

In our analysis of genetic predisposition to acute coronary syndrome, we compared 1,399 consecutive patients from five coronary care units in Prague to controls selected from 1% population sample of the same Czech population polymorphism in four genes. Polymorphism in connexin-37, stromelysin-1, PAI-1, and lymphotoxin-α were proved in predisposition to MI in Japanese population. Although our groups were larger and well defined, no association of any of these four genes was documented in our project [27].

We analyzed environmental interaction with the most frequently studied candidate gene for MI – apolipoprotein E [20, 28, 29]. Apolipoprotein E is a cell-surface protein of triacylglycerol-rich lipoproteins, and it is important ligand for apolipoprotein B/E receptor (LDL receptor) on the surface of human tissue cells [17]. Polymorphism of this gene (alleles 2, 3, and 4) influences lipoprotein metabolism, and individuals possessing E4 allele display higher LDL concentration. Genotypes with this disadvantage allele (E3/4 and E4/4) are at higher risk of premature MI and this fact was confirmed in several already published studies [20, 28, 29], whereas some of them failed to find this negative effect. We compared the prevalence of E4+ genotypes in 1,066 male individuals admitted for MI in five coronary care units in Prague under 65 years of age and compared them with the same number of age-matched controls selected from 1% population sample [17]. Methods and protocols of the study from the WHO MONICA Project were applied.

Frequency of the apoE4+ genotype was significantly higher (22.38%) compared to controls (16.76%). Then we gradually decreased the patient group size, eliminating smokers in the first step, diabetics in second one, and hypertonics in the last step. Number of individuals included decreased to 350 (without smokers), then to 277 (after diabetics elimination), and to final group 129 (after additive elimination of hypertonics). OR increased gradually from 1.36 for the whole group to final 1.71, and this trend was statistically significant. The final group where most genetic influence was expected displays significantly higher prevalence of family history of cardiovascular disease (measured as CVD mortality in the first-line relatives). It is an example of interaction of environmental and metabolic effects with apolipoprotein E as a candidate gene in the risk of premature MI, and it might explain different results in different populations.

Conclusions

After almost two decades looking for "the gene" for premature MI, it is evident that this gene has not been identified yet. There is also very low chance to use molecular genetic methods to identify individuals with a high risk of MI at this moment and to apply this tool to clinical practice. Probably a gene score might be partly informative for individual risk bringing additional information to analysis of risk factors including family history of cardiovascular disease. On the other hand, with all data obtained and published we are able to understand that MI is a complex pathology with participation of a large number of candidate genes with a relatively small effect. Molecular genetics data enlarge our understanding of this problem and we learned a lot. In addition, further progress of whole gene scan might be useful to understand an adaptation of human genes to substantial change of the environmental long-lasting effects [30]. Still we lack a useful tool of molecular genetics for medical practice in MI predisposition.

References

1. Austin MA, Thalmud PJ, Luong LA, et al. Candidate-gene studies of the atherogenic lipoprotein phenotype: a sib-pair linkage analysis of DZ women twins. Am J Hum Genet. 1998;62:406–19.

2. Marenberg ME, Risch N, Berkman LF, et al. Genetic susceptibility to death from coronary heart disease in a study of twins. N Engl J Med. 1994;330:1041–6.

3. Kathiresan S, melander O, Anevski D, et al. Polymorphisms associated with cholesterol and risk of cardiovascular events. N Engl J Med. 2008;358:1240–9.

4. Frikke-Schmidt R, Nordestgaard BG, Jensen GB, et al. Genetic variation in ABCA1 predicts ischemic heart disease in the general population. Arterioscler Thromb Vasc Biol. 2008;28:180–6.

5. Elder SJ, Lichtenstein AH, Pittas AG, et al. Genetic and environmental influences on factors associated with cardiovascular disease and the metabolic syndrome. J Lipid Res. 2009;50:1917–26.

6. Després J-P, Lemieux I, Bergeron J, et al. Abdominal obesity and the metabolic syndrome: contribution to global cardiometabolic risk. Arterioscler Thromb Vasc Biol. 2008;28:1039–49.

7. Arsenault BJ, Lemieux I, Despres J-P, et al. The hypertriglyceridemic-waist phenotype and the risk of coronary artery disease: results from the EPIC-Norfolk Prospective Population Study. CMAJ. 2010;182:1427–32.

8. Talmud PJ, Smart M, Presswood E, et al. ANGPTL4 E40K and T266M effects on plasma triglyceride and HDL levels, postprandial responses, and CHD risk. Arterioscler Thromb Vasc Biol. 2008;28:2319–25.

9. Zimmermann E, Kring SI, Berentzen TL, et al. Fatness-associated FTO gene variant increases mortality independent of fatness – in cohorts of Danish men. PLoS ONE. 2009;4:e4428.

10. Poledne R, Lorenzova A, Staveke P, et al. Proinflammatory status, genetics and atherosclerosis. Physiol Res. 2009;25:S111–18.

11. Licastro F, Chiapellim M, Caldarera CM, et al. Acute myocardial infarction and proinflammatory gene variants. Ann N Y Acad Sci. 2007;1119:227–42.

12. Thompson SR, Macaskie PA, Beiby JP, et al. IL 188 haplotypes are associated with serum IL-18 concentrations in a population-based study and a cohort of individuals with premature coronary heart disease. Clin Chem. 2007;53:2078–85.

13. Hubacek JA, Stamek V, Gebauerova M, et al. A FTO variant and risk of acute coronary syndrome. Clin Chim Acta. 2010;100:1069–72.

14. Visvikis-Siest S, Marteau JB. Genetic variants predisposing to cardiovascular disease. Curr Opin Lipidol. 2006;17:139–51.

15. Humphries SE, Cooper JA, Thalmud PJ, et al. Candidate gene genotypes, along with conventional risk factor assessment, improve estimation of coronary heart disease risk in healthy UK men. Clin Chem. 2007;53:8–16.

16. Armendariz AD, Krauss RM. Hepatic nuclear factor 1-α:inflammation, genetics and atherosclerosis. Curr Opin Lipidol. 2009;20:106–11.

17. Poledne R, Hubacek JA, Stanek V, et al. Why we are not able to find the coronary heart disease gene – apoE as an example. Folia Biol (Praha). 2010;56:218–22.

18. Shiffman D, Kane JP, Louie JZ, et al. Analysis of 17,576 potentially functional SNP´s in three case-control studies of myocardial infarction. PLoS ONE. 2008;3:e2895.

19. Coronary Artery Disease Consortium. Large scale association analysis of novel genetic loci for coronary artery disease. Arterioscler Thromb Vasc Biol. 2009; 29:774–80.

20. McPherson R, Pertsemlidis A, Kavaslar N, et al. A common allele on chromosome 9 associated with coronary heart disease. Science. 2007;316:1488–91.

21. Humphries SE, Yinnakouris N, Talmud PJ, et al. Cardiovascular disease risk prediction using genetic information (gene scores): is it really informative? Curr Opin Lipidol. 2008;16:128–32.

22. Samani NJ, Erdmann J, Hall AS, et al. Genome-wide association analysis of coronary artery disease. N Engl J Med. 2007;357:443–53.

23. Helgadottir A, Thorleifsson G, Manolescu A, et al. A common variant on chromosome 9p21 affects the risk of myocardial infarction. Science. 2007;316:1491–3.

24. Ordovas JM, Tai ES. Why study gene-environment interactions? Curr Opin Lipidol. 2008;19:158–67.

25. Talmud PJ. Gene-environment interaction and its impact on coronary heart disease risk. Nutr Metab Cardiovasc Dis. 2007;17:148–52.

26. Stephens JW, Bain SC, Humphries SE, et al. Gene-environment interaction and oxidative stress in cardiovascular disease. Atherosclerosis. 2008;200:229–38.

27. Hubacek JA, Stanek V, Gebauerova M, et al. Lack of an association between connexin-37, stromelysin-1, plasminogen activator-inhibitor type 1 and lymphotoxin-alpha genes and acute coronary syndrome in Czech Caucasians. Exp Clin Cardiol. 2010;15:e52–6.

28. Liu S, Ma J, Ridker PM, et al. A prospective study of the association between APOE genotype and the risk of myocardial infarction among apparently healthy men. Atherosclerosis. 2003;166:323–9.

29. Schmitz F, Mevissen V, Krantz C, et al. Robust association of the APOE ε4 allele with premature myocardial infarction especially in patients without hypercholesterolaemia: the Aachen study. Eur J Clin Invest. 2007;37:106–8.

30. Parnell LD, Lee YC, Lai CQ, et al. Adaptive genetic variation and heart disease risk. Curr Opin Lipidol. 2010;21:116–22.

Genetic Background of Myocardial Infarction

Kouichi Ozaki and Toshihiro Tanaka

Abstract

Myocardial infarction (MI) is a common disease whose pathogenesis includes genetic factors, and it is among the leading causes of death. In 2000, we started a genome-wide association study (GWAS) for MI using nearly 90,000 gene-based single-nucleotide polymorphisms (SNPs), and identified lymphotoxin-a (LTA) conferring risk of MI in Japanese population. This was the first GWAS that identified a disease susceptibility gene in the world. Moreover, through examining the LTA cascade by combination of biological and genetic analyses, we have identified additional MI-susceptible genes, *LGALS2*, *PSMA6*, and *BRAP*, so far. We present here our recent work focused on identification and functional analyses of genes that confer risk of MI.

Keywords

Genetic risk factors • Myocardial infarction • Signaling molecule • Single-nucleotide polymorphism

Introduction

Coronary artery diseases (CADs), including myocardial infarction (MI), have been the major cause of mortality and morbidity among late-onset diseases in many industrialized countries with a Western lifestyle [1, 2]. MI often occurs without any preceding clinical signs and is followed by severe complications, especially ventricular fibrillation and cardiac rupture, which might result in sudden death. Although recent advances in treatment and diagnosis have greatly improved the quality of life for patients after MI, its morbidity is still high. MI is a disease of the vessel that feeds the cardiac muscle, called the coronary artery. Abrupt occlusion of the coronary artery results in irreversible damage to cardiac muscle. Plaque rupture with thrombosis is a well-established critical factor in the pathogenesis of MI [3, 4]. Although detailed mechanisms of plaque rupture are unknown, inflammation is thought to play an important role in its pathogenesis.

T. Tanaka (✉)
Laboratory for Cardiovascular Diseases, Center for Genomic Medicine, RIKEN, Yokohama, Japan
e-mail: toshitan@src..jp

B. Ostadal et al. (eds.), *Genes and Cardiovascular Function*,
DOI 10.1007/978-1-4419-7207-1_12, © Springer Science+Business Media, LLC 2011

Inflammatory mediators like cytokines are involved in atheroma formation; rapid evolution of the atheromatous injury, leading to rupture of the plaque; and intraluminal thrombosis [5]. Epidemiological studies revealed that coronary risk factors include type 2 diabetes mellitus, hypercholesterolemia, hypertension, and obesity. Some studies reported a genetic factor; one reported that first-degree relatives of patients who have had an acute MI before age 55 have a two to seven times higher risk of MI [6]. A twin study indicated an eightfold increase in risk of death from MI when a first twin dies of MI before age 55 [7]. Common genetic variants are believed to contribute to the genetic risk of disease [8–10]. In this context, we started genome-wide association studies (GWAS) of this disorder using nearly 90,000 gene-based SNPs (http://snp.ims.u-tokyo.ac.jp/) [11] by high-throughput multiplex PCR invader assay system [12], and identified several genes conferring risk of MI including LTA [13–15]. Although the roles of these susceptible genes in MI pathogenesis are under investigation, these findings showed the potent power of GWAS, which is hypothesis-free, to identify unexpected anchors to further understand the disease. Through examining the LTA cascade by combination of biological and genetic analyses, we have identified additional MI-susceptible genes [16–18]. In this chapter, we focus on our genetic association results and show that our initial hypothesis-free strategy unexpectedly revealed the importance of inflammation in the pathogenesis of MI.

Genome-Wide Association Study (GWAS): Identification of LTA as a Susceptibility Gene for MI

Through a large-scale case-control association study using 92,788 SNP markers, one SNP in the LTA, encoding an inflammatory cytokine lymphotoxin-a, (6p21.3) was identified as a candidate susceptibility locus for MI[13]. Following linkage disequilibrium, haplotype mapping and further functional analyses revealed that two

Table 1 Confirmation of association between MI and LTA exon3 SNP

Genotype	MI(%)	CO(%)	χ^2 (P value)
Exon3 804 C/A, T26N			
CC	1,028 (36.3)	1,333 (39.2)	AA vs. CC+CA
CA	1,318 (46.5)	1,630 (48.0)	23.31
AA	487 (17.2)	436 (12.0)	(0.0000014)
Total	2,833	3,399	

functional SNPs (LTA intron 1 252A > G and exon 3 804 C > A) were in complete linkage disequilibrium in this locus and conferred risk of MI. Recently, we have further confirmed an association between MI and LTA exon 3 804 C > A SNP using larger sample sizes (approximately 2,833 case and 3,399 control subjects), and we obtained a similar association result ($P < 0.001$; recessive association model) (Table 1). Furthermore, among white Europeans (in the Precocious Coronary Artery Disease [PROCARDIS] study), a transmission disequilibrium test analysis of 447 trio families with CAD demonstrated that the LTA 804 C allele (26 N-LTA) was excessively transmitted to affected offspring ($\chi^2 = 8.44$, $P = 0.002$, recessive association model) [19].

Association of the SNP in *LGALS2*: Encoding Galectin-2 that Interacts with LTA

After identifying LTA as a novel genetic risk factor for MI, we searched for proteins that interact with LTA to better understand its role in the pathogenesis of this disease. Using both the *Escherichia coli* two-hybrid system and a phage-display method, we identified a protein, galectin-2, as a binding partner of LTA [16]. Because galectin-2 was shown to bind to LTA, we examined whether variations on *LGALS2* (encoding galectin-2) were also associated with susceptibility to MI. We found one SNP (3279 C > T) in intron 1 of *LGALS2;* this substitution represses the level of galectin-2 expression and shows a significant association with MI [16]. This genetic substitution seemed to affect the transcriptional level of

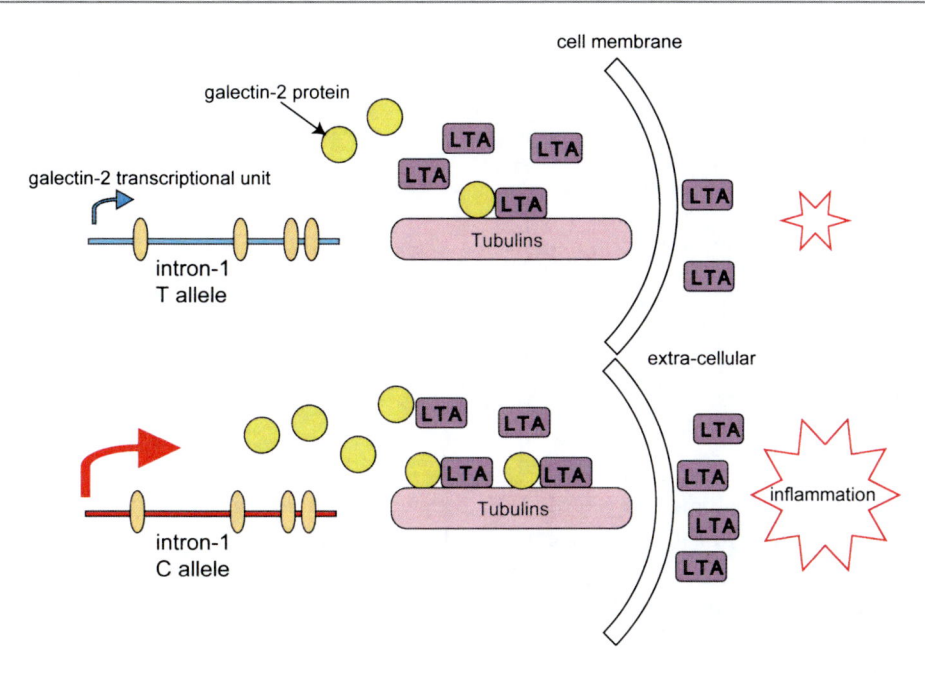

Fig. 1 Hypothetical roles of the SNP in *LGALS2* in the inflammatory process in the pathogenesis of MI

galectin-2, which led to altered secretion of LTA, thereby affecting the degree of inflammation. We also found that galectin-2 binds to tubulins, which are important components of microtubules, suggesting a role in intracellular trafficking. It is likely that LTA is another molecule that uses the microtubule cytoskeleton network for translocation, and galectin-2 mediates LTA trafficking through binding to microtubules [20, 21], although the precise role of galectin-2 in this trafficking machinery complex has yet to be elucidated (Fig. 1).

A Functional SNP in *PSMA6*: Encoding Intercellular LTA Signaling Molecule Associated with MI

Because LTA binding to its receptor strongly activates nuclear factor κB (NFκB) by proteasomal degradation of its inhibitory partner (IκB) protein [22], we hypothesized that the variation(s) in the genes encoding proteasomal proteins could confer risk of MI. The 20S proteasome, which is composed of 7α- and 10β-subunits, is the core particle for 26S proteasome system [23]. We selected tagSNPs with minor allele frequencies of more than 10% that covered most of haplotypes in the genomic region of genes encoding these subunits and found that one SNP (rs1048990) in the 5′-untranslated region of exon 1 (5′UTR -8 C > G) of *PSMA6*, encoding proteasome subunit alpha type 6 was significantly associated with MI (Table 2) [17]. The SNP, located within 5′UTR of exon 1 in this gene, enhanced the transcriptional level of *PSMA6*. Moreover, suppression of *PSMA6* expression level using siRNA in cultured coronary vascular endothelial cells as well as T-lymphocyte cell line reduced activation of NFκB, a central mediator of inflammation, by stabilizing phosphorylated IκB. Thus, the levels of *PSMA6* protein influence the degree of inflammation, indicating that *PSMA6* SNP is a novel genetic risk factor for MI [17].

SNPs in *BRAP* Associated with Risk of MI

To further understand the molecular mechanism that confers risk of MI, we searched proteins that interact with galectin-2. By means of tandem affinity purification, followed by matrix-assisted

Table 2 Association between MI and exon1 SNP in *PSMA6*

Genotype	Numbers of MI	Numbers of MI (%)	Numbers of control	Numbers of control (%)
PSMA6 exon1–8 C>G (rs1048990)				
CC	1,134	43.8	1,382	48.5
CG	1,137	43.9	1,216	42.7
GG	321	12.4	253	8.9
Total	2,592	100	2,851	100
	χ^2	P	Odds ratio	95% CI
Allele frequency	21.1	0.0000044	1.21	1.11–1.31
Recessive model	17.7	0.000025	1.45	1.22–1.73
Additive model	19.2	0.000012	1.48	1.24–1.77

laser desorption/ionization-time of flight (MALDI/TOF) mass spectrometry analysis, we identified the *BRAP*, *BRCA1*-associated protein, as a possible binding partner of galectin-2 (Fig. 2a) [18]. We confirmed their interaction by coimmunoprecipitation experiments (Fig. 2b) and examined whether genetic variation in *BRAP* was associated with susceptibility to MI by resequencing of genomic DNA and followed by association study of selected tag SNPs. As an initial association study, we compared genotype frequencies of these tag SNPs in about 450 individuals with MI and 450 controls and found that one SNPrs3782886, in exon 5 (90A>G, R241R) of *BRAP* was significantly associated with MI (*P* = 0.0014). Haplotypes based on these tag SNPs showed a less significant association with MI. rs11066001 was in very strong LD (r^2 = 0.96) with rs3782886, so we examined these two SNPs in 2,475 cases and 2,778 controls, and found strong associations with MI (χ^2 = 83.6, *P* = 3.0 × 10^{-18}, OR = 1.48, by comparison of allele frequency of rs11066001; Table 3). To further confirm the association, we examined two additional panels, 862 cases and 1,113 controls from the Japanese population, and 349 cases and 994 controls from the Taiwanese population, and confirmed the association of rs11066001 and rs3782886 with MI in these two sets (Table 3).

According to HapMap data (http://www.hapmap.org) [24], minor allele frequencies of rs3782886 were 0.239 in Japanese in Tokyo and 0.148 in Han Chinese in Beijing, but this allele was observed in neither CEPH individuals (Utah residents with ancestry from northern and western Europe) nor Yoruba individuals from Ibadan, Nigeria. No information was available for rs11066001. We additionally examined a panel of 50 CEPH individuals and found that there was no variation at these two SNP loci. These results indicate that these SNPs are likely to be present only in Asian populations. However, the possibility cannot be excluded that other variations in this gene confer risk of MI in other populations. Because rs1041981 in LTA and rs7291467 in *LGALS2* were associated with MI, as described above, we also performed logistic regression analysis for the combinatorial effect of rs11066001 (*BRAP*), rs1041981 (LTA exon 3 804 C>A SNP), and rs7291467 (*LGALS2*) on MI susceptibility. We did not find any evidence of gene–gene interactions as addition of a statistical interaction term showed no significance. The combinatorial effect was consistent with a multiplicative odds ratio model [18]. We also examined the possibility of confounding effects by age, gender, and classical risk factors within cases and found no obvious relationships between genotype and these factors. These results indicated that the significant SNP in *BRAP* is an independent risk factor of MI [18]. Using antibodies directly labeled with fluorescein (*a*-galectin-2) or rhodamine (*a-BRAP*), we examined subcellular localization of native galectin-2 and *BRAP* in human coronary artery smooth muscle cells (HCASMC) and found that these proteins colocalized in the cytoplasm and nucleus (Fig. 2c). We also investigated whether the *BRAP* protein is

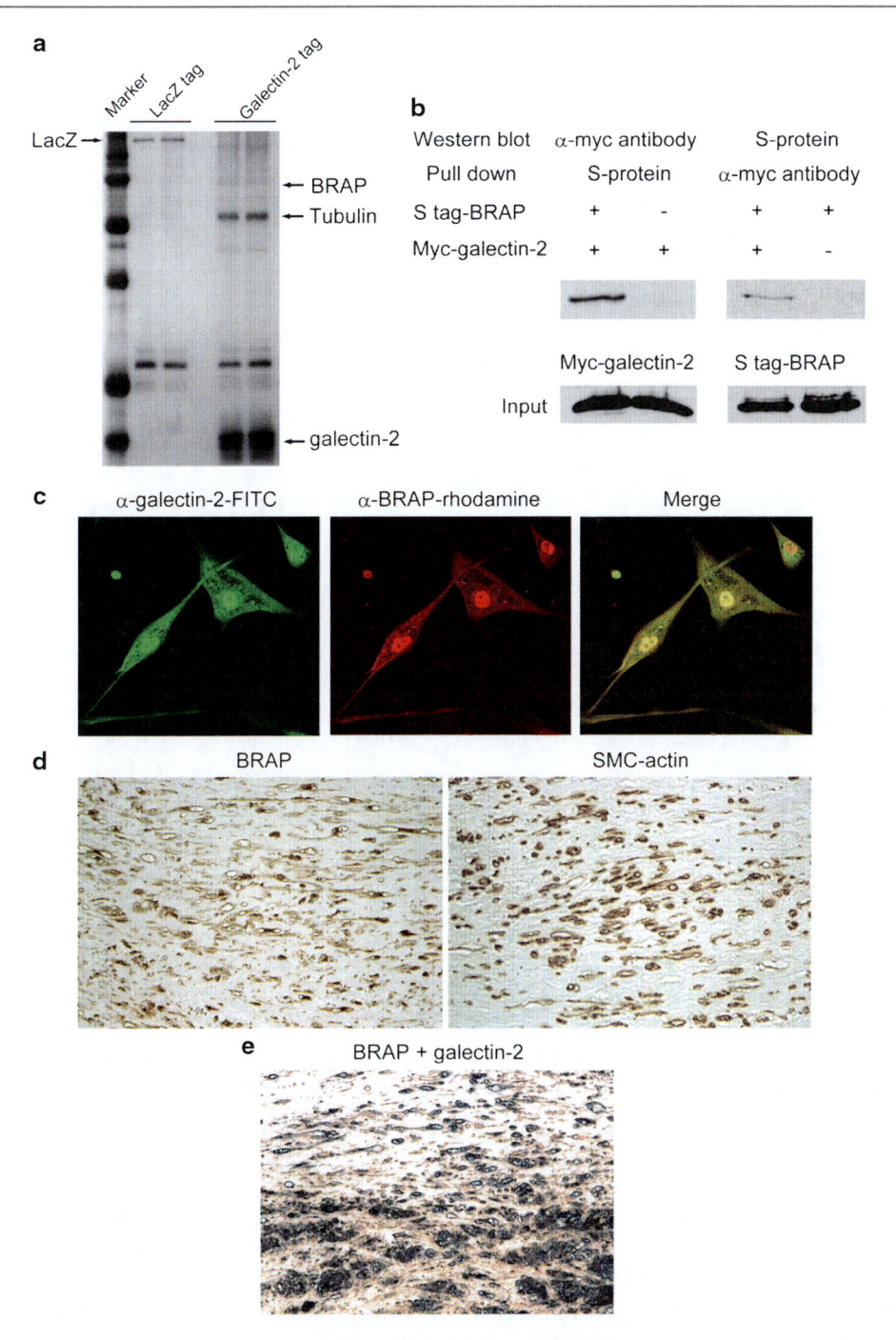

Fig. 2 Galectin-2 interacts with *BRAP*. (**a**) Isolation of TAP-tagged galectin-2 and interacting proteins. (**b**) Co-immunoprecipitation of Myc-tagged galectin-2 and S-tagged *BRAP* in COS7 cells. (**c**) Co-localization of endogenous galectin-2 with *BRAP* in HCASMC. (**d**) Expression and co-localization of galectin-2 and *BRAP* in the coronary atherectomy specimen. Single-labeled immunohistochemistry of serial sections of primary atherosclerotic lesions from human coronary arteries obtained by directional coronary atherectomy, stained with antihuman *BRAP* or antihuman SMC-actin. Magnification, ×65.5 (*BRAP*) and ×90 (SMC-actin). (**e**) Double-labeled immunohistochemical staining with anti-*BRAP* (*brown*) and galectin-2 (*blue*) antibodies. Magnification, ×89.5

Table 3 Association of the two *BRAP* SNPs (rs11066001 and rs3782886) with MI

Study population	rs11066001				rs3782886			
	MAF[a]		Comparison of allele frequency		MAF[a]		Comparison of allele frequency	
	Cases	Controls	OR[b] (95% CI)	P value[c]	Cases	Controls	OR[b] (95% CI)	P value[c]
Japanese								
First panel	0.34	0.26	1.48 (1.36–1.61)	3.0×10^{-18}	0.35	0.28	1.42 (1.31–1.54)	2.8×10^{-15}
Replication panel	0.34	0.26	1.46 (1.27–1.67)	4.4×10^{-6}	0.36	0.27	1.50 (1.31–1.71)	1.8×10^{-7}
Combined	0.34	0.26	1.47 (1.37–1.56)	1.3×10^{-24}	0.35	0.27	1.44 (1.34–1.55)	7.0×10^{-23}
Taiwanese	0.33	0.27	1.31 (1.09–1.58)	4.7×10^{-3}	0.33	0.28	1.26 (1.05–1.52)	1.5×10^{-2}

[a] Minor allele frequency
[b] Odds ratio
[c] Adjusted for Bonferroni's correction in Japanese cohorts

in fact expressed in the myocardial infarction lesion, that is, the atherosclerotic lesion of the coronary artery. Immunoreactivities for *BRAP* were detected in the SMCs and macrophages in atherosclerotic plaques (Fig. 2d). Co-expression of *BRAP* and galectin-2 was also observed in the majority of polymorphic SMCs and activated macrophages by double-labeled immunohistochemistry (Fig. 2e).

The two SNPs in *BRAP* showing very strong associations did not cause amino acid substitutions. Therefore, we investigated whether these SNPs, rs11066001 (intron3 270A>G) and rs3782886 (exon5 90A>G; R241R), would affect *BRAP* expression by reporter gene analysis. A clone containing the intron3 270A allele showed approximately half of the transcriptional activity of the 270G allele or that of the *BRAP* promoter only. No allelic difference was observed in constructs containing the exon5 SNP [18]. To confirm these results, we cloned three tandem copies of the genomic segment including these SNPs, and obtained similar results. These results indicate that the substitution in intron3, but not the one in exon5, affected the transcription level of *BRAP*. We subsequently looked for nuclear factor(s) that might bind to oligonucleotides corresponding to genomic sequences of the 270A allele. No known protein was predicted to bind to this DNA segment by TFSEARCH program (http://www.cbrc.jp/research/db/TFSEARCHJ.html) based on the TRANSFAC database. Using nuclear extracts from HCASMC, we observed

one band in the lane corresponding to the A allele, indicating binding of a nuclear protein(s) to the A allele [18]. This result suggested that an unidentified nuclear factor(s) interacting with this genomic region might suppress transcription of *BRAP* and thereby play a role in the pathogenesis of MI. *BRAP* was originally identified as a protein that binds to the signal peptide of breast cancer suppressor protein *BRCA1* [25], and is known to be an E3 ubiquitin ligase that associates with Ras and modulates mitogen-activated protein (MAP) kinase signaling through regulation of the scaffolding activity of KSR (kinase suppressor of Ras) [26]. The MAP kinase signaling pathway is well known as a regulator of cell survival, growth, differentiation, transformation, and production of proinflammatory factors [27, 28]. Galectin-2 was also implicated in the inflammatory pathway through interactions with lymphotoxin-*a* and tubulin proteins [16]. Thus, we examined whether the cellular level of *BRAP* protein could influence NFκB, a central transcription factor of inflammation [29]. An siRNA against *BRAP* significantly suppressed *BRAP* mRNA, and resulted in inhibition of NFκB activation in HCAEC [18]. This result implied that altered expression of *BRAP* might influence the expression levels of genes involved in the NFκB-dependent inflammatory pathway. Thus, it is conceivable that a higher expression level of *BRAP* with a minor allele of intron3 (G allele) might enhance the degree of inflammation through activation of NFκB protein, thereby playing an important role in the

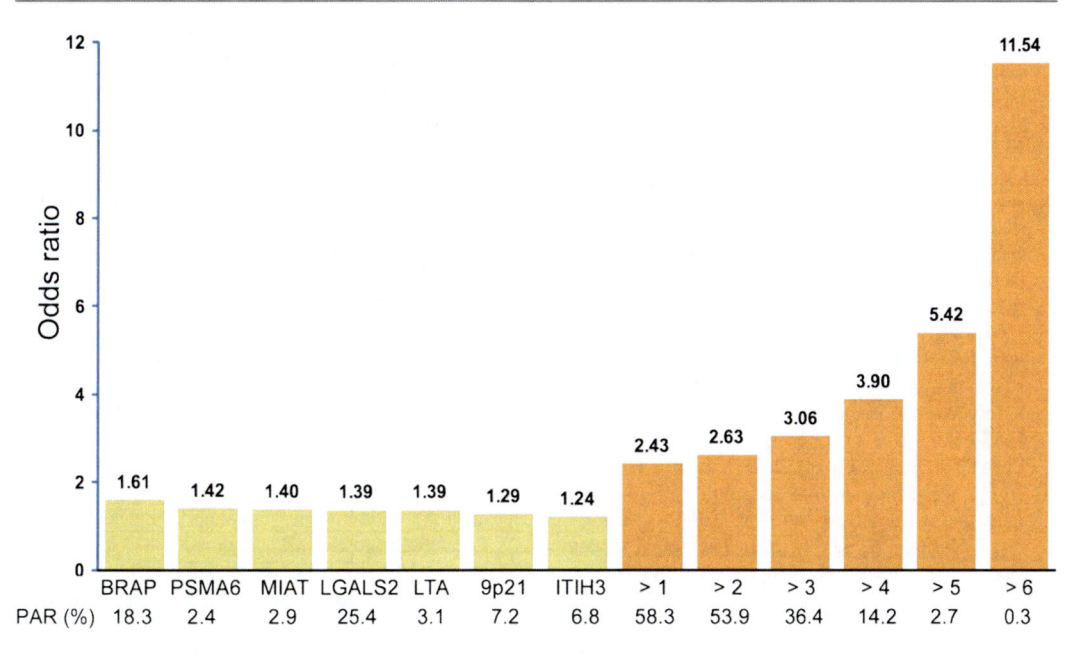

Fig. 3 Odds ratios according to the number of genetic risk factors *PAR* population attributable risk

pathogenesis of MI, although the relationship of *BRAP* protein with activation of coronary artery endothelial cells involved in plaque instability and/or rupture remains to be tested.

methods) and clarification of the molecular mechanism in the pathogenesis of causative genes (for therapeutics) for this common but serious disorder.

Conclusion

To date, we have identified two other loci (SNPs in *MIAT, ITIH3*) [14, 15] that confer increased risk of MI, and also have replicated the association for SNP locus on 9p21 previously identified by European GWAS [30, 31]. Each odds ratio of these genetic risk factors described here is relatively small (Fig. 3); however, by combination of these genetic risk factors, the odds ratio has risen by about 11 (Fig. 3). This result suggests that the combination of genetic risk factors strongly contributes to the pathogenesis of MI. Coronary artery disease attributable to atherosclerosis is a leading cause of MI in many countries. We believe that knowledge of genetic factors contributing to its pathogenesis provides a useful clue for development of diagnostic methods, treatments, and preventive measures through combinations of risk variants (for diagnostic

References

1. Breslow JW. Cardiovascular disease burden increases, NIH funding decreases. Nat Med. 1997;3:600–1.
2. Braunwald E. Shattuck lecture – cardiovascular medicine at the turn of the millennium: triumphs, concerns and opportunities. N Engl J Med. 1997;337:1360–9.
3. Falk E, Shah PK, Fuster V. Coronary plaque disruption. Circulation. 1995;92:657–71.
4. Libby P. Molecular bases of the acute coronary syndromes. Circulation. 1995;91:2844–50.
5. Ross R. Atherosclerosis – an inflammatory disease. N Engl J Med. 1999;340:115–26.
6. Lusis AJ, Mar R, Pajukanta P. Genetics of atherosclerosis. Annu Rev Genomics Hum Genet. 2004;5:189–218.
7. Marenberg ME, Rish N, Berkman LF, et al. Genetic susceptibility to death from coronary heart disease in a study of twins. N Engl J Med. 1994;330:1041–6.
8. Lander ES. The new genomics: global views of biology. Science. 1996;274:536–9.
9. Risch N, Merikangas K. The future of genetic studies of complex human diseases. Science. 1996;273:1516–7.
10. Collins FS, Guyer MS, Charkravarti A. Variations on a theme: cataloging human DNA sequence variation. Science. 1997;278:1580–1.

11. Haga H, Yamada R, Ohnishi Y, et al. Gene-based SNP discovery as part of the Japanese Millennium Genome Project: identification of 190,562 genetic variations in the human genome. J Hum Genet. 2002; 47:605–10.

12. Ohnishi Y, Tanaka T, Ozaki K, et al. A high-throughput SNP typing system for genome-wide association studies. J Hum Genet. 2001;46:471–7.

13. Ozaki K, Ohnishi Y, Iida A, et al. Functional SNPs in the lymphotoxin-alpha gene that are associated with susceptibility to myocardial infarction. Nat Genet. 2002;32:650–4.

14. Ishii N, Ozaki K, Sato H, et al. Identification of a novel non-coding RNA, *MIAT*, that confers risk of myocardial infarction. J Hum Genet. 2006;51: 1087–99.

15. Ebana Y, Ozaki K, Sato H, et al. A functional SNP in *ITIH3* is associated with susceptibility to myocardial infarction. J Hum Genet. 2007;52:220–9.

16. Ozaki K, Inoue K, Sato H, et al. Functional variation in *LGALS2* confers risk of myocardial infarction and regulates lymphotoxin-alpha secretion in vitro. Nature. 2004;429:72–5.

17. Ozaki K, Sato H, Iida A, et al. A functional SNP in *PSMA6* confers risk of myocardial infarction in the Japanese population. Nat Genet. 2006;38:921–5.

18. Ozaki K, Sato H, Inoue K, et al. SNPs in *BRAP* associated with risk of myocardial infarction in Asian populations. Nat Genet. 2009;1:329–33.

19. PROCARDIS Consortium. A trio family study showing association of the lymphotoxin-alpha N26 (804A) allele with coronary artery disease. Eur J Hum Genet. 2004;12:770–4.

20. Ozaki K, Tanaka T. Genome-wide association study to identify SNPs conferring risk of myocardial infarction

21. and their functional analyses. Cell Mol Life Sci. 2005;62:1804–13.

21. Tanaka T, Ozaki K. Inflammation as a risk factor for myocardial infarction. J Hum Genet. 2006;51: 595–604.

22. Beinke S, Ley SC. Functions of NF-kappaB1 and NF-kappaB2 in immune cell biology. Biochem J. 2004;382:393–409.

23. Coux O, Tanaka K, Goldberg AL. Structure and functions of the 20S and 26S proteasomes. Annu Rev Biochem. 1996;65:801–47.

24. International HapMap Consortium. A haplotype map of the human genome. Nature. 2005;437:1299–320.

25. Li S, Ku CY, Farmer AA, et al. Identification of a novel cytoplasmic protein that specifically binds to nuclear localization signal motifs. J Biol Chem. 1998; 273:6183–9.

26. Matheny SA, Chen C, Kortum RL, et al. Ras regulates assembly of mitogenic signaling complexes through the effector protein IMP. Nature. 2004;427:256–60.

27. Ory S, Morrison DK. Signal transduction: implications for Ras-dependent ERK signaling. Curr Biol. 2004;14:R277–8.

28. O'Neill LA. Targeting signal transduction as a strategy to treat inflammatory diseases. Nat Rev Drug Discov. 2006;5:549–63.

29. Karin M, Delhase M. The I kappa B kinase (IKK) and NF-kappa B: key elements of proinflammatory signaling. Semin Immunol. 2000;12:85–98.

30. Helgadottir A, Thorleifsson G, Manolescu A, et al. A common variant on chromosome 9p21 affects the risk of myocardial infarction. Science. 2007;316:1491–3.

31. McPherson R, Pertsemlidis A, Kavaslar N, et al. A common allele on chromosome 9 associated with coronary artery disease. Science. 2007;316:1488–91.

Angiotensin Converting Enzyme I/D Polymorphism and Cardiovascular Risk: Disclosed Story

Anna Vasku, Jiri Blahak, Daniel Baumgartner, and Julie Bienertova-Vasku

Abstract

The renin–angiotensin system (RAS) plays an important role in regulating the main characteristics of cardiovascular functions. The aim of the study is to test possible associations of ACE I/D polymorphism with coronary artery disease (CAD) and diabetes evaluated together in 600 persons with coronarography. Four groups of patients (the CAD+DM+patients with both CAD and diabetes, the CAD+DM−patients with CAD, the CAD−DM+with only diabetes, and the CAD−DM−without CAD as well as diabetes) were compared in ACE I/D polymorphism, intermediate phenotypes (hemodynamic and metabolic parameters), and pharmacological therapy. We proved a number of significant differences especially between the CAD+DM+and CAD−DM−groups. Although the patients had been treated according to their clinical state, we were able to prove significant differences between ACE I/D genotypes (in the model of heterozygote advantage) in these groups (hypertension, obesity, BMI, renal insufficiency, more cardiovascular risk factors, some inflammatory factors, glycemia, and lipid profile). The drugs were administered more frequently to the DD+II carriers, which further supports the heterozygote advantage hypothesis tested in the study. We proved a heterozygote advantage model for ACE I/D polymorphism, CAD, and diabetes mellitus confirmed by associations with intermediate phenotypes and by therapy schedule.

Keywords

CAD • Diabetes mellitus • ACE I/D

A. Vasku (✉)
Department of Pathophysiology, Faculty of Medicine,
Masaryk University, Brno, Czech Republic
e-mail: avasku@med.muni.cz

B. Ostadal et al. (eds.), *Genes and Cardiovascular Function*,
DOI 10.1007/978-1-4419-7207-1_13, © Springer Science+Business Media, LLC 2011

Introduction

In many biological processes, evolutionary adaptations, and thus also complex diseases, there are certain gene pattern combinations together with environmental factors that correspond to what we can call a general predisposition. This makes the understanding of the underlying mechanisms very complicated. In contrast to monogenic disorders, the basic principles of genetics of complex disorders still remain to be elucidated. This is why the attitude of clinicians toward the results of genetic studies focused on genetics of complex diseases often suffers from unsubstantiated expectation over suspect "big factor genes" to severe scepticism to genetic background in diseases, such as essential hypertension or ischemic heart disease. It can be rather supposed that a certain allelic combination of frequent polymorphisms will be found in the population (possibly various loci in different patients with the same disease) that will be possible to be successfully associated with a disease.

Pathophysiological Features of the RAS System

The renin–angiotensin system (RAS) plays an important role in regulating the main characteristics of cardiovascular functions, arterial pressure, and blood volume [1]. In the classical (systemic) system, the enzyme renin is released into the circulation from kidney juxtaglomerular cells in response to sympathetic stimulation, renal artery hypotension, or decreased levels of sodium in the distal tubules [2]. Renin converts angiotensinogen (AGT) from the liver to the decapeptide angiotensin (Ang) I, which in turn undergoes proteolytic cleavage to the biologically active octapeptide, Ang II. The latter step is carried out by the angiotensin-converting enzyme (ACE), which is highly expressed in vascular endothelium, particularly in the lungs. Alternatively, a recently identified carboxypeptidase, ACE2, cleaves one amino acid from either Ang I or Ang II [3–7], decreasing Ang II levels and increasing

the metabolite Ang 1–7, which has vasodilator properties. Thus, the balance between ACE and ACE2 seems to be an important factor controlling Ang II levels. Ang II is further degraded by aminopeptidases to Ang III (Ang 2–8) and Ang IV (Ang 3–8) with their specific receptors Mas and IRAP [3–7]. Ang II has many important functions, including increasing arterial pressure by constricting resistance vessels, stimulating thirst center in the brain, stimulating aldosterone release from the adrenal cortex, thus increasing sodium and fluid retention by the kidney; stimulating release of antidiuretic hormone from the posterior pituitary to increase fluid retention; enhancing sympathetic adrenergic function by facilitating norepinephrine release from sympathetic nerves and inhibiting its reuptake; and causing cardiac and vascular remodeling [1, 8]. These actions mostly result from activation of AT_1, a 7-transmembrane (7-TM) receptor that mainly couples to the G_q/G_{11} family of heterotrimeric G-proteins and activates multiple signaling pathways. AT_1 can function independently of Ang II as a mechanical stress receptor [9]. Binding of Ang II to its receptors mediates intracellular free radical generation which promotes mitochondrial dysfunction [10]. The type 2 receptor, AT_2, couples to hetero-trimeric G_i/G_o proteins. Although originally thought to simply oppose the physiological actions of AT_1, AT_2 seems to act in some conditions like AT_1 in having growth stimulatory and proinflammatory actions [11]. Insulin receptor transinactivation by AT_2 was recently shown to require expression of a novel protein, AT_2-interacting protein (ATIP1) that constitutively interacts with the C-terminal tail of AT_2 [12].

In addition to the systemic RAS, "local" RAS that generates Ang II to act in an autocrine and paracrine manner, was described for a number of tissues in the 1990s, including heart, vessels, adipose tissue, adrenals, brain, and kidney [13, 14]. The local production of Ang II plays an important role in regulating a number of physiological processes, including blood pressure, vasopressin release, drinking behavior, sodium reabsorption, and sympathetic outflow. Activation of a local RAS has been implicated in cardiac remodeling.

Mechanical stress, for instance, enhances expression of cardiac renin and AGT genes [15].

The local hematopoietic bone marrow (BM) renin–angiotensin system (RAS) was shown to mediate alterations of hematopoiesis [16]. A close interrelationship between cardiac RAS and the hematopoietic bone marrow RAS was reported earlier [17]. In relation to atherogenesis, Strawn et al. proposed a lipid–angiotensin system connection within the bone marrow that participates in atherosclerosis initiation [18, 19]. The "bone marrow response to lipid" hypothesis supposes that pro-atherogenic properties of hematopoietic and non-hematopoietic progenitors are determined by the local actions of modified low-density lipoprotein (LDL) on the expression of local RAS genes [19]. According to our results, ACE inhibitors are able to modify the red blood cell count as well as mean corpuscular volume of erythrocytes in patients with essential hypertension, which also seems to reflect involvement of local RAS system in bone marrow [20, 21].

Angiotensin-Converting Enzyme (ACE)

ACE is a zinc metalloendopeptidase, which functions as a C-terminal peptidyl dipeptidase and converts the biologically inactive Ang I to the potent vasoconstrictor and cardiovascular trophic factor, Ang II. A single gene encodes two different ACE proteins through transcription from alternative promoters [22]. The ubiquitous somatic ACE is highly expressed in vascular endothelial cells and has two tandem, independent catalytic sites with distinct properties. Somatic ACE is produced by various other cells as well, including activated macrophages, tubular epithelium, and proximal gut epithelium. Developing male germ cells produce a different ACE isoezyme, germinal or testis ACE, which has a single active site [23].

Somatic ACE is a major contributor to cardiovascular homeostasis, and randomized studies have shown that ACE inhibitors improve symptoms and survival in all grades of heart failure

when given with diuretics [24]. The beneficial effects of ACE inhibitors are in large part due to the prevention of events downstream of Ang II formation, such as elevated vascular tone, heart and vessel remodeling, and salt and water retention. However, ACE also hydrolyzes bradykinin, a potent vasodilator and cardioprotective agent. Since bradykinin is more readily hydrolyzed by ACE than Ang I [25], the net therapeutic effect of ACE inhibitors may reflect both diminished Ang II and increased bradykinin levels. In addition, the tetrapeptide N-acetyl-seryl-aspartyl-lysyl-proline (AcSDKP), which is normally present in mammalian plasma and many tissues, is hydrolyzed almost exclusively by ACE [26]. AcSDKP is generated from the N-terminus of thymosin $\beta 4$ (the main G-actin sequestering peptide in eukaryotic cells) and has antifibrotic actions in the heart and kidney that may result in part from inhibition of cellular proliferation and TGF-β signaling [27, 28].

ACE Gene (17q23)

In the last decades, ACE gene has been cloned that allowed the identification (1) of two isoenzymes, one called somatic ACE resulting from gene duplication and primarily expressed in endothelial cells, and the other, called germinative or testicular ACE, resulting from the transcription in the male reproductive system of a more simple gene, (2) of an hydrophobic C-terminal peptide for membrane-anchoring and specifically cleaved by a metalloprotease to release soluble forms of both isoenzymes, and (3) of several allelic polymorphisms, one of them consisting of an insertion/deletion (I/D) polymorphism in a short intronic Alu sequence that could account for half the variance in plasma ACE level and resulting in a large interindividual variability; moreover this I/D polymorphism was proposed as a genetic marker for identifying individuals at high risk of ischemic heart disease and of anticipating in one individual the efficacy of the antihypertensive therapy [29]. In 1992, PCR method for simple detection of ACE I/D polymorphism was published [30].

Case-Control Studies: ACE I/D and Cardiovascular Diseases

No evidence was found to support an association between ACE genotype and heart failure [31]. ACE genotype distributions were similar between the patients with and without symptomatic CHF in CAD [32]. There was no evidence that ACE gene I/D polymorphism plays a role in the development of CHF in CAD or any influence on exercise capacity in treated patients with ischemic CHF [33].

ACE DD genotype is associated with decreased exercise tolerance in CHF, possibly mediated by altered pulmonary function. Pharmacological strategies effecting more complete inhibition of serum and tissue ACE and/or potentiation of bradykinin may improve exercise capacity in patients with CHF and ACE DD genotype [34].

The higher incidence of hypertension in 684 healthy subjects, which had completed 6 years of follow-up, was observed in the older age groups (36–45 and 46–55 years) with DD and ID genotypes [35].

A total of 4,264 normotensive and 2,174 hypertensive participants of the Rotterdam Study (a population-based prospective cohort study) were available for follow-up from 1990 until 2000. Incidence rates (IR) of heart failure in normotensive subjects were the same over all genotype strata (10 per 1000 person-years) in ACE I/D polymorphism. In hypertensive subjects, the IR increased with the number of D-alleles present. Hypertensive subjects carrying the II-genotype did not have an increased risk of heart failure compared to normotensive II subjects. However, hypertensive subjects carrying one or two copies of the D-allele did have a significantly increased risk of heart. The findings suggest that the ACE I/D polymorphism may play a modifying role in the development of heart failure in hypertensive subjects [36].

The ACE gene polymorphism distribution was found to be similar in CHF patients and control subjects. However, ACE gene DD polymorphism was associated with a more severe condition, greater LVDD, and higher plasma Ang II level [37].

Case-Control Studies: ACE I/D and Diabetes Mellitus

Recently, a meta-analysis of results from 14 studies with 1,985 patients with T2D and 4,602 controls was performed [38]. The D allele carriers in ACE I/D polymorphisms were evaluated to have an increased risk for T2D compared to the I allele carriers, with the highest significance for recessive model for DD genotype [38].

Genotype-Phenotype Studies: ACE Activity in Plasma

Plasma ACE activity measured in 197 unrelated healthy Caucasian (Czech) subjects was correlated with sex, ABO blood groups, and ACE I/D polymorphism. Marked differences in plasma ACE activity levels were observed both among the blood groups and among ACE phenotypes; the highest activity was observed in DD genotype and blood group B. The I/D polymorphism and the ABO system turned out to be two independent (additive) factors influencing plasma ACE activity. Together, they are responsible for 9.56% of the phenotypic variability of ACE in Czech population [39].

A marked difference in the plasma Ang II levels was observed among the three genotypes (DD, ID, and II). The levels of plasma Ang II in the DD genotype class were the highest [37]. ACE gene DD polymorphism was associated with greater LVDDs, higher plasma Ang II levels, and the greatest decreased magnitude of plasma Ang II levels after treatment in patients with chronic heart failure where ACE gene DD polymorphism might be a marker of a higher level of activation of the renin–angiotensin system (RAS) [37].

Genotype-Phenotype Studies: Systolic and Diastolic Dysfunction

Higher heart rate variability was associated with ACE DD genotype [40]. Both systolic and diastolic cardiac dysfunctions coexist in various degrees in the majority of patients with heart failure. Endogenous bradykinin seems to contribute to the cardioprotective effect of the ACE inhibitor, improving left ventricular diastolic dysfunction rather than systolic dysfunction, via modification of NO release and Ca^{2+} handling and suppression of collagen accumulation [41]. In 1,200 male military recruits, LV dimensions and mass were compared at the start and end of a 10-week physical training period. LV mass increased with training by 8.4 g overall, but with DD men showing roughly three-fold greater growth than II men. It clearly demonstrates the importance of the ACE–renin–angiotensin system in determining LV dimensions in situations of high cardiac demand, which may also be important in pathology such as hypertension and heart failure. The use of these "stress-the-genotype" approaches to explore gene–environment interactions are likely to be the key to understanding the causes determining both coronary artery disease and other multifactorial disorders [42].

DD significantly and early affected myocardial diastolic properties in the total group of 684 healthy subjects, which had completed 6 years of follow-up, also when stratified for age [35]. The ACE genotype was determined in 171 patients selected with idiopathic dilated cardiomyopathy (IDC) in New York Heart Association functional class II to III heart failure and with a LV ejection fraction of 40%. The frequency of ACE gene ID alleles was not different in the study versus non-age-matched and age-matched control groups. The ejection fraction was found to be worse in patients with the DD genotype. The LV end-systolic and end-diastolic diameters were increased in patients with the DD genotype. Multifactor regression analysis showed the ACE genotype to be an independent predictor of both ejection fraction and end-diastolic diameter. This indicates that the DD genotype of the ACE gene is independently associated with both a reduced LV systolic performance and an increased LV cavity size in patients with IDC [43].

The ACE gene polymorphism was evaluated in 90 patients after heart transplantation because of end-stage dilated cardiomyopathy compared to the population sample. A decrease of heterozygote ID carriers in the patients was proved [44].

ACE I/D, Coronary Artery Disease, and Diabetes: Continuing Story

Abnormality of the microvascular system causing impared tissue perfusion is referred to be common among cardiovascular risk factors, including hypertension, diabetes, and obesity [45]. If it is so, reading descriptive characteristics of cardiovascular association studies, everybody must mention different numbers of comorbidities and/or risk factors which can unpredictably modify their results. Therefore, we decided to evaluate possible association of ACE I/D polymorphism with CAD and diabetes evaluated together. In this manner we have obtained four groups of patients (CAD + DM + patients with both CAD and diabetes, CAD + DM – patients with CAD, CAD – M + with only diabetes, and CAD – DM – without CAD as well as diabetes. Further, significant differences in intermediate phenotypes (hemodynamic and metabolic parameters, drug therapy) were analyzed in the groups.

Methods

Patient Population

The study comprised 600 consecutive patients with suspected or known CAD referred to the 1st Department of Internal Medicine/Cardioangiology for coronary angiography between October 2005 and February 2007, 417 men (median age 63, range 25–87 years) and 183 women (median age 67, range 27–91 years). During the short-term hospitalization, the patients underwent full cardiological investigation (history, physical examination, electrocardiography, laboratory examination, coronary angiography, echocardiography in patients with unclear diagnosis). Coronary angiography was performed using the standard technique. The coronary lesions were visually analyzed in multiple projections. Based on the morphology of coronary arteries, two patient groups were defined: (1) patients with significant coronary atherosclerosis (at least one coronary artery with luminal diameter narrowing by 50% or more, CAD group) and (2) patients with normal smooth coronary arteries. Patients with insignificant coronary atherosclerosis (stenoses with luminal diameter narrowing below 50% or luminal irregularities) were excluded from the study (N=59).

Other diseases, such as diabetes, hypertension, obesity, and hyperlipidemia, were evaluated at the same time according to clinical guidelines. The study was approved by the institutional ethics committee; informed consent of all patients is archived.

Genotyping

Genomic DNA was isolated from peripheral leukocytes by a standard technique using proteinase K. The ACE I/D genotypes of all subjects were detected using a PCR method according to Rigat (1992). The reaction mixture contained 12.9 µL of PCR water, 2.5 µL of KCl buffer, 2.5 µL of $MgCl_2$, 1.25 µL of each primer (P1: 5'-CTGGAGACCACTCCCATCCTTT, P2:5'-GATGTGGCCATCACATTCGT), 0.5 µL of dNTPs, 0.1 µL of Taq polymerase 5U, and finally 4 µL of genomic DNA. The amplification products were separated on 2% agarose gel, containing ethidium bromide (EtBr, 1.2 µL per 10 mL) and visualized under UV light. The PCR yields amplification products of 490 bp/490 bp in case of II genotype; in DD genotype it is a 190 bp/190 bp pattern and heterozygous ID genotype gives products of 490 bp/190 bp.

Statistical Analyses

In all groups of subjects, distributions of genotype and allelic frequencies and their differences were calculated using χ^2 tests and Fisher's exact test. Consistency of genotype frequencies with the Hardy–Weinberg equilibrium was tested using the χ^2 test on a contingency table of observed versus predicted genotype frequencies.

Kruskal–Wallis ANOVA test by Ranks was used to compare continuous parameters in groups. Odds ratio (OR) and 95% confidence interval were calculated to estimate the risks related to detected polymorphisms. To calculate the significance of OR, Fisher's exact test was used. The program package Statistica v. 8.0 (Statsoft Inc., Tulsa, OK) was employed.

Results

We did not observe any difference in genotype distribution (Pg) and allelic frequency (Pa) in ACE I/D polymorphism between patients with and without CAD (Table 1). Similarly, no differences were observed after patients' division according to diabetes (Table 1). No significant results were observed when the presence of both diseases has been evaluated (Table 2).

Another possibility, how to search expected interaction of CAD, DM, and ACE I/D polymorphism, was to test different models of inheritance. No significant difference was observed either in the DD-recessive model, or in the (DD+ID) codominant models (data not shown).

Finally, a "heterozygote advantage" model was calculated. No difference for CAD has been found (Table 3). However, when the groups of patients with and without diabetes were been compared, a significant difference between these two groups was observed (Table 3). Odds ratio (OR) for the ID

Table 1 ACE I/D polymorphism, CAD, diabetes: case-control study

CAD	N	ACE I/D – DD	ACE I/D – ID	ACE I/D – II	Pg	D allele (%)	Pa
CAD+	484	162	206	116	0.486	54.8	0.552
CAD–	116	33	56	27		52.6	
All grps	601	195	263	143			
Diabetes							
DM+	171	61	62	48	0.06	53.8	0.818
DM–	430	134	201	95		54.5	
All grps	600	195	263	143			

Pg = probability of a diference in genotype distribution
Pa = probability of a diference in allelic frequency

Table 2 ACE I/D polymorphism, CAD and diabetes: case-control (CAD – DM –) study

CAD DM	N	ACE – DD	ACE – ID	ACE – II	Pg	D allele (%)	Pa
CAD+DM+	153	58	53	42	0.09	55.2	0.880
CAD+DM–	331	104	153	74	0.924	54.5	0.997
CAD–DM+	17	3	8	6	0.357	41.2	0.149
CAD–DM–	99	30	48	21		54.5	
All grps	600	195	263	143			

Pg = probability of a diference in genotype distribution
Pa = probability of diference in allelic frequency

Table 3 ID advantage model, CAD and diabetes: case-control study

CAD	N	ACE – ID (%)	ACE – (II + DD)	P
CAD+	484	206 (43)	278	0.156
CAD–	116	56 (48)	60	
All grps	601	263	338	
Diabetes				
DM+	171	62 (36)	109	0.01
DM–	430	201 (47)	229	
All grps	600	263	338	

P = probability of a diference between ID and (II + DD) frequencies

Table 4 ID advantage model, CAD and diabetes: case-control (CAD – DM –) study

CAD DM	N	ACE – ID	ACE – (II + DD)	ID genotype (%)	P
CAD+DM+	153	53	100	53.0	0.02
CAD+DM–	331	153	178	46.2	0.389
CAD–DM+	17	8	9	47.1	0.561
CAD–DM–	99	48	51	48.5	
All grps	600	263	143		

P = probability of a diference between ID and (II + DD) frequencies

genotype in diabetic patients was 0.65; 95% confidential interval (CI) was 0.45–0.93. When both diseases had been evaluated together, a significant difference was found between CAD+DM+ and CAD–DM–persons. This significance disappeared after correction for multiple comparison by Bonferoni's correction (Pcorr=0.06, Table 4).

The heterozygote advantage model was used for comparison of eight groups (including ACE I/D genotype as ID or II+DD). We proved several highly significant differences in some hemodynamic (EF LV, plasma creatinine), proinflammatory (leukocyte number and fibrinogen),

and especially in metabolic parameters (BMI, glycemia, total cholesterol, LDL, HDL, triglycerides). The significance of these differences is sufficiently high to "survive" multiple comparisons (Tables 5 and 6), although the parameters had to be modified by different therapy.

Table 7 summarizes comorbidities and risk factors in all groups. Generally, in most cases, we proved significant differences between the CAD+DM+ and CAD–DM–groups. Moreover, we observed a higher frequency of ID genotype in CAD+DM+with hypertension compared to CAD–DM–group (OR=6.42, 95% CI 2.17–19.04,

Table 5 Significant differences among groups and ACE genotype (heterozygote advantage model)

Group × ACE	N	EF LV median (range, %)	Leu median (range, ×10⁹/L)	Fibrinogen median (range, g/L)	BMI median (range, kg/m²)	Creatinine median (range, μmol/L)
CAD+DM+(ID)	53	50 (18–70)	7.7 (4.3–13.9)	4.4 (2.8–5.6)	30 (22–40)	94.5 (5.6–180.0)
CAD+DM+(II+DD)	100	50 (20–75)	7.5 (3.5–12.7)	4.1 (2.5–5.6)	29 (21–43)	104 (70–200)
CAD+DM−(ID)	153	55 (20–75)	7.6 (4.0–16.9)	4.0 (2.1–218.0)	28 (18–43)	98 (71–176)
CAD+DM−(II+DD)	178	55 (18–75)	7.9 (3.6–127.0)	4.0 (1.05–5.90)	28 (18–43)	99 (66–189)
CAD−DM+(ID)	8	60 (55–70)	7.0 (4.9–9.8)	4.1 (2.6–5.4)	31 (20–38)	107 (69–117)
CAD−DM+(II+DD)	9	50 (20–60)	7.5 (2.8–10.6)	3.7 (3.1–5.4)	30 (21–42)	92 (83–116)
CAD−DM−(ID)	48	60 (15–75)	6.35 (3.1–10.0)	3.7 (2.24–5.60)	29 (21–36)	94 (60–161)
CAD−DM−(II+DD)	51	60 (37–70)	6.75 (3.8–10.9)	3.6 (2.7–5.4)	27 (21–42)	91 (66–131)
All groups	600	55 (15–75)	7.5 (2.8–127)	4.0 (1.05–218)	29 (18–43)	98 (5.6–200)
Kruskal–Wallis ANOVA by Ranks		H=50.98161 P=0.0000	H=33.97776 P=0.0000	H=37.81505 P=0.0000	H=25.39687 P=0.0006	H=35.49770 P=0.0000

Table 6 Significant differences among groups and ACE genotype (heterozygote advantage model)

Group × ACE	N	Glycemia (median, range, mmol/L)	Cholesterol (median, range, mmol/L)	LDL (median, range, mmol/L)	HDL (median, range, mmol/L)	Triglycerides (median, range, mmol/L)
CAD+DM+(ID)	53	7.4 (3.3–13.9)	4.49 (2.12–9.80)	2.52 (0.86–101.00)	1.06 (0.63–1.83)	1.63 (0.53–6.33)
CAD+DM+(II+DD)	100	6.8 (3.4–17.4)	3.97 (2.61–9.43)	2.12 (1.19–4.96)	0.98 (0.59–1.89)	1.87 (0.68–10.50)
CAD+DM–(ID)	153	5.2 (3.5–10.7)	4.29 (2.51–8.18)	2.40 (0.91–102.00)	1.08 (0.58–2.38)	1.40 (0.54–6.64)
CAD+DM–(II+DD)	178	5.1 (3.6–8.1)	4.40 (2.25–8.39)	2.48 (0.65–101.00)	1.09 (0.60–2.18)	1.44 (0.46–6.36)
CAD–DM+(ID)	8	6.8 (5.1–12.1)	4.67 (2.95–7.47)	2.40 (1.19–4.85)	1.13 (0.86–1.76)	1.96 (0.80–3.00)
CAD–DM+(II+DD)	9	5.6 (4.2–8.0)	3.97 (2.97–6.11)	2.82 (1.12–4.10)	1.09 (0.73–1.52)	1.09 (0.93–2.72)
CAD–DM–(ID)	48	4.9 (3.9–6.8)	4.65 (2.25–6.40)	2.79 (0.83–4.15)	1.28 (0.50–2.54)	1.19 (0.43–3.02)
CAD–DM–(II+DD)	51	4.9 (3.8–8.3)	4.98 (3.49–7.90)	2.87 (1.67–5.54)	1.38 (0.81–2.59)	1.37 (0.63–4.23)
All groups	600	5.6 (3.3–17.4)	4.42 (2.12–9.8)	2.47 (0.65–102.00)	1.09 (0.50–2.59)	1.48 (0.43–10.5)
Kruskal–Wallis ANOVA by Ranks		H=150.2524 P=0.0000	H=30.08967 P=0.0001	H=30.80595 P=0.0001	H=79.14303 P=0.0000	H=35.63787 P=0.0000

Table 7 Significant differences among groups and ACE genotype (heterozygote advantage model)

Group × ACE	N	Hypertension (%)	Obesity (%)	Hyperlipidemia (%)	Renal insufficiency (%)	No risk factors - more than 1 (%)	Current smoking (%)
CAD+DM+(ID)	53	49 (92)	24 (45)	33 (62)	17 (32)	11 (21)	4 (8)
CAD+DM+(II+DD)	100	84 (84)	37 (37)	55 (55)	26 (27)	28 (28)	6 (6)
CAD+DM−(ID)	153	120 (78)	41 (27)	91 (59)	26 (17)	25 (16)	32 (25)
CAD+DM−(II+DD)	178	137 (77)	43 (24)	97 (54)	27 (15)	28 (16)	29 (16)
CAD−DM+(ID)	8	7 (88)	4 (50)	5 (63)	2 (25)	1 (13)	1 (13)
CAD−DM+(II+DD)	9	7 (78)	4 (44)	6 (67)	1 (11)	2 (22)	1 (11)
CAD−DM−(ID)	48	29 (60)	9 (19)	30 (63)	3 (6)	8 (17)	7 (15)
CAD−DM−(II+DD)	51	39 (76)	14 (27)	38 (75)	1 (1)	4 (8)	5 (10)
All groups	600	472 (79)	176 (29)	355 (59)	103 (17)	107 (18)	85 (14)

Table 8 Differences among groups and ACE genotype (heterozygote advantage model) — drugs

Group × ACE	N	Aspirin (%)	Other antiaggregation t. (%)	ACEI (%)	Beta-blockers (%)	Statins (%)	Other antilipid t. (%)	AT1R antagonists (%)	Antivitamin K t.
CAD+DM+(ID)	53	46 (87)	28 (53)	31 (58)	50 (94)	52 (98)	2 (4)	23 (43)	1 (2)
CAD+DM+(II+DD)	100	89 (89)	57 (57)	73 (73)	97 (97)	100 (100)	2 (2)	18 (18)	2 (2)
CAD+DM−(ID)	153	130 (85)	98 (64)	107 (70)	143 (93)	145 (95)	5 (3)	19 (12)	5 (3)
CAD+DM−(II+DD)	178	160 (90)	109 (61)	124 (70)	166 (93)	168 (94)	1 (1)	21 (12)	6 (3)
CAD−DM+(ID)	8	0 (0)	0 (0)	5 (63)	2 (25)	2 (25)	0 (0)	2 (25)	1 (13)
CAD−DM+(II+DD)	9	2 (22)	0 (0)	6 (66)	6 (66)	3 (33)	0 (0)	2 (22)	2 (22)
CAD−DM−(ID)	48	13 (27)	0 (0)	17 (35)	27 (56)	12 (25)	0 (0)	5 (10)	3 (6)
CAD−DM−(II+DD)	51	6 (12)	0 (0)	22 (43)	25 (49)	15 (29)	0 (0)	11 (22)	3 (6)
All grps	600	446 (74)	292 (49)	385 (64)	516 (86)	497 (83)	10 (2)	101 (17)	23 (4)

P = 0.0003). Similarly, a significant increase of ID carriers in obese CAD + DM + compared with obese CAD – DM – group was proved (OR = 3.59, 95% CI 1.45–8.86, P = 0.004) which was not observed between (II + DD) carriers. A higher risk of renal insufficiency between CAD + DM + and CAD – DM – group was also observed. However, the highest OR was calculated for the (II + DD) genotype (OR = 17.69, 95% CI 2.32–134.73, P = 0.00007) in CAD + DM + group.

The CAD + DM + patients with genotype (II + DD) had more cardiovascular risk factors compared to (II + DD) CAD – DM – subjects (OR = 4.57, 95% CI 1.51–13.87, P = 0.003). No differences for hyperlipidemia and current smoking among the groups were observed; the state of lipids had to be substantially influenced by therapy.

Then we evaluated the drug administration schedule in the groups (Table 8). Aspirin was applied much more frequently in patients with CAD + DM + compared to those with CAD – DM –, especially in the (II + DD) carriers (OR = 60.68, 95% CI 21.08–174.60, P = 0.0000001). No differences in other anti-aggregation therapy administration were observed. ACE inhibitors were prescribed more frequently to CAD + DM + patients, especially with II + DD genotype (OR = 3.56, 9 5% CI 1.75–7.24, P = 0.0003). A similar situation was repeated in beta-blockers [OR for CAD + DM + and (II + DD) ACE genotype was 33.63, 95% CI 9.41–120.15, P = 0.0000001], statins [OR for CAD + DM + (II + DD) = 237.6, 95% CI 30.29–1864.03, P = 0.0000001], and warfarin prescription (OR = 14, 95% CI 1.71–114.86, P = 0.03). On the opposite, the AT1R antagonists were administered more frequently to patients with the ID genotype and CAD + DM + compared to patients with CAD – DM – with the same genotype (OR = 6.38, 95% CI 2.18–18.63, P = 0.0002). It is necessary to mention that drug prescription could not be influenced by genotype knowledge because genotyping was performed independently of clinical decisions.

When we evaluate the number of affected coronary arteries, diabetes, and ACE I/D polymorphism, a highly significant heterozygote advantage can be observed in patients with two affected coronary arteries and diabetes mellitus compared to those without diabetes. In these patients, OR for ID genotype, CAD with two affected coronary arteries and diabetes is 0.27, 95% CI 0.12–0.59, P = 0.0005.

Conclusions

The main task of the study was to summarize clinical and genetic results and to do it as simply as possible to prevent statistical artefacts (or doubts about statistical correctness).

We proved a lot of significant differences especially between CAD + DM + and CAD – DM – groups. Although the patients had been treated according to their clinical state, we were able to prove significant differences between ID and (II + DD) ACE genotypes in hypertension, obesity, and renal insufficiency prevalence, in BMI values, in the number of cardiovascular risk factors, in some inflammatory factors, glycemia, and lipid profile. Generally, the drugs were administrated more frequently to the II + DD carriers that support the heterozygote advantage hypothesis tested in the study. We were able to find only one study with a similar design [46] which did not confirm association of ACE I/D with diabetes mellitus type 2. Unfortunately, a different evaluation of a significance of coronary artery stenosis for patients' exclusion of the study was used. The results of both studies are not fully comparable; in Grammer's study, the heterozygote advantage hypothesis has not been tested.

The most important conclusion of the study is the necessity to define generally accepted association study design for complex diseases with respect to precise description of the clinically valid parameters, comorbidities, and risk factors including their "standard" prevalence.

Acknowledgments The study was supported by the project IGA NS10206-3/2009 of the Ministry of Health of the Czech Republic.

Special thanks to Prof. Jaroslav Meluzín, MD, CSc. and Vladimír Kincl, MD from the 1st Department of Internal Medicine/Cardioangiology, St. Ann's Faculty Hospital Brno, Faculty of Medicine, Masaryk University for providing clinical data databases.

References

1. Dostal DE, Baker KM. The cardiac renin–angiotensin system: conceptual, or a regulator of cardiac function? Circ Res. 1999;85:643–50.
2. Hall JE. Historical perspective of the renin–angiotensin system. Mol Biotechnol. 2003;24:27–39.
3. Crackower MA, Sarao R, Oudit GY, et al. Angiotensin-converting enzyme 2 is an essential regulator of heart function. Nature. 2002;417(6891):822–8.
4. Chappell MC, Modralt JG, Diz DI, et al. Novel aspects of the renal renin-angiotensin system: angiotensin-(1-7), ACE2 and blood pressure regulation. Contrib Nephrol. 2004;143:77–89.
5. Raizada MK, Ferreira AJ. ACE2: a new target for cardiovascular disease therapeutics. J Cardiovasc Pharmacol. 2007;50:112–19.
6. Fyhrquist F, Saijonmaa O. Renin-angiotensin system revisited. J Intern Med. 2008;264:224–36.
7. Iwai M, Horiuchi M. Devil and angel in the renin-angiotensin system: ACE-angiotensin II-AT1 receptor axis vs. ACE2-angiotensin-(1-7)-Mas receptor axis. Hypertens Res. 2009;32:533–6.
8. Booz GW, Baker KM. Intracellular signaling and the cardiac renin angiotensin system. In: De Mello WC, editor. Renin angiotensin system and the heart. West Sussex: John Wiley & Sons; 2004. p. 1–17.
9. Zou Y, Akazawa H, Qin Y, et al. Mechanical stress activates angiotensin II type 1 receptor without the involvement of angiotensin II. Nat Cell Biol. 2004;6:499–506.
10. Benigni A, Cassis P, Remuzzi G. Angiotensin II revisited: new roles in inflammation, immunology and aging. EMBO Mol Med. 2010;2:247–57.
11. Lévy BI. Can angiotensin II type 2 receptors have deleterious effects in cardiovascular disease? Implications for therapeutic blockade of the renin-angiotensin system. Circulation. 2004;109:8–13.
12. Nouet S, Amzallag N, Li JM, et al. Trans-inactivation of receptor tyrosine kinases by novel angiotensin II AT2 receptor-interacting protein ATIP. J Biol Chem. 2004;279:28989–97.
13. Re RN. Tissue renin angiotensin systems. Med Clin North Am. 2004;88:19–38.
14. Pohl M, Kaminski H, Castrop H, et al. Intrarenal renin angiotensin system revisited: role of megalin-dependent endocytosis along the proximal nephron. J Biol Chem. 2010;285(53):41935–46.
15. Malhotra R, Sadoshima J, Broscius FC, et al. Mechanical stretch and angiotensin II differentially upregulated the renin angiotensin system in cardiac myocytes in vitro. Circ Res. 1999;85:137–46.
16. Haznedaroglu IC, Ozturk MA. Towards the understanding of the local hematopoietic bone marrow renin-angiotensin system. Int J Biochem Cell Biol. 2003;35:867–80.
17. Haznedaroglu IC, Tuncer S, Gursoy M. A local renin-angiotensin system in the bone marrow. Med Hypotheses. 1996;46:507–10.
18. Strawn W, Richmond R, Ferrario C. A new understanding of atherosclerosis: The bone marrow response-to-lipid hypothesis. In: Heart disease: pathogenesis, diagnosis and treatment. Washington, DC: 3rd World Congress on Heart Disease; 2003. p. 183–8.
19. Strawn WB, Ferrario CM. Angiotensin II AT(1) receptor blockade normalizes CD11b(+) monocyte production in bone marrow of hypercholesterolemic monkeys. Atherosclerosis. 2008;196:624–32.
20. Vasku A, Soucek M, Znojil V, et al. Does angiotensin I-converting enzyme inhibitor therapy have an anti-proliferative effect on blood-forming bone marrow? Exp Hematom. 1998;26:277–8.
21. Vasku A, Holla L, Znojil V. The best model of a cat is a cat, especially the same cat. Exp Hematol. 1999;27: 187–8.
22. Costerousse O, Jaspard E, Wei L, et al. The angiotensin I-converting enzyme (kininase II): molecular organization and regulation of its expression in humans. J Cardiovasc Pharmacol. 1992;20(Suppl. 9):S10–15.
23. Kessler SP, Rowe TM, Gomos JB, et al. Physiological non-equivalence of the two isoforms of angiotensin-converting enzyme. J Biol Chem. 2000;275:26259–64.
24. Waeber B. Combination therapy with ACE inhibitors/angiotensin II receptor antagonists and diuretics in hypertension. Expert Rev Cardiovasc Ther. 2003;1: 43–50.
25. Ryan MJ, Sigmund CD. ACE, ACE inhibitors, and other JNK. Circ Res. 2004;94:1–3.
26. Azizi M, Junot C, Ezan E, et al. Angiotensin I-converting enzyme and metabolism of the haematological peptide N-acetyl-seryl-aspartyl-lysyl-proline. Clin Exp Pharmacol Physiol. 2001;28:1066–106.
27. Kanasaki K, Koya D, Sugimoto T, et al. N-Acetyl-seryl-aspartyl-lysyl-proline inhibits TGF-beta-mediated plasminogen activator inhibitor-1 expression via inhibition of Smad pathway in human mesangial cells. J Am Soc Nephrol. 2003;14:863–72.
28. Pokharel S, Rasoul S, Roks AJ, et al. N-Acetyl-ser-asp-lys-pro inhibits phosphorylation of Smad2 in cardiac fibroblasts. Hypertension. 2002;40:155–61.
29. Baudin B. New aspects on angiotensin-converting enzyme: from gene to disease. Clin Chem Lab Med. 2002;40:256–65.
30. Rigat B, Hubert C, Corvol P, et al. PCR detection of the insertion/deletion polymorphism of the human angiotensin converting enzyme gene (DCP1) (dipeptidyl carboxypeptidase 1). Nucleic Acids Res. 1992; 20:1433.
31. Covolo L, Gelatti U, Metra M, et al. Angiotensin-converting-enzyme gene polymorphism and heart failure: a case-control study. Biomarkers. 2003;8:429–36.
32. Schunkert H. Polymorphism of the angiotensin-converting enzyme gene and cardiovascular disease. J Mol Med. 1997;75:867–75.
33. Akbulut T, Bilsel T, Terzi S, et al. Relationship between ACE gene polymorphism and ischemic chronic heart failure in Turkish population. Eur J Med Res. 2003;8:247–53.

34. Abraham MR, Olson LJ, Joyner MJ, et al. Angiotensin-converting enzyme genotype modulates pulmonary function and exercise capacity in treated patients with congestive stable heart failure. Circulation. 2002;106: 1794–9.

35. Di Pasquale P, Cannizzaro S, Scalzo S, et al. Cardiovascular effects of I/D angiotensin-converting enzyme gene polymorphism in healthy subjects. Findings after follow-up of six years. Acta Cardiol. 2005;60:427–35.

36. Deckers JW, Deinum J, van Duijn CM. Angiotensin converting enzyme insertion/deletion polymorphism and the risk of heart failure in hypertensive subjects. Eur Heart J. 2004;25:2143–8.

37. Huang W, Xie C, Zhou H, et al. Association of the angiotensin-converting enzyme gene polymorphism with chronic heart failure in Chinese Han patients. Eur J Heart Fail. 2004;6:23–7.

38. Niu W, Qi Y, Gao P, et al. Angiotensin converting enzyme D allele is associated with an increased risk of type 2 diabetes: evidence from a meta-analysis. Endocr J. 2010;57:431–8.

39. Abraham MR, Olson LJ, Joyner MJ, et al. Angiotensin-converting enzyme genotype modulates pulmonary function and exercise capacity in treated patients with congestive stable heart failure. Circulation. 2002;106: 1794–9.

40. Busjahn A, Voss A, Knoblauch H, et al. Angiotensin-converting enzyme and angiotensinogen gene poly-morphisms and heart rate variability in twins. Am J Cardiol. 1998;81:755–60.

41. Fujii M, Wada A, Tsutamoto T, et al. Bradykinin improves left ventricular diastolic function under long-term angiotensin-converting enzyme inhibition in heart failure. Hypertension. 2002;39:952–7.

42. Montgomery H, Brull D, Humphries SE. Analysis of gene-environment interactions by "stressing-the-genotype" studies: the angiotensin converting enzyme and exercise-induced left ventricular hypertrophy as an example. Ital Heart J. 2002;3:10–4.

43. Candy GP, Skudicky D, Mueller UK, et al. Association of left ventricular systolic performance and cavity size with angiotensin-converting enzyme genotype in idiopathic dilated cardiomyopathy. Am J Cardiol. 1999;83:740–4.

44. Vancura V, Hubacek J, Malek I, et al. Does angiotensin-converting enzyme polymorphism influence the clinical manifestation and progression of heart failure in patients with dilated cardiomyopathy? Am J Cardiol. 1999;83:461–2.

45. Levy BI, Schiffrin EL, Mourad JJ, et al. Impaired tissue perfusion: a pathology common to hypertension, obesity, and diabetes mellitus. Circulation. 2008;26:968–76.

46. Grammer TB, Renner W, von Karger S, et al. The angiotensin-I converting enzyme I/D polymorphism is not associated with type 2 diabetes in individuals undergoing coronary angiography. (The Ludwigshafen Risk and Cardiovascular Health Study). Mol Genet Metab. 2006;88:378–83.

PPARs and Myocardial Response to Ischemia in Normal and Diseased Heart

Tana Ravingerova, Adriana Adameova,
Slavka Carnicka, Tara Kelly, Martina Nemcekova,
Jana Matejikova, and Antigone Lazou

Abstract

Peroxisome proliferator-activated receptors (PPARs), ligand-activated transcription factors, belong to the nuclear hormone receptor superfamily regulating expression of genes involved in different aspects of lipid metabolism and inflammation, and all three isoforms of PPAR (α, β/δ, and γ) detected so far modulate cardiac energy production. The activation of PPAR-α by its natural ligands, long-chain fatty acids (FAs) and eicosanoids, promotes mitochondrial FA oxidation as the primary ATP-generating pathway in the normal adult myocardium. Moreover, under physiological and pathological conditions associated with acute or chronic oxygen deprivation, PPAR-α modulates the expression of genes that determine myocardial substrate selection (FA vs. glucose) aimed at the maintenance of energy production to preserve basic cardiac function. However, whether PPAR activation plays a beneficial or detrimental role in myocardial response to ischemia/reperfusion (I/R) is still a matter of debate. Although PPAR-α and PPAR-γ agonists, hypolipidemic and antidiabetic drugs, have been reported to protect the heart against I/R, the role of PPARs in cardioprotection, in particular in pathological models, is not completely elucidated. This chapter reviews some findings demonstrating the impact of PPAR activation on cardiac resistance to ischemia in normal and pathologically altered heart. Specifically, it addresses the issue of decreased susceptibility to ischemia in the experimental model of streptozotocin-induced diabetes, with particular regard to the role of PPAR gene expression and its modulation by concomitant pathology, such as hypercholesterolemia. Finally, the involvement of

T. Ravingerova ($\boxtimes$)
Institute for Heart Research, Slovak Academy
of Sciences and Centre of Excellence for Cardiovascular
Research of SAS, Bratislava, Slovakia
e-mail: usrdravi@savba.sk

B. Ostadal et al. (eds.), *Genes and Cardiovascular Function*,
DOI 10.1007/978-1-4419-7207-1_14, © Springer Science+Business Media, LLC 2011

PPAR in the mechanisms of pleiotropic lipid-independent cardioprotective effects of some hypolipidemic drugs in both normal and diseased heart is also discussed.

Keywords

Cardioprotection • HMG-CoA reductase inhibitors • Hypolipidemic drugs • Myocardial ischemia • Pleiotropic effects • PPAR

Introduction

Peroxisome proliferator-activated receptors (PPARs) are ligand-activated transcription factors that belong to the nuclear hormone receptor superfamily regulating expression of genes involved in different aspects of lipid metabolism [1, 2], energy production [3], and inflammation [4]. All three isoforms of PPAR detected so far, α (alpha), β/δ (beta/delta), and γ (gamma), encoded by separate genes, are expressed in many species including rodents [5] and humans [6]. They differ in their tissue distribution, ligand specificity, and cofactor interactions [7, 8]. Therefore, PPAR isoforms regulate different sets of genes, and there are different biological consequences of their stimulation. PPAR-α has been recognized as the central regulator of mitochondrial fatty acids (FAs) catabolism, whereas PPAR-γ is thought to regulate lipid anabolism or storage. Until recently, the function of PPAR-β/δ was relatively less explored. However, several lines of evidence suggest that all three isoforms modulate cardiac energy metabolism [1, 2]. Nevertheless, it is still a matter of debate whether PPAR activation plays a beneficial or detrimental role in the setting of ischemia/reperfusion (I/R), in particular in pathologically altered myocardium. Conflicting findings have documented both the negative impact of PPAR-α up-regulation on myocardial functional recovery upon I/R [9, 10], in particular during early reperfusion [11], and beneficial effects of PPAR-α and PPAR-γ agonists on I/R damage [12–15]. This contradiction is apparently related to the fact that PPAR activation may improve myocardial function via metabolic or other, metabolism-independent, activities.

Tissue Distribution and Function of PPAR

Table 1 illustrates the main tissue distribution and physiological effects of PPAR isoforms. Two of the three PPAR isoforms, PPAR-α and PPAR-β/δ, are abundantly expressed in tissues with high level of FA oxidation (FAO) including heart, liver, kidney, skeletal muscle, and pancreas [7, 16]. PPAR-γ (and its splice variants) is mainly associated with adipose tissue and macrophages, with a low level of more ubiquitous expression in liver, heart, skeletal muscle, and bone marrow [8]. PPAR-β/δ is abundantly and ubiquitously expressed at much higher levels than PPAR-γ and PPAR-α [5]. It is important to note that tissue expression of all three PPAR isotypes may vary under different physiological and/or pathological conditions. Figure 1 demonstrates

Table 1 Tissue distribution and physiological effects of PPAR isoforms

Tissue distribution	Effects
PPAR-alpha	FA metabolism,
Liver, skeletal muscle,	Cell cycle,
heart, kidney, adipose	Control of inflammation and
tissue	apoptosis
PPAR-beta/delta	FA metabolism,
Ubiquitously	Wound healing,
	Control of inflammation
PPAR-gamma	
• gamma1	Adipogenesis,
All tissues including	Lipid storage,
heart, muscle, kidney	Control of inflammation and
• gamma2	apoptosis,
Adipose tissue	Increased insulin sensitivity
• gamma3	and glucose disposal
Macrophages	

PPAR peroxisome proliferator-activated receptors, *FA* fatty acids

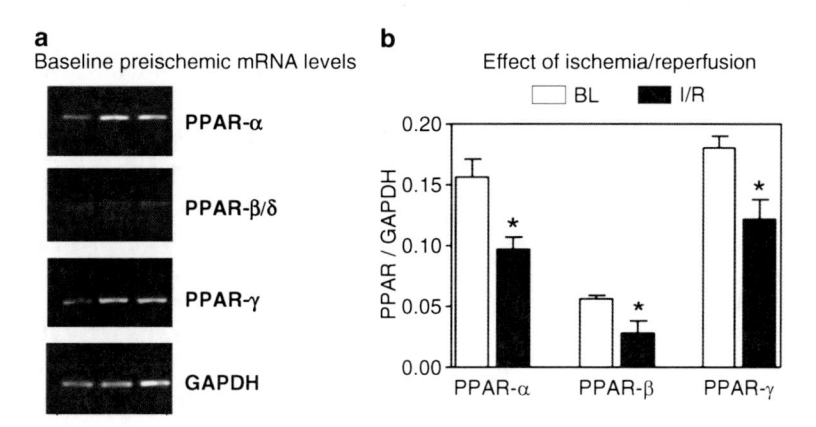

Fig. 1 Expression of PPAR-α, PPAR-β/δ and PPAR-γ mRNA in the heart of control rats at baseline (BL), and after 30 min-global ischemia and 2-h repefusion (I/R). (**a**) Total RNA was extracted and PPAR isoforms or GAPDH mRNA were amplified by RT-PCR. PCR products were analyzed by ethidium bromide/agarose gel electrophoresis. (**b**) PPAR mRNA was measured by quantative PCR. *Empty bars* –baseline levels; *filled bars* – PPAR levels after I/R. Results are presented as means ± S.E.M for at least four different hearts. *$P < 0.05$ relative to BL

that all three PPAR isoforms are present in the myocardial tissue of rats under normal conditions and that their gene expression is modified by ischemia/reperfusion (I/R) [17].

Heart tissue normally uses FA as the major energy source, and PPAR-α regulates genes encoding enzymes of FA transport/uptake and utilization via β(beta)-oxidation in mitochondria [18]. Activation of PPAR-α by its natural ligands (long-chain FA, eicosanoids) promotes mitochondrial FAO as the primary ATP-generating pathway in the normal adult myocardium [3, 18]. Moreover, under physiological and pathological conditions associated with acute or chronic oxygen deprivation, PPAR-α modulates expression of genes that determine myocardial substrate selection (FA vs. carbohydrates) in order to maintain adequate production of energy and preserve basic cardiac function [19]. In addition, involvement of PPAR in anti-inflammatory response in different tissues has also been recognized [20, 21].

Mechanisms of Action of PPAR

Natural and Synthetic PPAR Ligands

Upon binding to PPAR, different ligands can induce stimulatory or inhibitory responses depending on the nature of the specific target gene and its cellular location. Both natural and synthetic compounds have been recognized as PPAR ligands. Although many FA are capable of activating all three PPAR isoforms, some preference for specific FA by each PPAR has been demonstrated [22]. The long-chain polyunsaturated FA and their oxidized derivatives, especially eicosanoids such as 8-S-hydroxyeicosatetraenoic acid (8-S-HETE), leukotriene B4 (LTB4), and arachidonate monooxygenase metabolite epoxyeicosatrienoic acids, have been shown to potently activate PPAR-α with high affinity [23]. PPAR-γ can be activated by several prostanoids, such as 15-deoxy-Δ12,14-prostaglandin J2 (15d-PGJ2) and 12- and 15-hydroxyeicosatetraenoic acid (12- and 15-HETE), which are derivatives of arachidonic acid synthesized through the lipoxygenase pathway [24]. Prostaglandin 15d-PGJ2 is not only the most potent natural ligand for PPAR-γ identified to date, but also by far the most commonly used naturally occurring PPAR-γ agonist [25]. In addition to PPAR-γ naturally occurring agonists produced by human body, flavonoids ψ-baptigenin and hesperidin found in plants were identified as strong PPAR-γ agonists [26].

With respect to the synthetic ligands, hypolipidemic drugs fibrates (e.g., fenofibrate, clofibrate) are well-known ligands for PPAR-α [24]. Fibrates activate PPAR-α leading to increased expression of lipid-metabolizing enzymes that

Table 2 Naturally occurring and synthetic PPAR alpha and gamma modulators

Modulators	PPAR-α	PPAR-γ
Naturally occurring agonists	fatty acids eicosanoids leukotriene B4	fatty acids eicosanoids prostaglandin flavonoids ψ-baptigenin, hesperidin
Synthetic agonists	fibrates • fenofibrate • clofibrate WY 14643 GW7647	thiazolidinediones (glitazones) • rosiglitazone • pioglitazone • ciglitazone
Antagonists	MK-886	GW9662

PPAR peroxisome proliferator-activated receptors

effectively lower serum lipid levels, in particular triacylglycerols, in humans.

The most widely used PPAR-γ agonists belong to the thiazolidinedione (TZD) or glitazone class of anti-diabetic drugs used in the treatment of type-2 diabetes. The two available TZDs, rosiglitazone and pioglitazone, are currently used alone or in combination with other oral antidiabetic agents [24]. These drugs are known as insulin sensitizers, stimulating tissue uptake of glucose in the diabetics [27]; however, their action extends far beyond their hypoglycemic activity and involves limitation of lethal ischemic injury in the nondiabetic heart [13, 28–30]. Table 2 summarizes the most important PPAR modulators.

Regulation of PPAR Activity

Many proteins act as co-activators or corepressors that regulate the ability of PPAR to either stimulate or repress gene transcription. In the unbound state, PPAR/RXR heterodimers are associated with corepressors, which prevent gene transcription. However, once a ligand binds to the receptor, a conformational change occurs which not only facilitates corepressor dissociation, but also the recruitment of several positive co-activators that initiates a sequence of events ultimately leading to gene transcription [31].

Although co-activators and corepressors appear to be the major factors responsible for regulation of PPAR activity, these receptors can also be modulated by MAPK-induced phosphorylation. In fact, phosphorylation by extracellular signal-regulated kinases (ERKs) has been found to repress PPAR-α activity [3, 32], while phosphorylation induced by p38-MAPK enhances PPAR-α-mediated gene expression [33].

Transcriptional Transactivation

Upon activation by endogenous or synthetic ligands, PPARs form obligate heterodimers with the 9-cis-retinoic acid receptors (retinoid X receptor, RXR). The resulting complex undergoes a conformational change which allows binding of the heterodimer to a DNA sequence in the promoter region of target genes known as the peroxisome proliferator response element (PPRE), followed by the induction of gene transcription [25, 34] and synthesis of the respective gene products. When both PPAR and RXR are activated simultaneously, it results in significant synergistic enhancement of gene transcription [34]. The search for PPAR target genes with identified PPREs has led to the identification of numerous genes involved in lipid metabolism, oxidative stress, and the inflammatory response [1, 18, 20, 35].

Transcriptional Transrepression

In addition to PPAR transactivation, stimulation of PPAR can also negatively regulate gene expression in a ligand-dependent manner by inhibiting the activities of other transcription factors, such as activated protein-1 (AP-1), nuclear factor-kappaB (NF-κB), nuclear factor of activated T-cells (NFAT) or signal transducer and activator of transcription (STAT) via a mechanism known as ligand-dependent transrepression [36]. In contrast to transcriptional activation, transrepression does not involve binding of PPAR to the response element of the target genes but direct interaction with other transcription factors and corepressors or modulation of kinase activity.

Research suggests that PPAR may exert beneficial effects by negatively regulating the expression of pro-inflammatory genes in inflammation-related diseases including myocardial I/R [36]. Several mechanisms have been suggested to account for this activity including ligand-independent repression of the transcription of target genes via binding of PPAR to response elements in the absence of ligands and recruitment of the corepressor complexes [22].

PPAR Function and Outcome of Myocardial Ischemia/ Reperfusion Injury

Delivery of oxygen and metabolic substrates via coronary circulation is essential for normal cardiac function, and its cessation leads within minutes to irreversible cellular injury. The duration of ischemia and the extent of metabolic and structural alterations in the myocardium are the main factors that determine the progress toward cell death (by mechanisms of necrosis or apoptosis) or cell survival. Restoration of blood flow in the previously occluded coronary arteries is undoubtedly the main prerequisite of the heart rescue. However, reperfusion may have injurious components and limit the recovery of the tissue through the induction of "reperfusion injury" [37]. I/R injury represents a clinically relevant problem associated with reperfusion therapy, such as thrombolysis, percutaneous coronary intervention, and coronary artery bypass graft surgery [38, 39]. I/R injury is a complex cascade of events, where oxidative stress and inflammatory response play the pivotal role [40] and, besides other factors, it involves activation of nuclear factor-κB (NF-κB) as one of the central processes [41], in particular in the *ex vivo* perfused heart [42].

The role of PPARs in the pathogenesis of a variety of heart disorders, including myocardial damage due to acute myocardial I/R, is a matter of controversy and still remains unclear. Gene expression of PPAR-α declines in chronically hypoxic heart resulting in a substrate switch from FA to glucose, and down-regulation of PPAR-α has been considered as an adaptive response [32, 43]. In-line, experimental overexpression of PPAR-α was found to be related to impaired

cardiac recovery after ischemia [10]. It appears that in long-term processes, such as myocardial hypoxia and/or hypertrophy linked with limitations in oxygen supply, glucose as a fuel may be beneficial for the heart by decreasing oxygen consumption [32]. Moreover, chronic activation of PPAR-α (and increased rates of FAO at the expense of glucose oxidation) may be detrimental to the heart during postischemic reperfusion possibly due to FAO-induced oxidative stress [10].

On the other hand, other studies indicated that targeted deletion of PPAR-α resulted in increased serum levels of free FA and larger size of infarction in PPARα$^{-/-}$ mice subjected to ischemic challenge [14]. In acute settings, decrease of PPAR-α, in conjunction with the metabolic effects, was observed in a rat *ex vivo* model of 30-min ischemia/2-h reperfusion [44] and in the setting of acute I/R in the in vivo mice, in which reversal of down-regulation of PPAR-α and its target genes responsible for the metabolic fuel shifts (decreased FAO and increased glucose oxidation) improved postischemic myocardial contractile recovery and reduced the size of infarction [14]. Similarly, in our study of the isolated rat heart, we have also found that 30-min ischemia significantly decreased mRNA levels of all isoforms of PPARs and their further decline was observed following 2-h reperfusion (Fig. 1b) accompanied by the development of irreversible myocardial injury [45].

There is no clear consensus on whether attenuation of I/R-induced down-regulation of PPAR-α and FAO is beneficial or detrimental to the heart. The discrepancy in the results may arise from the different substrate availability in the different experimental models (ischemia/reperfusion, in vivo/in vitro protocols). Although FAO is an important source of energy production during the basic conditions, glucose uptake may be crucial during ischemia. It is believed that partial inhibition of FAO and a substrate switch from FA to glucose [3] improves functional recovery of the heart upon reperfusion [46] while overexpression of PPAR-α impairs postischemic cardiac recovery [10]. Thus, pharmacological interventions that increase glucose oxidation and suppress FAO appear to be beneficial for the recovery of the myocardium previously subjected to I/R [9, 11].

In the long term, however, this switch may become detrimental as less ATP is generated per mole of glucose oxidized, and lipid accumulation and lipotoxicity of the myocardium may develop [3]. The controversy regarding the role of PPAR-α in the heart suggests that the function of this transcription factor might not be the same in different cardiac pathologies or in their different stages and that effects other than lipid metabolism might also be involved.

PPAR and Endogenous Cardioprotection

The role of PPAR in the mechanisms of endogenous protection against I/R injury is less documented, although Takeda et al. [47] demonstrated that PPAR-γ agonists activated the ERK1/2 pathway of MAP-kinases in vascular smooth muscle cells through phosphatidylinositol 3-kinase (PI3K). Since ERK1/2 cascade and PI3K and its effector protein kinase B (Akt) are implicated in protective mechanisms of ischemic preconditioning and other forms of cardioprotection [48, 49], it has been hypothesized that pretreatment with the PPAR-γ agonist pioglitazone could confer preconditioning-like protection to the myocardium when given prior to myocardial I/R [50]. Indeed, pioglitazone induced significant anti-infarct protection comparable with the effect of classical ischemic preconditioning that appeared to involve both "survival"cascades (ERK1/2 and PI3K/Akt).

Moreover, it has been shown that PPAR-γ participates in a delayed effect of preconditioning with endotoxin (lipopolysaccharide, LPS) on myocardial and renal I/R injury in rats via a mechanism involving overproduction of endogenous PPAR-γ agonists, such as 15d-PGJ2 and others [51, 52].

PPAR Function in the Diseased Heart: Effects of Acute Diabetes

PPARs are up-regulated in the diabetic myocardium [19] that almost exclusively relies on FAO for energy production, resulting in increased myocardial oxygen consumption. The latter, along with high circulating levels and uptake of FA, as well as excess myocardial lipid accumulation may predispose the heart to contractile dysfunction and failure; therefore, the role of PPAR in myocardial injury in the diabetic myocardium still remains less clear [53].

In contrast to epidemiological studies demonstrating a higher risk of cardiovascular disorders in the diabetics, animal studies are not unequivocal and suggest that, besides higher myocardial vulnerability, diabetes mellitus may trigger adaptive processes leading to paradoxically enhanced ischemic tolerance that is now considered as a form of *metabolic* preconditioning suggested to share some molecular pathways with endogenous cardioprotection in the nondiabetic heart. Potential mechanisms of preconditioning-like protection in the diabetic myocardium may involve, besides antiapoptotic effects of high glucose itself acting as a preconditioning mimetic in the absence of insulin [54], a higher activity of "survival" protein kinases ERK1/2 and PI3K/Akt in acutely diabetic myocardium [55–58]. In addition, several other protective mechanisms, such as reduction in the levels of pro-inflammatory cytokines, increase in the cell survival factors (HIF1-α, VEGF) and angiogenesis, along with reduced fibrosis, have been found to be activated in the acute phase of streptozotocin (STZ)-induced diabetes [59].

Since the role of PPAR in cardioprotection, in particular in pathological models, such as the experimental model of STZ-induced diabetes mellitus, has not been sufficiently elucidated, we explored a potential link between cardiac response to I/R and gene expression of PPAR in the hearts of diabetic rats. One week after STZ administration (65 mg/kg, i.p.), despite high blood glucose levels (> 20 mmol/L) and reduced baseline functional parameters in the diabetic hearts [60], susceptibility to I/R in these hearts was decreased similarly to the effect of preconditioning in the normal nondiabetic hearts documented by reduced size of infarction, suppressed arrhythmogenesis, and lower myocardial ROS production during ischemia [60–62]. This was coupled with significantly enhanced baseline mRNA levels of all isoforms of PPAR that were preserved after

Fig. 2 Expression of PPAR-α, PPAR-β/δ and PPAR-γ mRNA in the heart of non-diabetic control (C) and diabetic (D) rats at baseline (BL), and after 30-min global ischemia and 2-h reperfusion (I/R). (**a**) Total RNA was extracted and PPAR isoforms or GAPDH mRNA were amplified by RT-PCR. PCR products were analyzed by ethidium bromide/agarose gel electrophoresis. (**b**) PPAR mRNA was measured by quantative PCR. *Empty bars* - non-diabetic hearts; *filled bars* - diabetic hearts. Results are presented as means ± S.E.M for at least four different hearts. *$P < 0.05$ relative to non-diabetics; † $P < 0.05$ relative to BL in the respective group

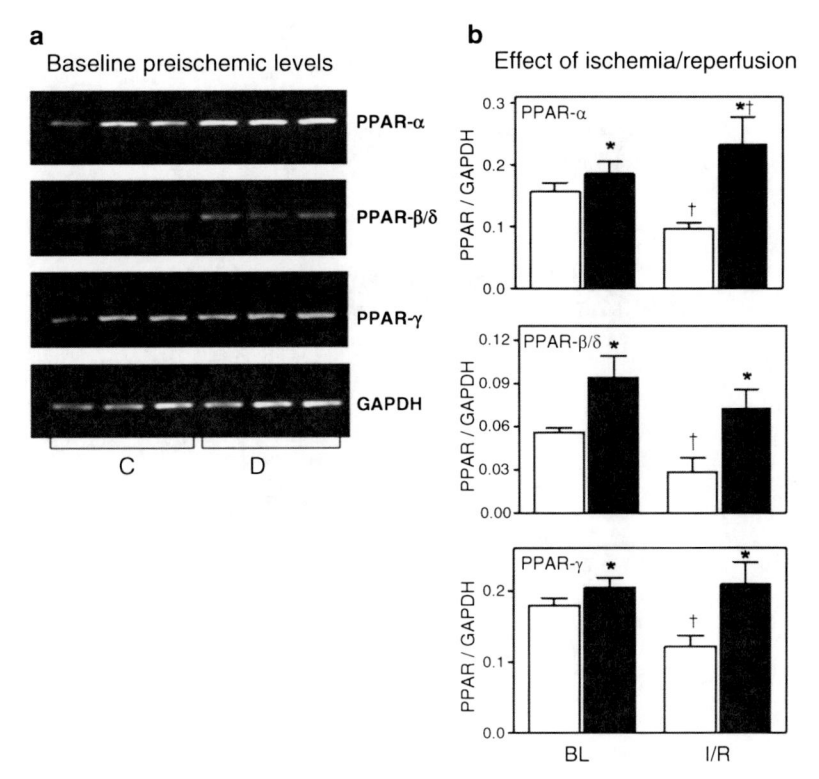

I/R in contrast to their marked down-regulation in nondiabetics (Fig. 2a, b), indicating that maintenance of enhanced PPAR gene expression during I/R may contribute to improved outcome of myocardial I/R injury in the diabetic heart [17]. The latter might possibly involve not only metabolic effects of PPARs but also their anti-inflammatory and anti-oxidative effects [20, 21] through negative regulation of NF-κB [36].

Effect of Hyperlipidemia on Ischemic Tolerance in the Diabetic Myocardium

Hyperlipidemia, especially hypercholesterolemia (HCH), is regarded as an independent risk factor for the development of ischemic heart disease. However, the controversy still remains on whether experimental HCH influences the severity of myocardial I/R injury per se and whether it interferes with the cellular mechanisms of endogenous cardioprotection. Most of the studies show that the major effect of preconditioning (infarct

size limitation) may be lost in cholesterol-fed animals [63], although molecular mechanisms of this effect are not completely clear. Recently, Kocsis et al. [64] demonstrated that HCH diet leads to alterations in preconditioning-induced gene expression in the mouse heart resulting in an enhanced oxidative/nitrosative stress signaling which, in turn, attenuates the cardioprotective effect of preconditioning. We addressed the issue of ischemic tolerance in the hearts of STZ-induced diabetic and simultaneously HCH rats (high fat-cholesterol diet, 1 week; 62) with the aim to explore a potential relationship between cardiac response to I/R in this model and gene expression of PPARs. Similar to the effect of HCH in the nondiabetic heart that abrogated the cardioprotective effect of preconditioning [63, 64], this comorbidity appeared to be one of the reasons for the loss of anti-infarct protection and the impaired post-ischemic recovery of ventricular function in the acutely diabetic Langendorff-perfused rat hearts, as well as the exacerbated severe ventricular arrhythmias in the

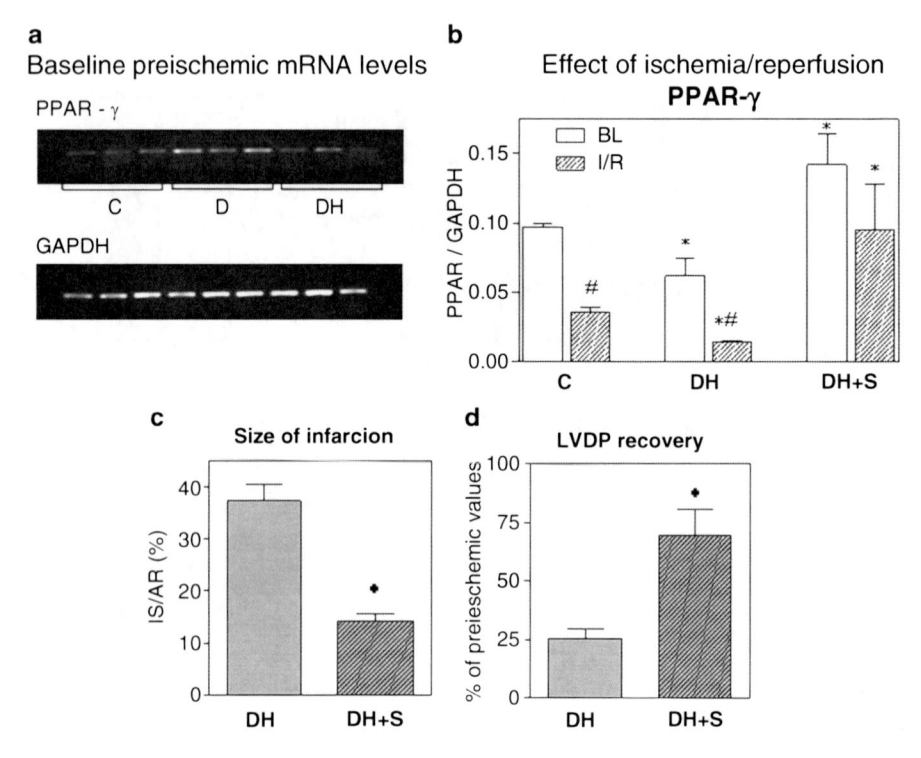

Fig. 3 Effect of 5-day treatment with simvastatin (S) on myocardial I/R injury and gene expression of PPAR-γ in the Langendorff-perfused hearts of diabetic and diabetic-hypercholesterolemic rats. (**a**) Expression of PPAR-γ mRNA in the heart of non-diabetic control (C), diabetic (D) and diabetic-hypercholesterolemic (DH) rats at baseline (BL). (**b**) Effect of simvastatin on the PPAR-γ gene expression at baseline and after 30-min global ischemia and 2-h repefusion (I/R). The results are presented as means ± S.E.M for at least four different hearts. *P < 0.05 relative to respective control groups; # P < 0.05 relative to

BL in the respective groups. (**c**) Effect of simvastatin on the size of myocardial infarction after 30-min regional ischemia and 2-h reperfusion in the hearts of D and DH rats. Infarct size (IS) is expressed in% of the area at risk (AR) size. Values are means ± S.E.M. from 12 hearts per group. * P < 0.05 vs. untreated group. (**d**) Recovery of left ventricular developed pressure (LVDP) after 30-min global ischemia and 2-h reperfusion expressed in% of preischemic values in simvastatin-treated and untreated hearts of D and DH rats. Values are means ± S.E.M. from 10 hearts per group. * P < 0.05 vs. untreated group

open-chest in vivo diabetic animals [62, 65], indicating that HCH might blunt endogenous cardioprotection in the diabetic heart. In addition, in this "double disease" model, we found that concurrent HCH suppressed gene expression of PPARs which were up-regulated in diabetics (Figs. 2 and 3a) and, in particular, decreased mRNA levels of PPAR-γ below those detected in normal controls both at baseline and after I/R (Fig. 3a, b). Cardioprotective effects (infarct size limitation, reduced arrhythmogenesis, and improved contractile recovery) and up-regulation of PPAR-γ mRNA levels in the diabetic hearts blunted by concurrent HCH were restored by simultaneous treatment of rats with simvastatin, a very effective hypolipidemic drug, (Fig. 3b, c, d)

without affecting the plasma cholesterol levels [65, 66]. These findings indicate that changes in PPAR gene expression might be involved in the adaptive protective mechanisms activated in the diabetic myocardium in the acute phase to counteract metabolic disorders, while loss of protection might be potentially related to concomitant HCH and down-regulation of PPAR promoting detrimental pro-inflammatory effects. Furthermore, cardioprotective effects of 3-hydroxy-3-methylglutaryl coenzyme A (HMG-CoA) reductase inhibitors, statins, independent of cholesterol lowering (pleiotropic effects), may be probably associated with the regulation of PPAR in this diabetic/hypercholesterolemic model since research has revealed that the positive impact of statins on inflammatory processes may be mediated through the activation and an increase in PPAR-α and PPAR-γ levels [67, 68].

Cardioprotective Effects of PPAR Agonists

Activation of PPAR-α with synthetic ligands has been shown to be cardioprotective in a setting of I/R, as manifested by a reduced infarct size and improved post-ischemic recovery of contractile function in different in vivo and *ex vivo* models of I/R [13, 14, 44]. In this context, treatment with PPAR-α selective and potent agonist GW7647 that reversed I/R-induced down-regulation of PPAR-α and its target genes attenuated myocardial contractile dysfunction and reduced the size of infarction [14]. Similar cardioprotective effects, in conjunction with the metabolic effects, were observed in a rat *ex vivo* model of 30-min ischemia/2-h reperfusion after treatment with the PPAR-α agonist clofibrate [44]. These studies do not support the view of the beneficial role of FAO inhibition in the mechanisms of protection against acute I/R, at least in this experimental setting.

Fibrates as PPAR-α agonists have shown protection against myocardial I/R injury beyond their lipid-lowering properties [13]. Other potent hypolipidemic drugs, statins, are being also intensively studied in this respect. By inhibition of the enzyme HMG-CoA reductase, statins have been shown to prevent the synthesis of isoprenoid intermediates of the cholesterol biosynthesis pathway involved in posttranslational modification of small GTP-binding proteins, such as Ras, Rho, and Rac, which modulate a variety of cellular processes [69], such as oxidative stress and inflammation [70–72], thrombogenesis [73], atherosclerotic plaque formation [74], vascular endothelial dysfunction [69], and the outcome of myocardial response to I/R [65, 75]. It is hypothesized that preconditioning-like effects of statins are attributed to up-regulation of "survival" pathways, such as PI3K/Akt, ERK1/2, and eNOS [76–78].

To get further insight into the potential regulatory effects of statins on PPAR activity, we focused on PPAR-α gene and protein expression in the hearts of normocholesterolemic rats

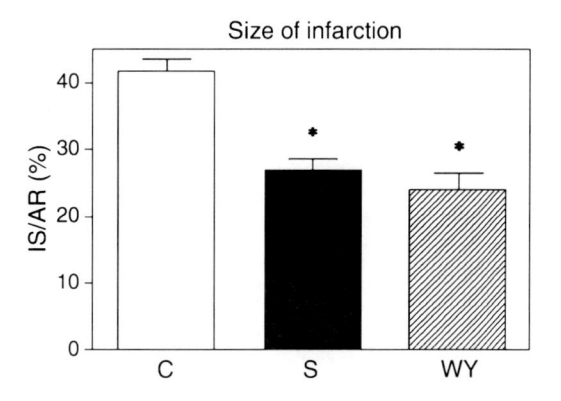

Fig. 4 Effects of simvastatin (S) and WY14643 (WY), a selective PPAR-α agonist, on the size of myocardial infarction after 30-min global ischemia and 2-h reperfusion in Langendorff-perfused rat hearts. Infarct size (IS) is expressed in % of the area at risk (AR) size. Values are means ± S.E.M. from 10-12 hearts per group. * $P < 0.05$ vs. untreated control (C) group

exposed to I/R after 5-day treatment with simvastatin [66]. A remarkable elevation in PPAR-α gene expression coupled with an enhanced protein expression (3.3-fold and 2-fold increase in mRNA and protein levels, respectively) was observed in the myocardium of these animals that was maintained after both ischemia and reperfusion and accompanied by a significant reduction of the infarct size, improved contractile recovery, and attenuation of severe ischemia- and reperfusion-induced ventricular arrhythmias [79]. In support of the view that PPAR-α activation may underlie the mechanisms of beneficial effects of statins against lethal myocardial injury in the hearts of normocholesterolemic animals, our studies confirmed that anti-infarct protection conferred by 5-day treatment with simvastatin in a rat *ex vivo* model of 30-min global ischemia and 2-h reperfusion was comparable with the effect of WY14643 (WY; Fig. 4), one of the most potent and selective PPAR-α agonists [25], a hypolipidemic compound that has been shown to protect rat myocardium against I/R injury [80].

Although statins are not specific PPAR ligands, they have been reported to up-regulate PPAR-α in some cell types, such as human HepG2 hepatoma cells [81] or mouse peritoneal macrophages [82], and to increase both PPAR-α expression and its protein levels in primary endothelial cells [67]. Our findings provide evidence of the

Fig. 5 Schematic representation of the potential mechanisms of PPAR activation by statins through the inhibition of HMG-CoA reductase-mevalonate pathway of cholesterol biosynthesis. For abbreviations, see the text

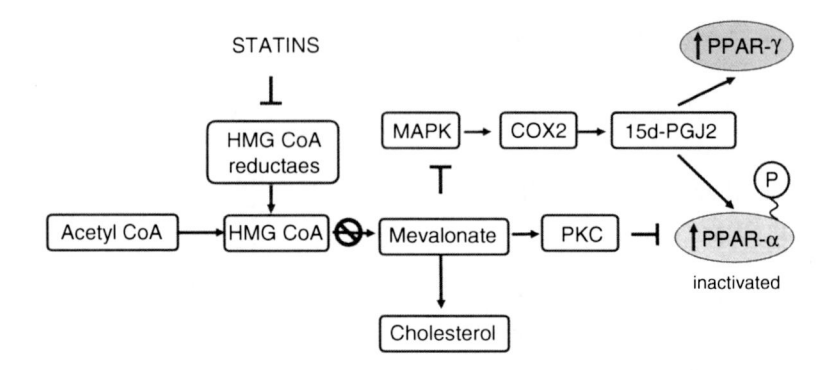

up-regulation of PPAR-α by statins in the myocardium, perhaps not via a direct agonistic mechanism. This is in agreement with the data documenting a beneficial effect of PPAR-α activation on cardiac I/R injury [13, 14, 44] and may indicate that preserved FAO is important for the maintenance of adequate energy production under the conditions of restored coronary flow, when oxygen supply is no longer rate-limiting.

PPAR and Inflammation

Beneficial effects of PPAR agonists may be attributed not only to modulation of cardiac metabolism but also to inhibition of inflammation with the salutatory effects on the cardiac muscle [21, 83]. In fact, in the experiments that have demonstrated beneficial effects of PPAR agonists on the myocardial, cerebral, and hepatal I/R injury, protection was attributed to the attenuation of oxidative stress and inflammatory response via inhibition of the activation of NF-kB [14, 15, 20, 52, 84–86]. Research indicates that the acute anti-inflammatory effect of simvastatin occurs through a mechanism involving inhibition of PKCα-induced phosphorylation (and inactivation) of PPAR-α and activation of PPAR-α (and PPAR-γ) via a cyclooxygenase (COX)-2–dependent increase in the levels of natural PPAR ligand 15d-PGJ$_2$, as well as decreased transactivation of NFκB [68, 82, 87, 88]. Figure 5 summarizes the potential mechanisms of PPAR activation as a part of pleiotropic effects of statins induced by the inhibition of the HMG-CoA reductase-mevalonate pathway. Moreover, a remarkable similarity between the pleiotropic

effects of statins (including anti-inflammatory and antioxidant effects) and the agonists of PPAR-α fibrates, which share a number of pharmacological properties with statins, suggests a mechanistic link between these two classes of drugs and similarity in their effects on PPAR-α [44, 89].

Thus, it is conceivable that an improved outcome of I/R injury in statin-treated normal and diabetic/hypercholesterolemic animals in our studies was linked to the anti-inflammatory effects of PPAR activation as well. In support of this, Planavila et al. [90] have reported that atorvastatin treatment prevented both the fall in the protein levels of PPAR-α and NF-kB activation in pressure-overload-induced cardiac hypertrophy.

Conclusions

The experimental data reviewed here suggest that changes in gene expression of PPARs are involved in the pathophysiological mechanisms of myocardial injury and may modulate it in a distinct way, dependent on the type and duration of cardiac pathology. Collectively, these data indicate that up-regulation of PPARs may underlie mechanisms of lipid-independent cardioprotective effects of hypolipidemic drugs in both normal and diseased heart. Thus, PPARs might represent an important therapeutic target in the management of ischemic heart disease in patients with or without metabolic disorders. However, a more detailed elucidation of the role of PPARs in myocardial ischemic injury and cardioprotection requires further investigation.

Acknowledgments Supported by grants VEGA SR 2/0173/08, 2/0054/11, 1/0620/10, APVV-LPP-0393-09, APVV 0538-07 and GSRT 5190/2005-759.

References

1. Desvergne B, Wahli W. Peroxisome proliferator-activated receptors: nuclear control of metabolism. Endocr Rev. 1999;20:649–88.

2. Kliewer SA, Xu HE, Lambert MH, et al. Peroxisome proliferator-activated receptors: from genes to physiology. Recent Prog Horm Res. 2001;56:239–63.

3. Barger PM, Kelly DP. PPAR signaling in the control of cardiac energy metabolism. Trends Cardiovasc Med. 2000;10:238–45.

4. Michalik L, Wahli W. Involvement of PPAR nuclear receptors in tissue injury and wound repair. J Clin Invest. 2006;116:598–606.

5. Kliewer SA, Forman BM, Blumberg B, et al. Differential expression and activation of a family of murine peroxisome proliferator-activated receptors. Proc Natl Acad Sci USA. 1994;91:7355–9.

6. Greene ME, Blumberg B, McBride OW, et al. Isolation of the human peroxisome proliferator activated receptor gamma cDNA: Expression in hematopoietic cells and chromosomal mapping. Gene Expr. 1995;4:281–99.

7. Braissant O, Foufelle F, Scotto C, et al. Differential expression of peroxisome proliferator-activated receptors (PPARs): tissue distribution of PPAR-alpha, -beta, and -gamma in the adult rat. Endocrinology. 1996;137:354–66.

8. Escher P, Braissant O, Basu-Modak S, et al. Rat PPARs: quantitative analysis in adult rat tissues and regulation in fasting and refeeding. Endocrinology. 2001;142:4195–202.

9. Panagia M, Gibbons GF, Radda GK, et al. PPAR-alpha activation required for decreased glucose uptake and increased susceptibility to injury during ischemia. Am J Physiol Heart Circ Physiol. 2005;288:H2677–83.

10. Sambandam N, Morabito D, Wagg C, et al. Chronic activation of PPARalpha is detrimental to cardiac recovery after ischemia. Am J Physiol Heart Circ Physiol. 2006;290:H87–95.

11. Kantor PF, Lucien A, Kozak R, et al. The antianginal drug trimetazidine shifts cardiac energy metabolism from fatty acid oxidation to glucose oxidation by inhibiting mitochondrial long-chain 3-ketoacyl coenzyme A thiolase. Circ Res. 2000;86:580–8.

12. Tabernero A, Schoonjans K, Jesel L, et al. Activation of the peroxisome proliferator-activated receptor alpha protects against myocardial ischaemic injury and improves endothelial vasodilatation. BMC Pharmacol. 2002;2:10.

13. Wayman NS, Hattori Y, McDonald MC, et al. Ligands of the peroxisome proliferator-activated receptors (PPAR-gamma and PPAR-alpha) reduce myocardial infarct size. FASEB J. 2002;16:1027–40.

14. Yue TL, Bao W, Jucker BM, et al. Activation of peroxisome proliferator-activated receptor-alpha protects the heart from ischemia/reperfusion injury. Circulation. 2003;108:2393–9.

15. Yeh CH, Chen TP, Lee CH, et al. Cardiomyocytic apoptosis following global cardiac ischemia and reperfusion can be attenuated by peroxisome proliferator-activated receptor alpha but not gamma activators. Shock. 2006;26:262–70.

16. Gilde AJ, van der Lee KA, Willemsen PH, et al. Peroxisome proliferator-activated receptor (PPAR) alpha and PPARbeta/delta, but not PPARgamma, modulate the expression of genes involved in cardiac lipid metabolism. Circ Res. 2003;92:518–24.

17. Ravingerová T, Adameová T, Kelly T, et al. The effect of diabetes mellitus on myocardial resistance to ischaemia/reperfusion injury and PPAR expression in the rat heart. Acta Physiol. 2007;191(S658):41.

18. Finck BN. The PPAR regulatory system in cardiac physiology and disease. Cardiovasc Res. 2007;73:269–77.

19. Huss JM, Kelly DP. Nuclear receptor signaling and cardiac energetics. Circ Res. 2004;95:568.

20. Delerive P, Fruchart JC, Staels B. Peroxisome proliferator-activated receptors in inflammation control. J Endocrinol. 2001;169:453–9.

21. Smeets PJH, Planavila A, van der Vusse GJ, et al. Peroxisome proliferator-activated receptors and inflammation: take it to heart. Acta Physiol. 2007;191:171–88.

22. Collino M, Patel NSA, Thiemermann Ch. PPARs as new therapeutic targets for the treatment of cerebral ischemia/reperfusion. Ther Adv Cardiovasc Dis. 2008;2:179–97.

23. Feige JN, Gelman L, Michalik L, et al. From molecular action to physiological outputs: peroxisome proliferator-activated receptors are nuclear receptors at the crossroads of key cellular functions. Prog Lipid Res. 2006;45:120–59.

24. Theocharis S, Margeli A, Vielh P, et al. Peroxisome proliferator-activated receptor-gamma ligands as cell-cycle modulators. Cancer Treat Rev. 2004;30:545–54.

25. Forman BM, Chen J, Evans RM. Hypolipidemic drugs, polyunsaturated fatty acids, and eicosanoids are ligands for peroxisome proliferator-activated receptors alpha and delta. Proc Natl Acad Sci USA. 1997;94:4312–17.

26. Salam NK, Huang TH, Kota BP, et al. Novel PPAR-gamma agonists identified from a natural product library: a virtual screening, induced-fit docking and biological assay study. Chem Biol Drug Des. 2008;71:57–70.

27. Sidell RJ, Cole MA, Draper NJ, et al. Thiazolidinedione treatment normalizes insulin resistance and ischemic injury in the zucker fatty rat heart. Diabetes. 2002;51:1110–17.

28. Khandoudi N, Delerive P, Berrebi-Bertrand I, et al. Rosiglitazone, a peroxisome proliferator-activated receptor-gamma, inhibits the Jun NH(2)-terminal kinase/activating protein 1 pathway and protects the heart from ischemia/reperfusion injury. Diabetes. 2002;51:1507–14.

29. Shiomi T, Tsutsui H, Hayashidani S, et al. Pioglitazone, a peroxisome proliferator-activated receptor-gamma agonist, attenuates left ventricular remodeling and failure after experimental myocardial infarction. Circulation. 2002;106:3126–32.

30. Lee TM, Chou TF. Troglitazone administration limits infarct size by reduced phosphorylation of canine myocardial connexin43 proteins. Am J Physiol Heart Circ Physiol. 2003;285:H1650–9.

31. Shibata H, Spencer TE, Onate SA, et al. Role of co-activators and co-repressors in the mechanisms of steroid/thyroid receptor action. Recent Prog Horm Res. 1997;52:141–64.

32. Barger PM, Brandt JM, Leonem TC, et al. Deactivation of peroxisome proliferator-activated receptor-alpha during cardiac hypertrophic growth. J Clin Invest. 2000;105:1723–30.

33. Barger PM, Browning AC, Garner AN, et al. p38 mitogen-activated protein kinase activates peroxisome proliferator-activated receptor alpha: a potential role in the cardiac metabolic stress response. J Biol Chem. 2001;276:44495–501.

34. Kliewer SA, Umesono K, Noonan DJ, et al. Convergence of 9-cis retinoic acid and peroxisome proliferator signalling pathways through heterodimer formation of their receptors. Nature. 1992;358:771–4.

35. Tan NS, Michalik L, Desvergne B, et al. Multiple expression control mechanisms of peroxisome proliferator-activated receptors and their target genes. J Steroid Biochem Mol Biol. 2005;93:99–105.

36. Abdelrahman M, Sivaraja A, Thiemerman Ch. Beneficial effects of PPAR-gamma ligands in ischemia-reperfusion injury, inflammation and shock. Cardiovasc Res. 2005;65:772–81.

37. Braunwald E, Kloner RA. Myocardial reperfusion: a double-edged sword? J Clin Invest. 1985;76:1713–9.

38. Roberto A, Prado EA. Ischemia/reperfusion injury. J Surg Res. 2002;105:248–58.

39. Rodríguez-Sinovas A, Abdallah Y, Piper HM, et al. Reperfusion injury as a therapeutic challenge in patients with acute myocardial infarction. Heart Fail Rev. 2007;12:207–16.

40. Turer AT, Hill JA. Pathogenesis of myocardial ischemia-reperfusion injury and rationale for therapy. Am J Cardiol. 2010;106:360–8.

41. Hall G, Hasday JD, Rogers TB. Regulating the regulator: NF-kappaB signaling in heart. J Mol Cell Cardiol. 2006;41:580–91.

42. Li C, Browder W, Kao RL. Early activation of transcription factor NF-kappaB during ischemia in perfused rat heart. Am J Physiol. 1999;276:H543–52.

43. Razeghi P, Young ME, Abbasi S, et al. Hypoxia in vivo decreases peroxisome proliferator-activated receptor alpha-regulated gene expression in rat heart. Biochem Biophys Res Commun. 2001;287:5–10.

44. Tian Q, Grzemski FA, Panagiotopoulos S, et al. Peroxisome proliferator-activated receptor alpha agonist, clofibrate, has profound influence on myocardial fatty acid composition. Chem Biol Interact. 2006;160:241–51.

45. Ravingerová T, Adameová A, Kelly T, et al. Treatment with statins protects rat heart against ischemia/reperfusion injury independent of lipid-lowering effects. J Mol Cell Cardiol. 2008;44:787.

46. Fragasso G, Piatti PM, Monti L, et al. Short- and long-term beneficial effects of trimetazidine in patients with diabetes and ischemic cardiomyopathy. Am Heart J. 2003;146:E18.

47. Takeda K, Ichiki T, Tokunou T, et al. 15-Deoxy-delta 12,14-prostaglandin J2 and thiazolidinediones activate the MEK/ERK pathway through phosphatidylinositol 3-kinase in vascular smooth muscle cells. J Biol Chem. 2001;276:48950–5.

48. Hausenloy DJ, Tsang A, Mocanu MM, et al. Ischemic preconditioning protects by activating prosurvival kinases at reperfusion. Am J Physiol Heart Circ Physiol. 2005;288:H971–6.

49. Ravingerová T, Matejíková J, Neckář J, et al. Differential role of PI3K/Akt pathway in the infarct size limitation and antiarrhythmic protection in the rat heart. Mol Cell Biochem. 2007;297:111–20.

50. Wynne A, Mocanu M, Yellon DM. Pioglitazone mimics preconditioning in the isolated perfused rat heart: a role for the prosurvival kinases PI3K and P42/44MAPK. J Cardiovasc Pharmacol. 2005;46:817–22.

51. Sivarajah A, McDonald MC, Thiemermann C. The cardioprotective effects of preconditioning with endotoxin, but not ischemia, are abolished by a peroxisome proliferator-activated receptor-gamma antagonist. J Pharmacol Exp Ther. 2005;313:896–901.

52. Collino M, Patel NSA, Lawrence KM, et al. The selective PPAR-gamma antagonist GW9662 reverses the protection of LPS in a model of renal ischemia-reperfusion. Kidney Int. 2005;68:529–36.

53. Nikolaidis LA, Levine TB. Peroxisome proliferator activator receptors (PPAR), insulin resistance, and cardiomyopathy: friends or foes for the diabetic patient with heart failure? Cardiol Rev. 2004;2:158–70.

54. Ricci C, Jong CJ, Schaffer SW. Proapoptotic and antiapoptotic effects of hyperglycemia: role of insulin signaling. Can J Physiol Pharmacol. 2008;86:166–72.

55. Strnisková M, Barancik M, Neckar J, et al. Mitogen-activated protein kinases in the acute diabetic myocardium. Mol Cell Biochem. 2003;249:59–65.

56. Xu G, Takashi E, Kudo M, et al. Contradictory effects of short- and long-term hyperglycemias on ischemic injury of myocardium via intracellular signaling pathway. Exp Mol Pathol. 2004;76:57–65.

57. Ma G, Al-Shabrawey M, Johnson JA, et al. Protection against myocardial ischemia/reperfusion injury by short-term diabetes: enhancement of VEGF formation, capillary density, and activation of cell survival signaling. Naunyn Schmiedebergs Arch Pharmacol. 2006;373:415–27.

58. Tsang A, Hausenloy DJ, Mocanu MM, et al. Preconditioning the diabetic heart: the importance of Akt phosphorylation. Diabetes. 2005;54:2360–4.

59. Malfitano C, Alba Loureiro TC, Rodrigues B, et al. Hyperglycaemia protects the heart after myocardial

infarction: aspects of programmed cell survival and cell death. Eur J Heart Fail. 2010;20:659–67.

60. Matejiková J, Kucharská J, Pancza D, et al. The effect of antioxidant treatment and NOS inhibition on the incidence of ischaemia-induced arrhythmias in the diabetic rat heart. Physiol Res. 2008;57:S55–60.

61. Ravingerová T, Neckář J, Kolář F. Ischemic tolerance of rat hearts in acute and chronic phases of experimental diabetes. Mol Cell Biochem. 2003;249:167–74.

62. Adameová A, Kuželová M, Andelová E, et al. Hypercholesterolemia abrogates an increased resistance of diabetic rat hearts to ischemia-reperfusion injury. Mol Cell Biochem. 2007;295:129–36.

63. Giricz Z, Lalu MM, Csonka C, et al. Hyperlipidemia attenuates the infarct size-limiting effect of ischemic preconditioning: role of matrix metalloproteinase-2 inhibition. J Pharmacol Exp Ther. 2006;316:154–61.

64. Kocsis GF, Csont T, Varga-Orvos Z, et al. Expression of genes related to oxidative/nitrosative stress in mouse hearts: effect of preconditioning and cholesterol diet. Med Sci Monit. 2010;16:BR32–9.

65. Adameová A, Harcarová A, Matejíková J, et al. Simvastatin alleviates myocardial contractile dysfunction and lethal ischemic injury in rat heart independent of cholesterol-lowering effects. Physiol Res. 2009;58: 449–54.

66. Ravingerová T, Adameová A, Kelly T, et al. Changes in PPAR gene expression and myocardial tolerance to ischemia: relevance to pleiotropic effects of statins. Exp Clin Cardiol. 2008;13:150.

67. Inoue I, Goto S, Mizotani K, Awata T, et al. Lipophilic HMG-CoA reductase inhibitor has an anti-inflammatory effect: reduction of MRNA levels for interleukin-1beta, interleukin-6, cyclooxygenase-2, and p22phox by regulation of peroxisome proliferator-activated receptor alpha (PPARalpha) in primary endothelial cells. Life Sci. 2000;67:863–76.

68. Zelvyte I, Dominaitiene R, Crisby M, et al. Modulation of inflammatory mediators and PPARgamma and NFkappaB expression by pravastatin in response to lipoproteins in human monocytes in vitro. Pharmacol Res. 2002;45:147–54.

69. Takemoto M, Liao JK. Pleiotropic effects of 3-hydroxy-3-methylglutaryl coenzyme a reductase inhibitors. Arterioscler Thromb Vasc Biol. 2001;21: 1712–19.

70. Van Linthout S, Riad A, Dhayat N, et al. Anti-inflammatory effects of atorvastatin improve left ventricular function in experimental diabetic cardiomyopathy. Diabetologia. 2007;50:1977–86.

71. Zhou R, Xu Q, Zheng P, et al. Cardioprotective effect of fluvastatin on isoproterenol-induced myocardial infarction in rat. Eur J Pharmacol. 2008;586: 244–50.

72. Adameova A, Xu YJ, Duhamel TA, Tappia PS, Shan L, Dhalla NS. Anti-atherosclerotic molecules targeting oxidative stress and inflammation. Curr Pharm Des. 2009;15:3094–107.

73. Schafer A, Fraccarollo D, Eigenthaler M, et al. Rosuvastatin reduces platelet activation in heart failure: role of NO bioavailability. Arterioscler Thromb Vasc Biol. 2005;25:1071–7.

74. Shimizu K, Aikawa M, Takayama K, et al. Direct anti-inflammatory mechanisms contribute to attenuation of experimental allograft arteriosclerosis by statins. Circulation. 2003;108:2113–20.

75. Adameová A, Kuzelová M, Faberová V, et al. Protective effect of simvastatin and VULM 1457 in ischaemic-reperfused myocardium of the diabetic-hypercholesterolemic rats. Pharmazie. 2006;61:807–8.

76. Efthymiou CA, Mocanu MM, Yellon DM. Atorvastatin and myocardial reperfusion injury: new pleiotropic effect implicating multiple prosurvival signaling. J Cardiovasc Pharmacol. 2005;45:247–52.

77. Di Napoli P, Taccardi AA, Grilli A, et al. Simvastatin reduces reperfusion injury by modulating nitric oxide synthase expression: an ex vivo study in isolated working rat hearts. Cardiovasc Res. 2001;51:283–93.

78. Merla R, Ye Y, Lin Y, et al. The central role of adenosine in statin-induced ERK1/2, Akt and eNOS phosphorylation. Am J Physiol. 2007;293:H1918–28.

79. Ravingerová T, Adameová A, Kelly T, et al. Changes in PPAR gene expression and myocardial tolerance to ischaemia: relevance to pleiotropic effects of statins. Can J Physiol Pharmacol. 2009;87:1028–36.

80. Bulhak AA, Sjöquist PO, Xu CB, et al. Protection against myocardial ischaemia/reperfusion injury by PPAR-alpha activation is related to production of nitric oxide and endothelin-1. Basic Res Cardiol. 2006;101:244–52.

81. Martin G, Duez H, Blanquart Ch, et al. Statin-induced inhibition of the Rho-signaling pathway activates PPARα and induces HDL apoA-I. J Clin Invest. 2001;107:1423–32.

82. Paumelle R, Blanquart C, Briand O, et al. Acute anti-inflammatory properties of statins involve peroxisome proliferator-activated receptor-α via inhibition of the protein kinase C signaling pathway. Circ Res. 2006; 98:361–9.

83. Diep QN, Benkirane K, Amiri F, et al. PPAR alpha activator fenofibrate inhibits myocardial inflammation and fibrosis in angiotensin II-infused rats. J Mol Cell Cardiol. 2004;36:295–304.

84. Ogata T, Miyauchi T, Sakaiet S, et al. Myocardial fibrosis and diastolic dysfunction in deoxycorticosterone acetate-salt hypertensive rats is ameliorated by the peroxisome proliferator-activated receptor-alpha activator fenofibrate, partly by suppressing inflammatory responses associated with the nuclear factor-kappa-B pathway. J Am Coll Cardiol. 2004;43:1481–8.

85. Xu SQ, Li YH, Hu SH, et al. Effects of WY14643 on hepatic ischemia reperfusion injury in rats. World J Gastroenterol. 2008;14:6936–42.

86. Collino M, Aragno M, Mastrocola R, et al. Oxidative stress and inflammatory response evoked by transient cerebral ischemia/reperfusion: effects of the PPAR-alpha agonist WY14643. Free Radic Biol Med. 2006;41:579–89.

87. Inoue I, Itoh F, Aoyagi S, et al. Fibrate and statin synergistically increase the transcriptional activities of

PPARalpha/RXRalpha and decrease the transactivation of NFkappaB. Biochem Biophys Res Commun. 2002; 290:131–9.

88. Yano M, Matsumura T, Senokuchi T, et al. Statins activate peroxisome proliferator-activated receptor gamma through extracellular signal-regulated kinase 1/2 and p38 mitogen-activated protein kinase-dependent cyclooxygenase-2 expression in macrophages. Circ Res. 2007;100:442–1451.

89. Paumelle R, Staels B. Cross-talk between statins and PPARalpha in cardiovascular diseases: clinical evidence and basic mechanisms. Trends Cardiovasc Med. 2008;18:73–8.

90. Planavila A, Laguna JC, Vázquez-Carrera M. Atorvastatin improves peroxisome proliferator-activated receptor signaling in cardiac hypertrophy by preventing nuclear factor-kappa B activation. Biochim Biophys Acta. 2005;168:76–83.

Genes and Plasma Lipids in Czech Slavic Population

Jaroslav A. Hubacek and Rudolf Poledne

Abstract

Dyslipidemias are between the most important risk factors of the cardiovascular diseases. Studies with different designs show that the dyslipidemic pattern is clearly heritable and the heritability was estimated to be around 50%. We have analyzed the genetic background of elevated plasma lipids in three studies with different design, all originating from Czech Slavic population. We have examined two small groups of children (N ~ 90) selected from opposite part of the distribution curve of total cholesterol of 2,000 children; large population of 2,500 individuals selected according the WHO MONICA study criteria and finally 8 years cohort of 250 individuals where substantial decrease of the plasma lipids, as a consequence of the socioeconomic changes, was observed. Alltogether more than 100 variants within different candidate genes were analyzed. Our results showed that especially the variants within the genes for apolipoprotein E, apolipoprotein A5, hepatic lipase and HMGCo-A reductase play a significant role in the determination of the plasma lipid levels. Nutrigenetic analyses suggest an important role of gene environment interactions for variants within apolipoprotein A4, apolipoprotein A5, and cholesterol 7-alpha hydroxylase. However, we were not able to confirm some recent candidates, detected through the genome wide approach. For example the MLXIPL variants exhibit just very marginal effect on plasma triacylglycerols in our Slavic population. Our results point to some generally valid associations between genetic polymorphisms and plasma lipids and underline the importance of the analysis of the gene-gene and gene-environment interactions, as well as the intra-ethnic differences.

Keywords

Cholesterol • Dyslipidemia • Interaction • Nutrition • Polymorphisms • Slavic population • Triacylglycerols

J.A. Hubacek (✉)
Institute for Clinical and Experimental Medicine
and Centre for Cardiovascular Research,
Prague, Czech Republic
e-mail: jahb@ikem.cz

B. Ostadal et al. (eds.), *Genes and Cardiovascular Function*,
DOI 10.1007/978-1-4419-7207-1_15, © Springer Science+Business Media, LLC 2011

Introduction

Cardiovascular diseases are the main cause of mortality in industrial countries, and the dyslipidemias (elevated plasma levels of total or LDL-cholesterol and triacylglycerols, lower levels of HDL- cholesterol) are among the major risk factors of their development. External/environmental causes of dyslipidemias (at first unhealthy diet and low physical activity) have been known for decades. However, family and twin studies clearly show that a substantial part of the dyslipidemias have a significant genetic background [1]. The heritability (the proportion of phenotypic variance attributable to genetic variance) of the dyslipidemias was estimated to be around 50%, however, despite the intensive research and methodological efforts achieved recently, the exact causes remain undetected. Despite the fact that there are mutations (rare deleterious single-hit changes) in some genes (for example LDL receptor, apolipoproteins A5 and B, PCSK9, LPL maturation protein) causing the hypercholesterolemia/dyslipidemia [2], the vast majority of this pathology is based on a polygenic background. This means that it is caused by many variants within a lot of genes [3].

Soon after the first publications concerning the association between the individual genetic polymorphisms appeared [4], we have designed the first study. As the hypercholesterolemia is a result of both external and genetic factors, we supposed that pre-pubertal children are the best individuals to study the genetic predisposition – exposure to the negative external factors is shorter than in adults, they are non-smokers without alcohol consumption, and without lipid lowering medications; thus the genetic background could be more expressed.

Prague Children Study

In the late eighties, we have examined a total of 2,000 ten- to eleven-year-old children from complete biological families with at least one sibling, living in ten schools in the Prague 4 district [5].

Nonfasting total cholesterol was analyzed once from the blood obtained from the finger tip by dry chemistry method, with written agreement of the parents. The distribution curve of total cholesterol was constructed, to analyze the genetic predisposition of hypercholesterolemia; two groups, high-cholesterol (HCG, total cholesterol between 95 and 100 percentile) and low-cholesterol (LCG, total cholesterol between 5 and 10 percentile) were created. Individuals with the lowest total cholesterol, below 5-th percentile, were excluded because of the possibility of undetected and not examined metabolic disturbances, such as high level of thyroxine. These groups were repeatedly reexamined at intervals of 9–12 months and we excluded probands with at least two decreases (from the HCG group), or increases (from the LCG group) of total cholesterol over the desired values. Further, one proband with clinically confirmed diagnosis of familial hypercholesterolemia was also excluded from the HCG group. The final numbers of the probands within the groups were as follows: 82 probands in HCG with stable high total cholesterol levels and 86 probands in LCG with stable low total cholesterol levels.

Based on the candidate gene approach [6], almost 30 polymorphisms within the 13 genes with known functions in the metabolism and/or transport of plasma lipids were selected for the analysis during two decades. The overview of the variants is listed in Table 1.

As some of the polymorphisms were analyzed more than 20 years ago, Southern blotting and restriction fragment length polymorphism approach was used for a couple of variants. This makes the exact localization of the analyzed variant unclear and many of such variants are not characterized by the recent exact and unambiguous rs coding system. Later, we have analyzed the variants using the polymerase chain reaction and restriction analysis.

From the recent point of view, the protocol of the children study was underpowered – it was recognized that the relative by low number of individuals make such studies generally prone to false positive or false negative results. However, on the other hand, the several strengths of the study outweigh this problem. The unique and

Table 1 Complete list of the genes and variants analyzed in our studies

Gene	Variant	Protein function
APOE [a, b, c]	E2, E3, E4	Protein component of VLDL and HDL particles
APOB [a, c]	XbaI, C-516>T, Ins/del at signal peptide	Major constituent of LDL particles, major ligand for the interaction with LDL receptor
APOA1 [c]	G-75>A and C83>T	Major protein in HDL particles, cofactor for LCAT
APOA2 [a]	(CA)$_n$ repeat	The second most represented protein in HDL particles
APOA4 [c]	Thr347>Ser and Gln360>His	Structural component of chylomicrones and HDL particles
APOA5 [a, b, c]	T-1131>C, Ser19>Trp, Val153>Met	Modulates the activity of lipoprotein lipase and influenced the affinity of lipoprotein particles to cellular receptors;
APOC1 [a, b, c]	CGTT insertion/deletion	Constituent of triacylglycerol-rich particles, inhibitor of lipoprotein particles binding to cellular receptors
APOC3 [a, c]	C3238>G	Component of VLDL and HDL particles
CETP [a]	TaqI	Transfer insoluble cholesteryl esters among different lipoprotein particles
LPL [a]	Asp291>Ser	Key enzyme in lipoprotein metabolism, hydrolyses triacylglycerol in VLDL and chylomicrons
LDL receptor	PvuII	Major cell surface receptor that plays an key role in cholesterol homeostasis
CYP7A1 [a, b, c]	A-204>C *	The key enzyme in catabolism of cholesterol, catalyze the first step in bile acid synthesis
ABCG5 [a, c]	Gln604>Glu	Responsible for the secretion of cholesterol into bile, potentially influence the responsiveness to dietary changes
ABCG8 [a, c]	Asp19>His, Tyr54>Cys, Thr400>Lys, Ala632>Val	Responsible for the secretion of cholesterol into bile, potentially influence the responsiveness to dietary changes
HMGCoA reductase [a]	(TTA)$_n$ repeat	The key enzyme in cholesterol synthesis
Hepatic lipase [a, b, c]	C-480>T	Hydrolyses triacylglycerols in TG-rich particles
MLXIPL [b]	His241>Gln	Cellular transcription factor
Ghrelin [b]	Leu72>Met	Ligand for the growth hormone secretagogue receptor, regulates growth hormone release
INSIG2 [b]	G-102>A	Regulates lipid synthesis by blocking the activation of SREBPs by SCAP

[a]Analyzed in the children study
[b]Analyzed in MONICA study
[c]Analyzed in the nutrigenetic study

careful selection of the examined individuals from the opposite parts of the distribution curve with repeatedly confirmed phenotype allows us to detect the real effects of some of the analyzed variants who were simultaneously or later confirmed in large population studies.

The first analyzed gene was the gene for apolipoprotein E (*APOE*) [7]. Firstly, we have detected almost a four times higher frequency of the carriers of the *APOE4* allele in HCG compared to LCG and probands with *APOE2* allele were less common in this group. Importantly, analysis of the large population sample (see in more detail below) reveals the frequency of the *APOE4* allele carriers between the HCG and

LCG group. This association between the *APOE4* allele and elevated plasma LDL-cholesterol was 100 times confirmed in studies with different design and this confirms that our study is well designed and able to detect the real and significant effect of individual polymorphisms.

Until now, we have analyzed the effect of dozens other polymorphisms and were able to prove several significant differences in genotype frequencies between HCG and LCG groups (for a brief summary of the effects of individual polymorphisms see Table 2).

A significant difference was found in the frequencies of the genotypes of the ten + odd number of (TTA) repeats within the *HMGCoA*

Table 2 Complete list of the genes and variants analyzed in HCG and LCG children and their effects on plasma lipids

Gene	Variant	Different genotype frequency between the HCG and LCG	Association between polymorphisms and lipid traits within the HCG or LCH [a]
APOE	E2, E3, E4	E4 carriers more common in HCG	No
APOB	XbaI	No	No
	C-516>T	Not individually, yes in linkage –	No
	Ins/del at signal peptide	Carriers of the II genotype and T allele are more common within LCG	No
APOA2	(CA)$_n$ repeat	No	Carriers of the five and eight repeats have higher apoB and plasma cholesterol in HCG group
APOA5	T-1131>C	No	No
	Ser19>Trp	Yes, Trp carriers more common in HCG	No
	Val153>Met	No	No
APOC1	CGTT insertion/deletion	No	Yes
APOC3	C3238>G	No	No
CETP	TaqI	No	No
LPL	Asp291.Ser	Yes, carriers of the Ser291 were detected just within the LCG group	No
LDL receptor	PvuII	No	No
CYP7A1	A-204>C [b]	No	In HCG, CC individuals have higher total cholesterol than AA homozygotes
ABCG5	Gln604>Glu	No	In LCG Gln604 carriers have lower LDL cholesterol than Glu homozygotes
ABCG8	Asp19>His	No	In HCG, His19 carriers have lower total cholesterol than AspAsp homozygotes
	Tyr54C>ys	No	No
	Thr400>Lys	No	No
	Ala632>Val	No	No
HMGCoA reductase	(TTA)$_n$ repeat	Yes, carriers of the genotypes with odd alleles	No

[a]Recently specified as -203
[b]Possible gene-gene or gene-environment interactions necessary for the gene effect expression

reductase – these genotypes were almost twice more frequent in HCG than in LCG children [8]. However, this result was never confirmed or refitted in further studies.

Within the *APOB* gene, three variants have been investigated and strong, but not complete linkage disequilibrium (LD) was demonstrated between the variants within the regulatory part of the gene. Haplotype analysis suggests that deviations from LD are much higher in LCG children

than in HCG children [9]. Namely, the presence of the I/I genotype together with at least one T-516 allele was more than five times higher in LCG than in HCG.

Interestingly, we have detected a significant difference between the HCG and LCG group also within the *APOA5* gene. This gene, involved in the metabolism of triacylglycerol-rich particles was of outstanding interest, as we were participating on the description of the gene and have focused our research on this gene in a wide range of different aspects.

In HCG, there was more than a twice higher number of *APOA5* Trp19 carriers than in LCG, despite the fact that at the time of the first examination LCG and HCG did not differ in plasma triacylglycerol levels. It was a surprising result, as this gene was primarily detected as determinant of plasma triacylglycerol and not cholesterol. However, we have later confirmed this result [10] on a large population MONICA study (see below). In the population, the variant was associated with non-HDL cholesterol but not with total and/or LDL cholesterol – this fact can explain why this association was not detected before; despite the better risk prediction value, non/HDL cholesterol is usually not analyzed.

The gene for lipoprotein lipase is another gene primarily associated with triacylglycerol levels and exhibits also a different distribution of the variants between HCG and LCG groups. The carriers of the Ser291 allele seem to be protected from development of hypercholesterolemia.

The genotype of allelic frequencies of all other polymorphisms did not differ between the HCG and LCG significantly. For some of them, the exact role in the determination of plasma lipids remains unclear.

Interestingly, despite the fact that our groups represented a relatively narrow part of the population, for some analyzed variants we have observed also an association with plasma lipids within one group. From a recent point of view, it is likely that such observations represent a false positive result, but we cannot exclude (and we have not confirmed) that it could reflect the so-called variability gene effect. The variability gene effect [11] could be attributed to equilibrium with recently used epistasis (gene-gene) or gene-environment interactions [12]. We suppose that some other markers are necessary to be present for the expression of the allelic effect (for example, the consumption of a distinct kind of food in sufficient amount) on plasma lipids. According to our results, especially *APOA2* [13] and *CYP7A1* genes seem to be involved in such interactions. Similar effects at the *APOC1* locus almost surely reflect its allelic association (linkage disequilibrium) with different *APOE* alleles.

Based on the recent level of knowledge it is clear that the effects of individual polymorphisms on lipid traits need to be analyzed on large, well-selected population samples. The small studies are prone to both false positive and false negative results (type I and type II errors) and did not allow the adjustment to environmental and non-genetic factors (for example sex, age, smoking, BMI, alcohol intake, medication, dietary habits, physical activity…).

Large-Population-Based Study

To analyze the genetic determination of the plasma lipids in Czech Slavic population (primarily, later this sample was used also for the analysis of genetic predisposition to obesity, renal failure, osteoporosis,…), we have used the well defined and selected representative WHO MONICA (Multinational MONItoring of trends and determinants in CArdiovascular diseases) [14] study. The examined individuals were selected and collected in nine Czech districts – largest cities were avoided – as a 1% population sample to examine the cardiovascular risk factors. This study is based on the population register and we have reached very high response rate at the first examinations – between 70% and 85%. The DNA bank based on MONICA study includes DNA samples from 2,559 individuals (1,191 males and 1,368 females, aged 25–65 years at the time of the first examination – 1997/1998, response rate 63%).

More than 100 biochemical and anthropometric characteristics were collected for all individuals. All individuals were examined twice within the 3 years; the first examination was performed in 1997/8, the second in 2000/1. The availability of two independent values further enhances the strength of the genetic association studies, if the obtained results are the same or similar in both years.

During the last 10 years of research, we have analyzed more than 100 variants within about 30 genes. The first focus was to analyze the genes selected on the candidate gene approach (with known functions of gene products). Recently also the confirmatory studies of the SNPs detected

Table 3 Summary of the genes and variants analyzed in Czech MONICA sample with confirmed associations with plasma lipids

Gene	Variant	Detected association
APOE	E2, E3, E4	E4 allele carriers have higher, and E2 allele carriers have lower, levels of total and LDL cholesterol
APOCI	CGTT Ins/Del	Insertion allele is associated with elevated plasma TG levels
APOA5	T-1131>C	Carriers of the less common allele C have higher TG and non-HDL cholesterol levels
	Ser19>Trp	Carriers of the less common allele Trp have higher TG and non-HDL cholesterol levels
	Val153>Met	Higher HDL cholesterol was found in Val/Val homozygotes in females but not in males.
Hepatic lipase	C-480>T	Carriers of the T allele have higher levels of HDL cholesterol
MLXIPL	His241>Gln	Borderline association of the Gln allele with low plasma TG levels
INSIG2	G-102>A	Females, carriers of the GG genotype have higher levels of HDL cholesterol
Ghrelin	Leu72>Met	Met carriers have lower plasma HDL cholesterol

through genome wide analyses (GWAs) approach were performed.

In the Czech MONICA study we have so far analyzed the following genes/variants where we have expected some associations with plasma lipid traits – apolipoprotein E (E2, E3 and E4 alleles), apolipoprotein CI (promoter insertion/deletion), apolipoprotein A5 (T-1131 C, Ser 19Trp, Val153Met, 315 variants), hepatic lipase (similarly to lipoprotein lipase, hydrolyses triacylglycerols in TG-rich particles; C-480>T), and through GWAs discovered MLXIPL (cellular transcription factor; His241Gln). For more detail about some of the analyzed SNPs see Table 1.

In this population based study, we have confirmed major associations between the *APOE* and *APOA5* genes and plasma lipids. As expected, the plasma levels of total or LDL cholesterol were the lowest in carriers of the *APOE2* allele and highest in carriers of the *APOE4* allele but it needs to be mentioned that the lipid-lowering effect of the *APOE2* allele was more pronounced than the enhancing effect of the *APOE4* allele.

We were between the first, who described the effect of the common variants within the *APOA5* gene on the plasma levels of triacylglycerols [15, 16] and later also on plasma non-HDL cholesterol levels. For the *APOA5*, we have proved that the plasma levels of triacylglycerols are lowest in individuals with just common alleles and that there is linear enhancing effect of the less common alleles

(C-1131 and Trp19), which increase the plasma TG levels by about 0.25 mmol/L. The third examined *APOA5* variant (Val153>Met) was associated with HDL-cholesterol levels, in sex-dependent manner with ValVal homozygotes showing higher levels in females but not in males [17].

In addition, there is also a couple of variants, analyzed in the studies not primarily related to lipid metabolism but the association with a lipid parameter or another risk factor associated with CAD was detected in the "second phase data mining". This includes the gene for ghrelin (ligand for the growth hormone secretagogue receptor which also regulates growth hormone release) where the Leu72>Met variant is significantly associated with plasma levels of HDL-cholesterol both in males and females [18], promoter variant (G-102>A) within the *INSIG2* gene (regulates lipid synthesis by blocking the activation of SREBPs by SCAP) which exhibit a sex-specific effect on HDL-cholesterol levels – it is affected by the polymorphism just in females.

Surprisingly, we were not able to confirm the association between the His241>Gln variant within the *MLXIPL* gene and triacylglycerol levels [19], despite the fact that this GWA-approach-detected SNP was suggested to be the strongest genetic determinant of plasma triacylglycerol levels [20], even stronger than *APOA5* (for a brief summary of the effects of individual polymorphisms see Table 3).

Nutrigenetics in Population Based Study

One of the promising fields in the recent population-genetic research is the nutrigenetic. Here, the question how the individual genetic variants interact with diet in the determination of the plasma lipid levels is analyzed. More or less by chance we have the possibility to study the decrease of plasma lipids in the population after significant nation-wide changes in dietary habits. The possibility to study the interaction between the dietary changes and genes and plasma lipid changes was based on an unusual coincidence.

The 135 unrelated adult males and 155 adult females included in the "interventional" study represented a part of an 8-year cohort selected in 1988 and then reinvestigated in 1996 in one district according to the protocol of the MONICA study. All individuals have the lipid levels in both 1988 and 1996. Both data of cholesterol concentrations from the whole MONICA study and data of food consumption obtained from the Institute of Agricultural Economy in the Czech population were used as evidence of the changes between the years 1988 and 1996. From 1988 to 1996, the food intake and dietary composition in the Czech population changed dramatically. The major reason was probably that during the post communist economy transition, the subsistence on meat and dairy products was canceled in 1991. The most pronounced changes were found in the intake of animal fat and lard which decreased by 45%. Whereas the consumption of egg and beef and pork meat dropped by about 20%, the consumption of chicken and fish increased by 10%. Also the consumption of vegetables, fruits and vegetable oils increased – in 1988, the consumption was ~133 kg per capita and year, in 1996 it was already ~150 kg per capita and year. Reflecting these dietary changes, the mean cholesterol concentrations decreased in the population by ~ one-half mmol/L (about 10%). Importantly, there was no evidence for increase of physical activity and the body mass index remains unchanged between 1988 and 1996 [21].

As well as in the entire Czech population (results from the whole MONICA study), the cholesterol concentration in individuals form the district analyzed in detail decreased over the 8-year period by ~ 0.6 mmol/L. Interestingly, the decrease was not observed in all individuals. In fact, in 65% individuals total cholesterol decreased by more than 5%, in 25% remained unchanged and in 10% an increase by more than 5% was detected. Unfortunately, as we cannot in 1988 expect the political, socioeconomically and inferential life style changes, there are just the basic lipid/anthropometrical parameters available.

At this small cohort we have analyzed almost 30 variants within different genes (mostly the same variants as for the previous studies were selected) – apolipoprotein E, apolipoprotein C1, apolipoprotein A1 (major protein in HDL particles, cofactor for LCAT, which forms most of the cholesterol esters in plasma; G-75 > A and C83 > T), apolipoprotein A4 (structural component of chylomicrones and HDL particles; Thr347 > Ser and Gln360 > His) apolipoprotein A5, apolipoprotein B (just insertion/deletion within the signal peptide), hepatic lipase (C-480 > T), lipoprotein lipase (Ser447 > Ter), ABCG5 and ABCG8 transporters and finally cholesterol 7 alpha hydroxylase.

Of these analyzed variants, just five significantly influenced individual differences in the decrease of the plasma LDL-cholesterol. Interestingly, in all cases, the possible diet-induced changes were gender-specific [22–25]. According to our study greater profit from the dietary changes will be found in the male carriers of the following alleles (genotypes/haplotypes)

– Trp19 at *APOA5* gene
– C-204C at *CYP7A1* gene
– Gln360Gln + at least one TrpThr347 allele at *APOA4* gene
– Thr400Thr at *ABCG8* gene

In females, just the carriers of the Tyr54 allele within the ABCG8 transporter seem to have a better response to dietary changes.

Under the borderline of the statistical significance remains the apolipoprotein E variant where, in accordance with most of the published results, carriers of the *APOE4* allele seem to profit more from dietary interventions.

Other polymorphisms were not associated with significant changes in lipid parameters.

Again these negative results could be the result of the relatively low number of analyzed individuals and cannot be excluded as a candidates for the future nutrigenetic research.

Conclusions

Genetic polymorphisms within almost 100 genes encoding different proteins have been in the center of our attention for at least 20 years. A substantial part of them was analyzed in an effort to detect the putative association with plasma lipid traits. Apolipoproteins E and A5 genes and their variants belong to the most studied genetic factors in search of the genetic basis of dyslipidemia, and are undoubtedly linked to plasma levels of triacylglycerols and cholesterol. The hepatic lipase promoter is repeatedly associated with HDL-cholesterol not just in our study but also in other studies. Further, our results suggest that also genes for *HMGCoA* reductase, *CYP7A1* and *APOA4* could have some effects of plasma lipid levels of cholesterol and triacylglycerols. In the near future, we will focus on the analysis of the impact of gene – environmental interactions (most importantly, physical activity and dietary habits but also psychosocial factors and alcohol intake seem to be very important factors) on plasma lipids as well as on the detection of the significant gene-gene interactions.

References

1. Talmud PJ, Humphries SE. Genetic polymorphisms, lipoproteins and coronary artery disease risk. Curr Opin Lipidol. 2001;12:405–9.
2. Pullinger CR, Kane JP, Malloy MJ. Primary hypercholesterolemia: genetic causes and treatment of five monogenic disorders. Expert Rev Cardiovasc Ther. 2003;1:107–19.
3. Kathiresan S, Willer CJ, Peloso GM, et al. Common variants at 30 loci contribute to polygenic dyslipidemia. Nat Genet. 2009;41:56–65.
4. Rees A, Shoulders CC, Stocks J, Galton DJ, Baralle FE. DNA polymorphism adjacent tohuman apoprotein A-1 gene: relation to hypertriglyceridemia. Lancet. 1983;26:444–6.
5. Poledne R, Hubáček J, Píša Z, Pistulková H, Valenta Z. Genetic markers in hypercholesterolemic and normocholesterolemic Czech children. Clin Genet. 1994;46:88–91.

6. Hirschhorn JN. Genetic approaches to studying common diseases and complex traits. Pediatr Res. 2005;57(5 Pt 2):74R–7R.
7. Bennet AM, Di Angelantonio E, Ye Z, et al. Association of apolipoprotein E genotypes with lipid levels and coronary risk. JAMA. 2007;298:1300–11.
8. Hubáček JA, Pistulková H, Valenta Z, Poledne R. Repeat polymorphism in the HMG-CoA reductase gene and hypercholesterolemia. VASA. 1999;28:169–71.
9. Hubacek JA, Pistulková H, Škodová Z, Berg K, Poledne R. Association between apolipoprotein B promotor haplotypes and cholesterol status. Ann Clin Biochem. 2001;38:399–400.
10. Hubacek JA, Skodová Z, Lánská V, Adámková V. Apolipoprotein A-V variant (T-1131>C) affects plasma levels of non-high-density lipoprotein cholesterol in Caucasians. Exp Clin Cardiol. 2008;13:129–32.
11. Berg K. Level genes and variability genes in the etiology of hyperlipidemia and atherosclerosis. In: Berg K, Retterstól N, Refsum S, editors. From phenotype to genotype in common disorders. Copenhagen: Munksgaard; 1990. p. 77–91.
12. Phillips CM, Tierney AC, Roche HM. Gene-nutrient interactions in the metabolic syndrome. J Nutrigenet Nutrigenomics. 2008;1:136–51.
13. Hubáček JA, Pistulková H, Valenta Z, Poledne R. The variability gene effect of apo AII repeat polymorphism in high-cholesterolemic children. Med Sci Mon. 1999;5:605–8.
14. "MONICA Project", Manual of operations WHO/ MNC 82.2, 1983.
15. Hubáček JA, Škodová Z, Adámková V, Lánská V, Poledne R. The influence of APOAV polymorphisms (T-1131>C and S19>W) on plasma triglyceride levels and risk of myocardial infarction. Clin Genet. 2004;65:126–30.
16. Pennacchio LA, Olivier M, Hubacek JA, et al. An apolipoprotein influencing triglycerides in humans and mice revealed by comparative sequencing. Science. 2001;294:169–73.
17. Hubacek JA, Skodova Z, Adamkova V, Lanska V, Poledne R. Sex-specific effect of APOAV variant (Val153>Met) on plasma levels of high-density lipoprotein cholesterol. Metabolism. 2005;54:1632–5.
18. Hubáček JA, Bohuslavová R, Škodová Z, Adámková V. Variants vithin the ghrelin gene – association with HDL-cholesterol, but not with body mass index. Folia Biol (Praha). 2007;53:202–6.
19. Vrablik M, Ceska R, Adamkova V, et al. MLXIPL variant in individuals with low and high triglyceridemia in white population in Central Europe. Hum Genet. 2008;124:553–5.
20. Kooner JS, Chambers JC, Aguilar-Salinas CA, et al. Genome wide scan identifies variation in MLXIPL associated with plasma triglycerides. Nat Genet. 2008;40:149–51.
21. Poledne R, Skodová Z. Changes in nutrition, cholesterol concentration, and cardiovascular disease mortality in the Czech population in the past decade. Nutrition. 2000;16:785–6.

22. Hubacek JA, Skodova Z, Adamkova V, Lanska V, Pitha J. APOA5 variant Ser19Trp influences a decrease of the total cholesterol in a male 8 year cohort. Clin Biochem. 2006;39:133–6.

23. Hubacek JA, Bohuslavova R, Skodova Z, Pitha J, Bobkova D, Poledne R. Polymorphisms in the APOA1/C3/A4/A5 gene cluster and cholesterol responsiveness to dietary change. Clin Chem Lab Med. 2007; 45:316–20.

24. Hubacek JA, Berge KE, Štefková J, et al. Polymorphisms in *ABCG5* and *ABCG8* transporters and plasma cholesterol levels. Physiol Res. 2004;53:395–401.

25. Hubacek JA, Pitha J, Skodova Z, et al. Polymorphisms in CYP-7A1, not APOE, influence the change in plasma lipids in response to population dietary change in an 8 year follow-up; results from the Czech MONICA study. Clin Biochem. 2003;36:263–7.

Part V

Hypertension and Arrhythmias

Genetic Basis of Salt-Sensitive Hypertension in Humans

Frans H.H. Leenen, Md. Shahrier Amin,
Alexandre F.R. Stewart, and Frederique Tesson

Abstract

The genetic network responsible for blood pressure (BP) variation in the general population and specifically the hypertensive population remains elusive. Several recent genome-wide association studies (GWAS) have identified and confirmed loci associated with BP and hypertension. However, only a small fraction of the trait is currently explained. This apparent deficit relative to the estimates for heritability can be due to several factors, a major one being the poor assessment of the phenotype, i.e. BP. All GWAS have used so far office BPs, which are notoriously variable. Imputation of BP in treated subjects is done by a fixed number. In addition, BPs are usually being "adjusted" for e.g. age, gender or body mass index under the assumption that these do not alter BP systematically by genotype, an assumption that appears no longer valid.

A better approach may include more specific assessment of the actual BP level in a given individual for both cases and controls, preferably by 24-h ambulatory BP monitoring, for cases off antihypertensive therapy, and to stratify for factors such as sex, age and body mass index. This approach will likely provide better insight into the distinct genetic architectures contributing to different hypertension phenotypes and explain a substantially larger part of the BP variance. Further improvements will likely emerge when other environmental/lifestyle factors are incorporated, such as extent of alcohol intake, stress, salt intake or physical activity. In the ongoing Ottawa GWAS for BP response to salt, we hope to identify loci and genes associated with salt-sensitive versus salt-resistant hypertension.

Keywords

Blood pressure phenotypes • Candidates genes • Dietary salt • Genetics • Genome-wide association studies • Heritability • Hypertension • Salt resistance • Salt sensitivity • 24-h ambulatory blood pressure monitoring

F.H.H. Leenen (✉)
University of Ottawa Heart Institute,
Ottawa, ON, Canada
e-mail: fleenen@ottawaheart.ca

B. Ostadal et al. (eds.), *Genes and Cardiovascular Function*,
DOI 10.1007/978-1-4419-7207-1_16, © Springer Science+Business Media, LLC 2011

Introduction

Primary or essential hypertension affects 20–30% of the adult population in North America [1, 2], and represents a major risk factor for cardiovascular morbidity and mortality. There is a significant genetic contribution in the susceptibility to hypertension. Estimates for heritability – the proportion of variance in a trait that can be attributed to genetic variance – of systolic blood pressure (BP) range from 0.18 in the general population, 0.19–0.45 within families, 0.74 in young adult twins [3–5] to 0.80 in hypertensive adolescents with a family history of hypertension [6]. As will be reviewed in the next section, in spite of numerous studies the genetic network responsible for BP variation in the general population and specifically in the hypertensive population remains elusive.

Genome Scans for Essential Hypertension

A number of genetic linkage analyses have been performed in different populations around the world. Studies have used different sets of markers for genotyping and most were widely spaced (average inter-marker distance ~5–10 cm) which will miss variations in intermediate chromosomal segments. In the Family BP Program, the results from four individual studies incorporating >6,000 individuals of multiple ethnic origins were analyzed. In Whites with hypertension, high linkage was found on 2p11, 3p14, 14q32 and 16q12 for systolic BP and 3p14, 9q31, 14q32 and 16q12 for diastolic BP [7]. Interestingly, genetic linkage to BP has been weak in the larger studies for Caucasians, but strong when performed in small, possibly more homogeneous, populations (Framingham study – 17q; Dutch – 4p; Icelandic – 18q; Sardinian – 2p). Genome scan meta-analysis of nine studies in Caucasians demonstrated significant linkage to 2p12–q22.1 and 3p14.1–q172.3 loci [8]. The detection of BP alleles by genome-wide scans may also depend on their age. A hypertension allele that originated 100,000 years ago would by now be ubiquitous across the populations, making

its detection unlikely. For example, the aldosterone synthase (8q21) alleles C-344 and T-344 exist at an equal frequency in Caucasians (T/C ~0.53/0.47), TT homozygotes showing a 1.45 times higher risk of hypertension in Caucasians [9]. However, none of the linkage analyses showed significant linkage to this locus. On the other hand, regions with a significant impact might be found in a small population if the genes have emerged recently.

Linkage analysis, however, is best suited for monogenic disorders in which genes are more highly deterministic, with a major gene contribution and a minimum environmental contribution. Association studies are considered to be statistically more powerful than linkage analysis for complex traits.

The Wellcome Trust Case Control Consortium (WTCCC) study was the first attempt to identify SNPs associated with essential hypertension using a genome-wide association (GWA) approach [10]. The Affymetrix GeneChip 500 K Mapping Array Set was used. This study identified several loci for six common diseases but failed to spot one for hypertension [10]. The same year, the Framingham Heart Study was also negative for hypertension but the SNP density was low (~70,000) and probably insufficient to tag enough linkage disequilibrium blocks [11]. However, since the beginning of 2009, eight studies have yielded positive results in different populations including Caucasian [12–14], African-American [15] and Asian [16, 17] populations (Table 1). A few identified loci were reproducible; for example, eight loci associated with BP were found in both the Global BPgen and the CHARGE studies [12, 13]. Four were also associated with BP and hypertension in the Korean population [18] and two among Han Chinese [19]. Some genetic variations associated with BP and/or hypertension were located within genes making those genes sound as candidate genes [20, 21]. However, only a few of these polymorphisms have so far been associated with a function. A SNP associated with BP and located within an intronic conserved element of the STK39 gene has been shown to influence the expression of STK39 in vitro [22, 23].

Table 1 Most significant GWA findings with BP and hypertension phenotypes

Study population	Phenotyping	Major findings
The Wellcome Trust Case Control Consortium • 2,000 cases/3,000 non-phenotyped controls from Great Britain with Caucasian ancestry	History of hypertension diagnosed before 60 year of age, BP the mean of 1–3 BP recordings (BP not imputed for treatment)	Negative study
Framingham Heart Study 100 K Project • 1,260 subjects	For most subjects, BP the mean of 2 recordings (BP imputed for treatment)	Negative study
NFBC1966. 4,730 subjects with European ancestry	BP the mean of 2 recordings (BP not imputed for treatment)	Negative study
Global BPGen • 34,433 subjects with European ancestry	BP the mean of 2–4 recordings (BP imputed for treatment)	rs17367504 (CR1) and SBP rs11191548 (CR10) and SBP rs12946454 (CR17) and SBP ^a***rs16998073 (CR4) and DBP*** rs1530440 (CR10) and DBP rs653178 (CR12) and DBP rs1378942 (CR15) and DBP rs16948048 (CR17) and DBP
CHARGE • 29,136 subjects with European ancestry	BP the mean of 2 recordings (BP imputed for treatment)	rs1004467 (CR10) and SBP rs381815 (CR11) and SBP ^a***rs2681492 (CR12) and SBP*** ^a***rs2681472 (CR12) and DBP § HT*** ^a***rs3184504 (CR12) and SBP and DBP*** rs9815354 (CR3) and DBP rs11014166 (CR10) and DBP rs2384550 (CR12) and DBP rs6495122 (CR15) and DBP
KORA/HYPEST • 1,977 subjects with European ancestry	BP the mean of 2 recordings, subjects did not receive BP lowering medication	rs12153297 (CR5) and SBP rs11646213 (CR16) and HT
HUFS • 1,017 American subjects with African ancestry	BP the mean of 2 recordings (BP not imputed for treatment)	rs5743185 (CR2) and SBP rs16877320 (CR6) and SBP rs17365948 (CR8) and SBP rs12279202 (CR11) and SBP rs11160059 (CR14) and SBP

HT Hypertension
^aReplicated in another population

However, a replication study did not confirm the association of this SNP with BP [23]. A recent study looked at the association of 1,180 non-synonymous SNPs with systolic BP and hypertensive status [24]. Two SNPs, one in the arginine decarboxylase and another in the phospholipase D2 genes, were associated with both systolic BP and hypertension [24]. However, altogether, only a fraction of the trait (1–3%) is currently explained by haplotype-tagging SNPs [25].

Structural variations, such as CNVs, have been more recently characterized. CNVs are common in the human genome [26] and might alter gene dosage, disrupt coding sequences, or perturb long-range gene regulation [27]. SNPs and CNVs have been shown to capture 83.6% and 17.7% of the total detected genetic variation in gene expression, respectively [28]. The signals from the two types of variations have little overlap [28]. Therefore, both types of variants should be tested. So far, very few studies have explored the potential association of CNVs with BP/hypertension phenotypes [29, 30]. One of them found an association between a CNV and endothelin-1 expression [29].

Evaluation of Candidate Genes for Essential Hypertension

Loci suggested from a genome scan need to be further verified both by increasing the number of markers and assessing their physiological roles. Evaluation of candidate genes is therefore essential to investigate the effects of variants in relation to presence or absence of hypertension or more preferably to BP as a continuous variable. To date >150 genes have been studied for possible association with BP. We will only provide a brief summary of the main studies focusing on genes of possible interest for salt-sensitive hypertension particularly in Caucasians.

Single variants: A number of studies evaluated candidate genes in the RAAS, the sympathetic nervous system and relevant ion channels. Some variants in each category show major ethnic variability. The difference in frequency between normotensive and hypertensive populations is usually modest. Among the RAAS components that have been most widely studied, a meta-analysis for the angiotensinogen (*AGT*) M235T polymorphism including 45,267 subjects showed a stepwise increase in angiotensinogen levels and increased risk of hypertension by 8% in MT and 19% in TT homozygote Caucasians [31]. Homozygosity for the T allele of C-344T in aldosterone synthase promoter conferred a ~1.45 fold higher risk of hypertension in Caucasians [9]. A Mineralocorticoid Receptor gene variant showed marked protection [32], but this has not yet been reproduced. For other RAAS components (*ACE, AGTR1, AGTR2*) association has been weak or not always reproducible. In the sympathetic nervous system, variants contributing to hypertension have been identified in almost all steps. Most of these variants impart mild (<2 mmHg difference between groups) to moderate (2–6 mmHg difference) effects. Many ion channel mutations are causes of rare Mendelian forms of hypertension or hypotension. Recent studies showed that many common and rare variants of genes involved in sodium transport are present in the general population and loss-of-function mutation carriers exhibit lower BP [33]. The large number and diverse types of channels in neurons still need to be evaluated. Interestingly, variants of cytoskeletal components such as adducin, that might modulate ion channel activity have shown fairly consistent association with BP in different populations. The alpha adducin G460W substitution was found to be an important risk factor for hypertension in Caucasians [34, 35]. Variants of ion channel regulatory or interacting proteins have also been identified, and linked to greater change in BP over time.

Haplotypes: For several genes non-significant effects of individual variants attained significance when studied with co-inherited variants. In White siblings that shared two microsatellite marker alleles in chromosome 16p12 including the epithelial sodium channel (ENaC) β and γ subunits genes, the difference in systolic BP was half (7 mmHg) of those that did not share any alleles (14 mmHg) [36]. The estimated frequency of the *SCNN1G* haplotype (rs13331086, rs11074553, and rs4299163) was substantially greater in subjects with high (13.3%) than low (0.6%) systolic BP [37]. Homozygosity for the intron 6CC and exon 8CC/TT of the serum/glucocorticoid regulated kinase 1 gene (*SGK1*) compared to other genotypes was found to be responsible for 4/2 mmHg higher BP as well as a greater increase in BP [2.1/0.8 vs 1.6/0.4 mmHg/year] over a mean follow-up period of ~11 years [38]. In the same cohort, individuals with the *NEDD4L* haplotype (rs4149601GG + rs2288774 CC/CT) had 0.8/0.7 mmHg higher BP as well as greater increase in BP [1.7/0.4 vs 1.5/0.3 mmHg/year] [39]. Furthermore, multiple rare and common *WNK1* variants in haplotypes can contribute substantially to BP variation and hypertension [40, 41].

Gene-gene interactions: Few studies have assessed the effect of co-inherited mutations in different genes on BP. Genetic combinations might increase the risk of hypertension, nullify each other's effects or be protective and contribute to resistance to hypertension. For example carriers of the MM(*AGT*), AA(*AGTR1*), CC(*CYP11B2*), DD/ID(*ACE*) combination were found to have a substantially higher probability of being hypertensive [42]. In a cohort of 226 Chinese parents and 253 of their offsprings, synergism was noted for *ADD1* Trp and *ACE* I/D genotypes: 9.3 mmHg higher systolic BP in (*ADD1* TrpTrp+*ACE* DD) versus (*ADD1* TrpTrp+*ACE* II) [43]. Clear synergism for the *ADD1* variant and variants in other genes such as *ADD3*, *NEDD4L*, *WNK1* and AS have also been reported [34].

Assessment of Hypertensive Phenotype

Association studies indicate the possible contribution of a number of loci and genes to higher BP, but so far only a small fraction of the trait can be explained. Several factors may contribute to this apparent deficit relative to the estimates for heritability. A major factor may be the rather poor assessment of the phenotype, i.e. BP, particularly in the GWAS. In all GWAS, the BP was only quantified by office measurements (see Table 1). Even if measured properly, these BP values are notoriously variable and considering BP as a quantitative trait can markedly differ from the actual BP for a given individual. When considering BP as a qualitative trait (i.e. presence vs. absence of hypertension), office BP can readily lead to misdiagnosis, i.e. over-diagnosis ("white-coat hypertension"), or under-diagnosis ("masked hypertension"), and lead to high percentage of false positives or false negatives in cases and controls [44, 45]. No GWAS has so far employed the current gold standard for assessment of BP: 24 h ambulatory BP monitoring (ABPM).

A second confounder relates to the different approaches used to deal with the impact of antihypertensive drug therapy on BP in GWAS (Table 1). Tobin et al. [46] and Cui et al. [47] reviewed why some approaches are fundamentally

flawed. These include ignoring the problem altogether and analyzing observed BP in treated subjects as if it were underlying BP, or excluding treated subjects from the analysis. In studies evaluating BP as a quantitative trait, no appropriate correction for use of antihypertensive therapy can lead to substantial shrinkage in the estimated effect of the genetic determinants of BP as well as a marked reduction in statistical power. Correction relies upon imputation in treated subjects of the underlying BP from the observed BP. Newton-Cheh et al. [12] for the Global BP Gen consortium imputed BPs by adding 15 and 10 mmHg for systolic and diastolic BP. Levy et al. [13] for the CHARGE consortium added 10 and 5 mmHg to observed systolic and diastolic BPs. To account for the number of drugs, Cui et al. [47] proposed stepped increments of 8/4, 14/10 and 20/16 mmHg to the measured BPs of treated subjects taking 1, 2 and ≥ 3 drug classes. This appears to be a better approach rather than adding a fixed number irrespective of the intensity of antihypertensive therapy. However, none of these approaches take into account the marked inter-individual variability in BP responses to antihypertensive therapy. Figure 1 is an example of this large variability in BP response, in this particular study to hydrochlorothiazide. In addition, this study highlights that a major part of this variability can depend on the genetic background of the individual, in this study variants in three genes involved in sodium transport [34]. These variants may not only influence the antihypertensive response to the thiazide diuretic, but also may contribute to salt-sensitive increases in BP [34]. Imputing all treated BPs by adding a fixed number clearly would cause substantial shrinkage if not disappearance of the effect-size of these variants.

A third confounder relates to the presence of hypertension in controls for case control studies. Using an unphenotyped control sample from the general population may save resources [10], but clearly causes misclassification. According to the authors of the WTCC "the effect this has on power is modest unless the extent of misclassification bias is substantial: for example, if 5% of controls would meet the definition of cases as the

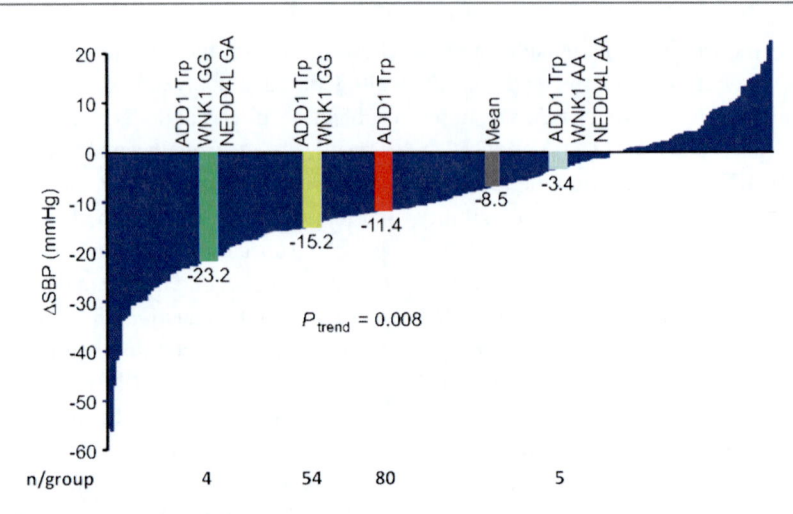

Fig. 1 Change in systolic BP after 1 month of treatment with hydrochlorothiazide (12.5 mg/day) in 193 hypertensive subjects. Mean decrease in BP −8.5 mmHg; −11.2 mmHg in carriers of the *ADD1*Trp allele (n=80); −15.2 mmHg in carriers of *ADD1*Trp and *WNK1*GG alleles (n=54); −23.2 mmHg in carriers of *ADD1*Trp, *WNK1*GG and *NEDD4L*G alleles (n=4), and only −3.4 mmHg in carriers of *ADD1*Trp with *WNK1*AA and *NEDD4L*AA alleles (n=5) (Reproduced from [34] with permission, Licence to publish # 2550841260089)

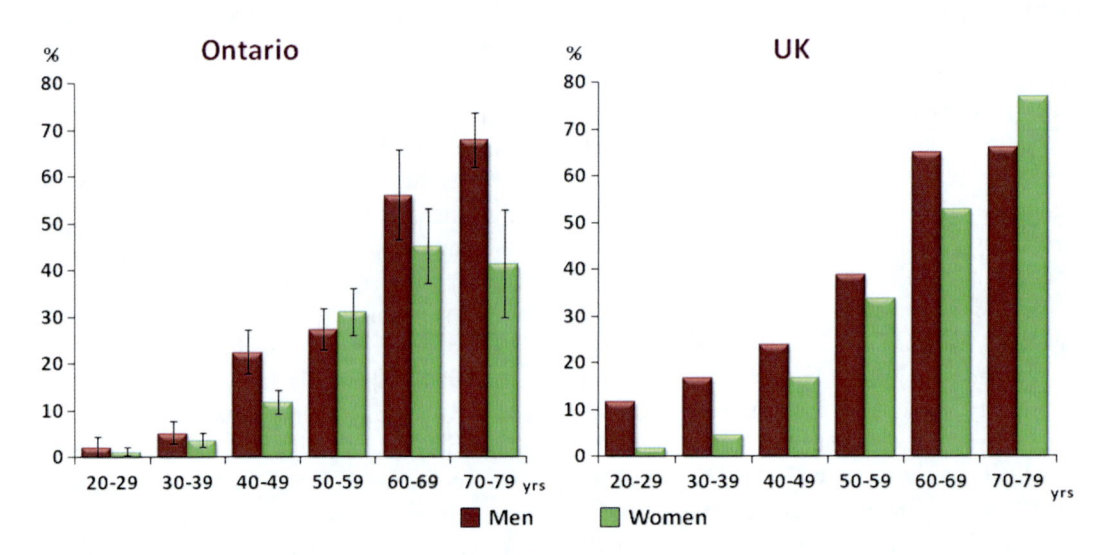

Fig. 2 Prevalence of hypertension in Ontario, Canada and in England by age and sex (Data derived from [2, 48])

same age, the loss of power is approximately the same as that due to a reduction of the sample size by 10%" [10]. Using a non-phenotyped control population may indeed be a valid approach for many diseases that are relatively rare in the general population, but not for hypertension. Figure 2 shows the increasing prevalence of hypertension by age, reaching up to 30–40% in the 50–59 year age-group, and 50–60% above 60 years of age [2, 48]. Zhang et al. [49] recently re-estimated

the power for the WTCC hypertension case control study and estimated that the statistical power was likely minimal. In late onset diseases such as hypertension, additional ambiguity will arise when individuals with putative variant alleles develop hypertension later in life. Are these young individuals "controls"?

Taking the above three issues all together, we propose as a more optimal strategy to minimize misclassification bias that (a) 24-h ABPM be performed in both cases and controls; (b) antihypertensive therapy be discontinued for a short period if possible at all, and (c) controls not being age-matched, but rather selected from the older (>65–70 years), normotensive population, who less likely may still develop genetically determined hypertension. This approach will provide a more specific assessment of the actual BP level in a given individual, thereby providing a more accurate, and likely larger, effect-size of the genetic determinants of BP variation in the population. This approach will likely also provide higher explanatory power for the heritability of hypertension and, a closer step toward the understanding of the underlying genetic architecture.

Genotype by Environment Interactions

Whereas proper assessment of the BP phenotype appears an essential step toward understanding of the underlying genotype, there are a variety of factors which modulate this relationship. These factors are often ignored, as stated by Clark et al. [50]: "Despite a plethora of editorials and perspectives that expound on its importance, most studies make an early and prominent assumption that no genotype – environment interactions exist." Alternatively, BPs are being "adjusted" for parameters such as age, gender or body mass index [12, 13] under the assumption that these do not alter BP systematically by genotype. This assumption appears no longer valid. Shi et al. [51] re-evaluated the genome-wide linkage analysis of hypertensive siblings conducted by the HyperGEN study for gene-age interaction using a newly developed variance components method that incorporates age variation in genetic effects. Substantially improved linkage evidence, in terms of both the number of linkage peaks and their significance levels, was observed. Gene-gender interactions have been demonstrated as well. Rana et al. [52] reported gender-specific effects of single nucleotide polymorphisms (SNPs), haplotypes, and gene-by-gene interactions that determine BP in white Americans. In females, polymorphisms in beta-1 and alpha-2A

adrenergic receptor genes contributed to BP, whereas in men, polymorphisms in beta-2 adrenergic receptor and angiotensinogen genes were associated. Such sex-specific association may still show up in a traditional, sex-adjusted analysis. However, associations may also go in the opposite direction. Seda et al. [53] reported that in male French Canadians rs575121 GG homozygotes had the highest systolic BP (131 ± 4 mmHg) but the same allele in women was associated with the lowest BP (113 ± 4 mmHg). Different genetic variants may also contribute to hypertension relative to weight. Söber et al. [54] reanalyzed the discovery sample KORA S3 together with the replication samples stratified by weight. For the top 2 SNPs of this study, rs11195419 (*ADRA2A*) contributed to BP levels only among overweight subjects, whereas rs10889553 (*LEPR*) did only among normal-weight subjects. Some gene variants may contribute to increasing BP dependently or independently (e.g. *FTO*) of their effects on weight [55, 56].

Altogether, it appears that in order to truly understand the distinct genetic architectures contributing to the different hypertension phenotypes, existing GWAS should be re-analyzed after stratification by factors such as sex, body composition parameters and age. One may anticipate identification of distinct genotypes with likely large effect sizes. If future studies also include more precise assessment of actual BP levels, the cumulative effect of identified loci may explain a substantially larger part of the BP variance than the current 1–3%.

Further improvements will likely emerge when other environmental/lifestyle factors are incorporated, such as extent of alcohol intake, stress, salt intake, physical activity.

Genes and Salt-Dependent Hypertension

Among the many variables affecting BP, high sodium intake has a significant influence on BP and the increase in BP with age. Findings from the European Project on Genes in Hypertension (EPOGH) indicate that the phenotype-genotype

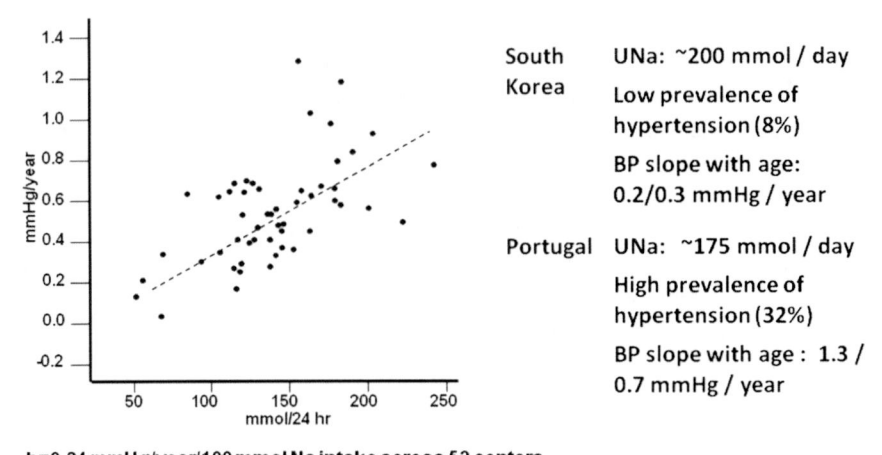

Fig. 3 Age-related increase in systolic BP relative to dietary salt intake across different populations in Intersalt (Data derived from [59])

relations strongly depend on host factors such as salt intake [57]. Indeed, in a Chinese population (n = 1,906) the estimate for heritability of systolic BP was 0.31 on regular dietary salt intake, and increased to 0.49 under low sodium intake [58]. Salt-sensitivity of BP has not yet been used in a genome scan to identify variants contributing to higher BP on high salt intake.

Salt and BP: In both INTERSALT and WHO-CARDIAC – two large multi-center cross-sectional studies, sodium intake was found to affect BP in most parts of the world. In INTERSALT [59] a significant linear relation was found between 24-h urinary sodium excretion and slope of systolic BP with age (0.3 mmHg/year/100 mmol Na) and diastolic BP (0.2 mmHg/year/100 mmol Na) across all populations in 52 centers (Fig. 3). When analyzed within individual centers, a significant positive coefficient for sodium and BP was found in 8 (3–8 mmHg systolic BP/100 mmol Na) and 3 (~4 mmHg diastolic BP/100 mmol Na) centers, while a negative coefficient was noted in 2 (−3 to −6 mmHg systolic BP/100 mmol Na) and 3 (−3 to −4 mmHg diastolic BP/100 mmol Na) centers. Similar differences were also present in populations in WHO-CARDIAC [60].

Assessment of salt-sensitivity: Several measures have been used to assess the BP response to salt – ranging from high versus low salt intake per se

to volume/saline loading and salt depletion with diuretics. These methods do not address the same mechanisms and the latter can misclassify as many as 50% of individuals by activating the sympathetic nervous and renin angiotensin systems [61]. Office versus ambulatory BP also classifies different sets of patients as salt-sensitive (SS) or salt-resistant (SR) [62] with the latter giving better estimates [62–64]. Meta analyses of lifestyle interventions showed that decreasing sodium intake by 70–100 mmol/day decreases BP by about 3–4/2–3 mmHg in hypertensives and by only 1/0.5 mmHg in normotensives [e.g. 65]. INTERSALT and controlled trials of low versus high salt diet [59, 62, 66] indicate the presence of several phenotypes – SS, SR and counterregulators, but overall the BP response to salt appears to be normally distributed (Fig. 4). The correlation coefficient for difference in BP between periods of regular versus low salt intake in Whites ranged from ~0.25 (parent offspring), to ~0.50 (sib-sib) and ~0.7 (twin-twin) [Ref 67].

Age and SS: The BP response to salt intake can be seen at all ages but prevalence of SS increases in older age groups. Hurwitz et al. [68] demonstrated that there is an increment of 2.4 mmHg to the SS component of systolic BP for each decade of age. Analysis of data involving 47,000 individuals from 24 communities showed that the

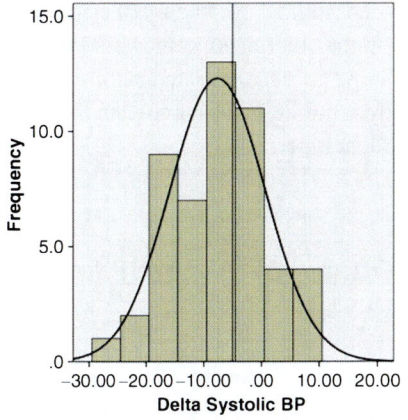

		Mean	SE	
Salt	**LS**	68	± 9.7	**mmol Na⁺/ 24 hr**
Resistant	**HS**	347	± 17.0	
(n=19)	**Delta**	0.8	± 1.0	**mmHg**
37%	**SBP**			
Salt	**LS**	82	± 6.9	**mmol Na⁺/ 24 hr**
Sensitive	**HS**	332	± 16.0	
(n=32)	**Delta**	−12.6 ± 1.0		**mmHg**
63%	**SBP**			

Fig. 4 Difference in day systolic BP on 24-h ambulatory BP monitoring after 3 weeks of high (~300 mmol/day) or low (~100 mmol/day) salt diet in subjects with mild hypertension. Average decrease in systolic BP: −7.8±1.2 mmHg. Salt-sensitivity was defined as a decrease in systolic BP≥5 mmHg on low vs high salt diet. (Leenen et al. unpublished data)

decrease in both systolic BP and diastolic BP in response to sodium restriction is positively related to age. The decreases in BP with 100 mmol/day reduction in sodium intake increase from 5.0/1.8 mmHg at 10–19 years to 10.3/4.3 mmHg at 60–69 years [68]. Reductions in BP varied from 5.3 mmHg in individuals <45 years to 7.5 mmHg in those >45 years. The mechanisms responsible for this increase in salt sensitivity of BP with age have not yet been determined, but less reactive increase in renin release with ageing likely plays a major role.

Gender and SS: Both epidemiological observations and controlled trials show a clear gender difference in the BP response to salt [69]. In premenopausal females, estrogens appear to blunt the effect of high salt on BP [70]. Exacerbated hypertension develops in ovariectomized mRen [2] Lewis rats on high salt diet [71]. Otherwise healthy women previously classified as being SR were found to become SS following surgical menopause [72], whereas transdermal 17β-estradiol reduces salt sensitivity in post-menopausal women [73].

Candidate gene studies for salt-sensitive hypertension: Based on studies in animal models of SS hypertension and human monogenic forms, candidate genes have been studied for possible association with SS in case-control and sib-pair analyses. However, there is a paucity of

such studies and most are limited in sample size. In larger samples from the general population, assessment of SS and the relationship to genotype has been limited to casual measurements of BP, urinary sodium (U_{Na}), or questionnaires on average food intake. The lack of universal definition of SS and use of different strategies to classify individuals makes comparisons difficult. Short cross-over trials (<2 weeks on each diet) may also underestimate the actual effect [66]. In a 2004 review, Beeks et al. [74] found only 28 potential studies that assessed genetic contribution to SS by some intervention, of which only 23 provided sufficient details. Moreover, of these 23 only 15 assessed effects of dietary salt. A pooled analysis could not be performed due to heterogeneity in methods. Since this review, only 4 more studies were reported, 1 in Chinese, 1 in Japanese and 2 in Caucasian populations.

Studies of single variants and haplotypes: Among the studies reviewed by Beeks et al. [74] only the α-adducin G460W and *HSD11B2* G534A and CA repeat variants showed reproducible positive association to SS in different populations. Homozygosity for the ADD1 WW was associated with ~two-fold greater response to sodium versus ADD1 G carriers. ADD1 WW is also associated with higher serum ouabain levels and higher increments of BP (2.2/1.4 mmHg per

50 mmol increase in U_{Na}) in carriers taking a high salt diet [75]. Contrary to association studies in essential hypertension, both positive and negative associations with SS were noted for *GNB3* C825T, *ACE* I/D and *AGT* M235T. In whites, mostly negative associations were found for *AGTR1* A1166C, *CYP11B2* C344T, and *SCNN1G* intron 2 conversion polymorphism. In Whites, the G protein-coupled receptor kinase 4 (*GRK4*) 486 V was associated with lower BP (~4.6 mmHg vs A486) [76]. In Japanese hypertensives (n = 83), the increase in BP with change in salt intake from ~50 to ~340 mmol/day varied according to the number of *GRK4* variant alleles: 25 subjects with none were all salt-resistant whereas the 29 subjects with ≥ 3 alleles were all salt-sensitive [77]. In a cohort of 171 hypertensive and 48 normotensive White individuals the *ADRB2* genotype was not associated with hypertension, but the difference in MAP between periods of low and high salt intake was higher for 46AA [16.5 mmHg] and 79CC [13.6 mmHg] homozygotes and individuals with the 46AA/79CC diplotype [16.5 mmHg] compared to 10.4 mmHg in the other genotypes [78]. *WNK1* or *KCNJ1* have not yet been studied.

Gene-gene interactions in salt-sensitive hypertension: Few studies assessed the simultaneous effect of several candidate genes on SS of BP. In a cohort of Spanish essential hypertensive patients, the II allele of *ACE* was found to be significantly associated with SS (odds ratio 2.23, 95% CI 1.34–3.71) and 9.8 mmHg increase in 24-h systolic BP on high salt in II vs 1.2 mmHg in DD [79]. However, no associations or interactions were found with *AGTR1* and *AGT*. In contrast, clear interactions were reported for *ADD1*, *WNK1* and *NEDD4L* variants and the change in systolic BP in response to a 2 h i.v. Na load in 341 Caucasian hypertensives, in a pattern opposite to the BP response to diuretic therapy [34]. It remains to be assessed whether the BP response to dietary salt follows this pattern.

In summary, little is known so far about the genes that are responsible for salt-sensitive hypertension. Most candidate genes associated with essential hypertension or changes in BP over time have shown little relation to SS or have not yet

been studied for their effect on salt sensitivity. On the other hand, some genes that have not been found to be associated with essential hypertension might have significant impact on the SS phenotype.

Ottawa GWAS for BP Response to Salt

There have been no GWAS in humans assessing the genetic contribution to salt sensitivity of BP. Genes that are responsible for imparting salt resistance have so far been largely ignored. Given the fact that the genetic constitution of the body is evolutionarily programmed to preserve salt within a narrow physiological range (intake < 50–100 mmol/day) and high salt in the diet has been a relatively recent introduction [74], emergence of SR genes appears to be a more recent event that might be detected more easily than SS genes which are probably more ancient in origin. Indeed, it is likely that the five-fold greater salt intake in the average Western diet would have naturally predisposed everyone to chronic elevation of BP had it not been due to the emergence of yet to be identified salt resistant genes. In a few populations, such as the indigenous Kuna of Panama, there is primary evidence that the protective factor is genetic rather than environmental. In this population, the low prevalence of hypertension and age-related rise in BP do not change significantly following migration to an urban environment and an increased salt intake [80].

The aim of the Ottawa GWAS is to identify novel genes that might be responsible for BP response to salt by performing GWA studies of subjects with essential hypertension of Caucasian origin from Eastern Ontario and Western Quebec. This population is not genetically homogeneous, and is a fair representation of the diversity seen in many parts of Canada. In order to enrich for risk alleles, individuals from families with a history of early onset hypertension will be chosen. The subjects will be carefully phenotyped for BP responses to high vs. low salt intake using 24-h ABPM. We propose a two-phase GWAS using both the Affymetrix Genome-Wide Human SNP Array 6.0 and the Affymetrix Axiom Genome-Wide Human Array. The Affymetrix Genome-Wide Human SNP Array 6.0 presents advantages of featuring 1.8 million genetic markers, including more than 906,600 SNPs and more than 946,000 probes for the detection of CNVs. On the more recent Affimetrix Axiom array, genotyping accuracy, haplotype coverage, and inter-plate variation have been improved as compared to the 6.0 arrays and allow the exclusive genotyping of SNPs specific for the European ancestry (Caucasian) population. However, the Axiom arrays do not provide CNV information because of the nature of the reaction, a hybridization followed by single nucleotide chain termination at the polymorphism. In contrast, the 6.0 arrays rely on hybridization to generate the primary signal and have over 946,000 non-polymorphic CNV probes covering the entire genome. The two methods are only partially redundant (only ~150,000 SNPs are common to the two arrays).

The GWAS has two major goals:

1. To identify genetic variants associated with SS versus SR hypertension by performing the first GWAS for salt sensitivity/resistance of hypertensive subjects (Phase I).

2. To identify/confirm genetic variants associated with hypertension/salt sensitivity by performing the first GWAS of younger (< 60 years of age) hypertensives compared to older (> 65 years of age) normotensive controls, whose BP status is confirmed by 24-h Ambulatory BP Monitoring (Phase II).

For the phase I population, healthy Caucasian males and post-menopausal women between 20 and 60 years of age are eligible, if they have a family history for early onset hypertension defined as ≥ 1 family member who developed persistent hypertension before 60 years of age, and have a resting BP $\geq 130/85$ and $\leq 160/100$ mmHg after stopping antihypertensive drug therapy for 2 weeks. To exclude subjects with white-coat hypertension, (pre)–hypertension needs to be present on the day-time BP on 24-h ABPM. Eligible subjects are randomized to a 3-week period of either low or high salt intake, and then cross-over to the alternative level of salt intake.

Current levels of salt intake are being assessed by food questionnaire and 24-h urine collection. For the low salt period, subjects receive personalized instructions how to lower their salt intake to ~100 mmol Na^+/day over a 1–2 week run in period. At the end, a second 24-h urine collection is done to ensure that the target is reached. If still > 130 mmol/day, then more instructions are given to further low salt intake, how salt diet is then maintained for 3 weeks. For the high salt period, subjects take a sodium supplement of up to 200 mmol/day to achieve a high salt diet of ~300 mmol/day. The supplement is gradually increased to diminish the chance of adverse GI side-effects. "Double-blinding" with placebo is of little value, since subjects will taste the salt. Instead, the study is single-blind, i.e. all measurements are done blinded for the level of salt intake. At the end of each 3-week period specific assessment include: 24-h urine collection to confirm target levels of sodium intake, BP in the office and by 24-h ABPM and blood sampling for assessment of explanatory variables such as parameters of the circulatory RAAS, plasma catecholamines and endogenous Na^+, K^+-ATPase inhibitors, "ouabain" and marinobufagenin.

The sample size requirement for Phase 1 of the study was calculated based on the quantitative trait change of systolic BP. Following the principles of sample size recalculation within an ongoing clinical trial [81, 82], the sample size needed was updated based on the hypertensive patients recruited having a standard deviation of 9.6 for systolic BP in place of the general initial estimate of 11.5 . Recalculating the sample size based on an additive genetic model, a minor allele frequency of 0.20, a minimal clinically important difference is the systolic BP change of 5.0 mmHg and the standard deviation of 9.6, a sample size of 230 patients will allow us to detect the systolic BP change of at least 5.0 mmHg with a level of significance of 0.001 and power of 90%.

SNPs identified to associate with salt sensitivity or resistance will be examined further in a phase II independent population of 1,500 hypertensive individuals compared to 1,500 older normotensive controls. Salt induced increases in BP occur in more than 50% of hypertensives, but in fewer than 10% of normotensive controls [66, 68, 83, 84]. Thus, the phase II population using cohorts enriched for individuals sensitive to salt (hypertensive) versus those resistant to salt (normotensive) will permit replication of SNPs identified in the phase I population. The same inclusion criteria apply as described for the Phase I Population. For the purpose of this study, for the control population normotensive is defined as an average day $BP \leq 130/80$ mmHg on 24-h ABPM. Older (>65 years) normotensive subjects are collected as controls to minimize the possibility of phenotypic misclassification. After discontinuation of antihypertensive drug therapy for 1–2 weeks, subjects meeting the in- and exclusion criteria have the following measurements: level of salt intake by 24-h urine collection, office BP and 24-h ABPM.

We will repeat GWA using both arrays, seeking to replicate variations for salt-sensitive hypertension in the case control phase II population. In Phase II, only variations showing an association with a p value of <0.0001 will be considered significant (after correction for false discovery rate). This Phase II population also provides an opportunity to replicate BP loci identified in previous GWAS.

For the second independent population of Phase II, which is used to ascertain replication of the initial loci showing associations with the systolic BP change in a case control study, a sample size of 1,500 cases and 1,500 controls is needed. This is based on an additive genetic model to detect an odds ratio of 1.5, for a minor allele frequency of 0.15, a level of significance of 0.00001 and power of 90%. The difference in genotype frequencies between cases and controls will be considered significant at $p < 0.00001$ for each SNP.

Conclusions

From a public health perspective, high salt intake has a clear effect on BP and thereby cardiovascular morbidity and mortality. Lowering the amount of salt added to foods is an important public health strategy. From an individual perspective, the impact of high salt intake on his/her cardiovascular system can vary from minimal to substantial and appears to a large extent to be genetically determined. Genetic diagnosis would be an ideal method of choice to advice life-style interventions for a particular individual. Studies performing careful assessment of phenotype and genotypes are essential to achieve this goal and, in addition, will very likely provide important new insights into novel mechanisms contributing to salt sensitivity or resistance of BP.

Acknowledgments The authors would like to acknowledge Mrs. Danielle Oja for her excellent skills in assisting in the preparation and formatting of the chapter.

The authors' research discussed in this chapter is being supported by operating grants from the Canadian Institutes of Health Research.

Frans H. H. Leenen is supported by the Pfizer Chair in Hypertension Research, an Endowed Chair supported by Pfizer Canada, University of Ottawa Heart Institute Foundation and the Canadian Institutes of Health Research.

References

1. Ong KL, Cheung BMY, Man YB, et al. Prevalence, awareness, treatment, and control of hypertension among United Stated adults 1999–2004. Hypertension. 2006;46:69–75.
2. Leenen FH, Dumais J, McInnis NH, et al. Results of the Ontario survey on the prevalence and control of hypertension. CMAJ. 2008;178:1441–9.
3. van Rijn MJE, Schut AFFC, Aulchenko YS, et al. Heritability of blood pressure traits and the genetic contribution to blood pressure variance explained by four blood-pressure-related genes. J Hypertens. 2007; 25:565–70.
4. Saunder CL, Gulliford MC. Heritabilities and shared environmental effects were estimated from household clustering in national health survey data. J Clin Epidemiology. 2006;59:1191–8.
5. Zeegers M, Fruhling R, Pak F, et al. The contribution of risk factors to blood pressure heritability estimates in young adults: the East Flanders prospective twin study. Twin Res. 2004;7:245–53.
6. Robinson RF, Batisky DL, Hayes JR, et al. Significance of heritability in primary and secondary pediatric hypertension. Amer J Hypertens. 2005;18:917–21.
7. Wu X, Kan D, Province M, et al. An updated meta-analysis of genome scans for hypertension and blood pressure in the NHLBI family blood pressure program (FBPP). Amer J Hypertens. 2006;19:122–7.
8. Koivukoski L, Fisher SA, Kanninen T, et al. Meta-analysis of genome-wide scans for hypertension and blood pressure in Caucasians shows evidence of susceptibility regions on chromosomes 2 and 3. Hum Mol Genet. 2004;13:2325–32.

9. Sookoian S, Gianotti TF, González CD, et al. Association of the C-344T aldosterone synthase gene variant with essential hypertension: a meta-analysis. J Hypertens. 2006;25:5–13.

10. Wellcome Trust Case Control Consortium. Genome-wide association study of 14,000 cases of seven common diseases and 3,000 shared controls. Nature. 2007; 447:661–78.

11. Levy D, Larson MG, Benjamin EJ, et al. Framingham heart study 100K project: genome-wide associations for blood pressure and arterial stiffness. BMC Med Genet. 2007;8:S3.

12. Newton-Cheh C, Johnson T, Gateva V, et al. Genome-wide association study identifies eight loci associated with blood pressure. Nat Genet. 2009;41: 666–76.

13. Levy D, Ehret KB, Rice K, et al. Genome-wide association study of blood pressure and hypertension. Nat Genet. 2009;41:677–87.

14. Org E, Eyheramendy S, Juhanson P. Genome-wide scan identifies CDH13 as a novel susceptibility locus contributing to blood pressure determination in two European populations. Hum Mol Genet. 2009;18: 2288–96.

15. Adeyemo A, Gerry N, Chen G, Herbert A, et al. A genome-wide association study of hypertension and blood pressure in African Americans. PLoS Genet. 2009;5:e1000564.

16. Cho YS, Go MJ, Kim YJ, Heo JY, et al. A large-scale genome-wide association study of Asian populations uncovers genetic factors influencing eight quantitative traits. Nat Genet. 2009;41:527–34.

17. Yang HC, Liang YJ, Wu YL, et al. Genome-wide association study of young-onset hypertension in the Han Chinese population of Taiwan. PLoS ONE. 2009; 4:e5459.

18. Hong KW, Jin HS, Lim JE, et al. Recapitulation of two genomewide association studies on blood pressure and essential hypertension in the Korean population. J Hum Genetics. 2010;55:336–41.

19. Niu W, Zhang Y, Ji K, et al. Confirmation of top polymorphisms in hypertension genome wide association study among Han Chinese. Clin Chim Acta. 2010;411:1491–5.

20. Hong KW, Go MJ, Jin HS. Genetic variations in ATP2B1, CSK, ARSG and CSMD1 loci are related to bood pressure and/or hypertension in two Korean cohorts. J Hum Hypertens. 2010;24:367–72.

21. Kato N, Miyata T, Tabara Y, et al. High-density association study and nomination of susceptibility genes for hypertension in the Japanese national project. Hum Mol Genet. 2009;17:617–27.

22. Wang Y, O'Connell JR, McArdle PF, et al. Whole-genome association study identifies STK39 as a hypertension susceptibility gene. Proc Natl Acad Sci USA. 2009;106:226–31.

23. Cunnington MS, Kay C, Avery PJ, et al. STK39 polymorphisms and blood pressure: an association study in British Caucasians and assessment of cis-acting influences on gene expression. BMC Med Genet. 2009;10:135.

24. Hong KW, Jin HS, Lim JE, Cho YS, Go MJ, Jung J, Lee JE, et al. Non-synonymous single-nucleotide polymorphisms associated with blood pressure and hypertension. J Hum Hypertens. 2010;24:763–74.

25. Harrap SB. Blood pressure genetics: time to focus. J Am Soc Hypertens. 2009;3:231–7.

26. McCarroll SA, Hadnott TN, Perry GH, et al. International HapMap consortium. Common deletion polymorphisms in the human genome. BMC Nat Genet. 2006;38:86–92.

27. Kleinjan DA, van Heyningen V. Long-range control of gene expression: emerging mechanisms and disruption in disease. Am J Hum Genet. 2005;76:8–32.

28. Stranger BE, Forrest MS, Dunning M, et al. Relative impact of nucleotide and copy number variation on gene expression phenotypes. Science. 2007;315:848–53.

29. Sun YV, Peyser PA, Kardia SL. A common copy number variation on chromosome 6 association with the gene expression level of endothelin 1 in transformed B lymphocytes from three racial groups. Circ Cardiovasc Genet. 2009;2:483–8.

30. Wellcome Trust Case Control Consortium. Genome-wide association study of CNVs in 16,000 cases of eight common diseases and 3,000 shared controls. Nature. 2010;464:713–20.

31. Sethi AA, Nordestgaard BG, Tybjæg-Hansen A. Angiotensinogen gene polymorphism, plasma angiotensinogen, and risk of hypertension and ischemic heart disease. Arterioscler Thromb Vasc Biol. 2003;23: 1269–75.

32. Martinez F, Mansego ML, Escudero JC, et al. Association of a mineralocorticoid receptor gene polymorphism with hypertension in a Spanish population. Am J Hypertens. 2009;22:649–55.

33. Ji W, Foo JN, O'Roak BJ, Zhao H, Larson MG, Simon DB, et al. Rare independent mutations in renal salt handling genes contribute to blood pressure variation. Nat Genet. 2008;40:592–9.

34. Manunta P, Lavery G, Lanzani C, et al. Physiological interaction between α-adducin and WNK1-NEDD4L pathways on sodium-related blood pressure regulation. Hypertension. 2008;52:366–72.

35. Province MA, Arnett DK, Hunt SC, et al. Association between the α-adducin gene and hypertension in the HyperGEN study. Am J Hypertens. 2000;13: 710–8.

36. Wong ZYH, Stebbing M, Ellis JA, et al. Genetic linkage of β and γ subunits of epithelial sodium channel to systolic blood pressure. Lancet. 1999;353:1222–5.

37. Büsst CJ, Scurrah KJ, Ellis JA, et al. Selective genotyping association between the epithelial sodium channel {gamma}-subunit and systolic blood pressure. Hypertension. 2007;50:672–8.

38. von Wowern F, Berglund G, Carlson J, et al. Genetic variance of SGK-1 is associated with blood pressure, blood pressure change over time and strength of the insulin-diastolic blood pressure relationship. Kidney Int. 2005;68:2164–72.

39. Fava C, von Wowern F, Berglund G, et al. 24-h ambulatory blood pressure is linked to chromosome 18q21-22 and genetic variation of NEDD4L associates with

cross-sectional and longitudinal blood pressure in Swedes. Kidney Int. 2006;70:562–9.

40. Tobin MD, Raleigh SM, Newhouse S, et al. Association of WNK1 gene polymorphisms and haplotypes with ambulatory blood pressure in the general population. Circulation. 2005;112:3423–9.

41. Newhouse S, Farrall M, Wallace C, et al. Polymorphisms in the WNK1 gene are associated with blood pressure variation and urinary potassium excretion. PLoS ONE. 2009;4:e5003.

42. Siani A, Russo P, Cappuccio FP, et al. Combination of renin-angiotensin system polymorphisms is associated with altered renal sodium handling and hypertension. Hypertension. 2003;43:598–602.

43. Wang J, Liu L, Zagato L, et al. Blood pressure in relation to three candidate genes in a Chinese population. J Hypertens. 2004;22:937–44.

44. Banegas JR, Segura J, Sobrino J, et al. Effectiveness of blood pressure control outside the medical setting. Hypertension. 2007;49:62–8.

45. Kotsis V, Stabouli S. The definition of true normotension needs out of office blood pressure measurements. J Hypertens. 2010;28:1778–9.

46. Tobin MD, Sheehan NA, Scurrah KJ, et al. Adjusting for treatment effects in studies of quantitative traits: antihypertensive therapy ad systolic blood pressure. Statist Med. 2005;24:2911–35.

47. Cui JS, Hopper JL, Harrap SB. Antihypertensive treatments obscure familial contributions to blood pressure variation. Hypertension. 2003;41:207–10.

48. Falaschetti E, Chaudhury M, Mindell J, et al. Continued improvement in hypertension management in England. Results From the health survey for England 2006. Hypertension. 2009;53:480–6.

49. Zhang K, Weder AB, Eskin E, et al. Genome-wide case/control studies in hypertension: only the tip of the iceberg. J Hypertension. 2010;28:1115–23.

50. Clark AG, Boerwinkle E, Hixson J, et al. Determinants of the success of whole-genome association testing. Genome Res. 2005;15:1463–7.

51. Shi G, Gu CC, Kraja AT, et al. Genetic effect on blood pressure is modulated by age. the hypertension genetic epidemiology network study. Hypertension. 2009;53:35–41.

52. Rana GK, Insel PA, Payne SH, et al. Population-based sample reveals gene–gender interactions in blood pressure in white Americans. Hypertension. 2007;49:96–106.

53. Šeda O, Tremblay J, Gaudet D, et al. Systematic, genome-wide, sex-specific linkage of cardiovascular traits in French Canadians. Hypertension. 2008;51:1156–62.

54. Sõber S, Org E, Kepp K, et al. Targeting 160 candidate genes for blood pressure regulation with a genome-wide genotyping array. PLoS ONE. 2009;4:e6034.

55. Pausova Z, Syme C, Abrahamowicz M, et al. A common variant of the FTO gene is associated with not only increased adiposity but also elevated blood pressure in French Canadians. Circ Cardiovasc Genet. 2009;2:260–9.

56. Melka M, Bernard M, Paterson A, et al. Genome-wide scan for genes of adolescent obesity-related high bood pressure. Hypertension. 2010;56:e64.

57. Kuznetsova T, Staessen JA, Brand E, et al. Sodium excretion as a modulator of genetic associations with cardiovascular phenotypes in the European project on genes in hypertension. J Hypertens. 2006;24:235–42.

58. Gu D, Rice T, Wang S, et al. Heritability of blood pressure responses to dietary sodium and potassium intake in a Chinese population. Hypertension. 2007;50:116–22.

59. INTERSALT. Intersalt: an international study of electrolyte excretion and blood pressure. Results for 24 hour urinary sodium and potassium excretion. BMJ. 1988;30:319–28.

60. Liu L, Liu L, Ding Y, et al. Ethnic and environmental differences in various markers of dietary intake and blood pressure among Chinese Han and three other minority peoples in China: results from the WHO cardiovascular diseases and alimentary comparison (CARDIAC) study. Hypertens Res. 2001;24:315–22.

61. He FJ, Markandu ND, MacGregor GA. Importance of the renin system for determining blood pressure fall with acute salt restriction in hypertensive and normotensive whites. Hypertension. 2001;38:321–5.

62. Gerdts E, Myking OL, Omvik P. Salt sensitive essential hypertension evaluated by 24 hour ambulatory blood pressure. Blood Press. 1994;3:375–80.

63. Gerdts E, Lund-Johansen P, Omvik P. Reproducibility of salt sensitivity testing using a dietary approach in essential hypertension. J Hum Hypertens. 1999;13:375–84.

64. Wilson DK, Sica DA, Miller SB. Ambulatory blood pressure nondipping status in salt-sensitive and salt-resistant black adolescents. Am J Hypertens. 1999;12:159–65.

65. Graudal NA, Galloe AM, Garred P. Effects of sodium restriction on blood pressure, renin, aldosterone, catecholamines, cholesterols, and triglyceride. JAMA. 1998;279:1383–91.

66. Obarzanek E, Proschan MA, Vollmer WM, et al. Individual blood pressure responses to changes in salt intake. Hypertension. 2003;42:459–67.

67. Miller JZ, Weinberger MH, Christian JC, et al. Familial resemblance in the blood pressure response to sodium restriction. Am J Epidemiol. 1987;126:822–30.

68. Hurwitz S, Fisher NDL, Ferri C, et al. Controlled analysis of blood pressure sensitivity to sodium intake: interactions with hypertension type. J Hypertens. 2003;21:951–9.

69. Yamori Y, Liu L, Ikeda K, et al. Different associations of blood pressure with 24-hour urinary sodium excretion among pre- and post-menopausal women. J Hypertens. 2001;19:535–8.

70. Barton M, Meyer MR. Postmenopausal hypertension, mechanisms and therapy. Hypertension. 2009;54:11–8.

71. Chappell MC, Yamaleyeva M, Westwood BM. Estrogen and salt sensitivity in the female mRen(2). Lewis rat. Am J Physiol. 2006;291:R1557–63.

72. Schulman IH, Aranda P, Raij L, et al. Surgical menopause increases salt sensitivity of blood pressure. Hypertension. 2006;47:1168–74.

73. Scuteri A, Lakatta EG, Anderson DE, et al. Transdermal 17 Beta-oestradiol reduces salt sensistivity of blood pressure in postmenopausal women. J Hypertens. 2003;21:2419–20.

74. Beeks E, Kessels AGH, Kroon AA, et al. Genetic predisposition to salt-sensitivity: a systematic review. J Hypertens. 2004;22:1243–9.

75. Wang JG, Staessen JA, Barlassina C, et al. Association between hypertension and variation in the α- and β-adducin genes in a white population. Kidney Internat. 2002;62:2152–9.

76. Zhu H, Lu Y, Wang X, et al. The G protein-coupled receptor kinase 4 gene affects blood pressure in young normotensive twins. Am J Hypertens. 2006;19:61–6.

77. Sanada H, Yatabe J, Midorikawa S, et al. Single-nucleotide polymorphisms for diagnosis of salt-sensitive hypertension. Clin Chem. 2006;52:352–60.

78. Pojoga L, Kolatkar NS, Williams JS, et al. β-2 adrenergic receptor diplotype defines a subset of salt-sensitive hypertension. Hypertension. 2006;48:892–900.

79. Giner V, Poch E, Bragulat E, et al. Renin-angiotensin system genetic polymorphisms and salt sensitivity in essential hypertension. Hypertension. 2000;35:512–7.

80. Hollenberg NK, Martinez G, McCullough M, et al. Aging, acculturation, salt intake, and hypertension in the Juna of Panama. Hypertension. 1997;29:171–6.

81. Wittes J, Brittain E. The role of internal pilot studies in increasing the efficiency of clinical trials. Stat Med. 1990;9:65–72.

82. Betensky RA, Tierney C. An examination of methods for sample size recalculations during an experiment. Stat Med. 1997;16:2587–98.

83. Wright JT, Rahman M, Scarpa A, et al. Determinants of salt sensitivity in black and white normotensive and hypertensive women. Hypertension. 2003;42:1087–92.

84. Weinberger MH, Finebert NS. Sodium and volume sensitivity of blood pressure: age and pressure change over time. Hypertension. 1991;18:67–71.

Gene–Environment Interactions: Their Role in Hypertension Development

Jaroslav Kunes, Michaela Kadlecova, and Josef Zicha

Abstract

Essential hypertension is a major risk factor for several cardiovascular diseases, the etiology of which is not yet completely understood. The problem is that blood pressure (BP) is a typical quantitative trait with multifactorial determination. The interactions of multiple genetic and environmental factors as well as gene–gene interactions cause modifications of various systems that adjust blood pressure to actual living conditions. Numerous environmental factors surrounding the organism could modify its development not only by the influence on the expression of genetic information but mainly by epigenetic mechanisms. However, despite considerable research effort, it is still difficult to identify all genes and/or other genetic determinants leading to essential hypertension and other cardiovascular diseases. This is mainly because these diseases usually become a medical problem in adulthood, although their roots might be traced back to earlier stages of ontogeny. The link between distinct developmental periods (e.g., birth and adulthood) should involve the changes in gene expression involving epigenetic phenomena. The purpose of the present paper is to bring some light on gene–environmental interactions potentially implicated in the pathogenesis of hypertension, with special attention to epigenetic inheritance.

Keywords

Cardiovascular system • Critical developmental periods • Dietary intervention • Epigenetics • Gene-environment interactions • Hypertension • Metabolic syndrome • Rat

J. Kunes (✉)
Institute of Physiology, Academy of Sciences
of the Czech Republic, Prague, Czech Republic
e-mail: kunes@biomed.cas.cz

B. Ostadal et al. (eds.), *Genes and Cardiovascular Function*,
DOI 10.1007/978-1-4419-7207-1_17, © Springer Science+Business Media, LLC 2011

Introduction

The understanding of the mechanisms for long-term regulation of blood pressure (BP) is the first prerequisite to elucidate the pathophysiology of hypertension. This has important clinical significance mainly in regard to human essential hypertension, one of the major risk factors for cardiovascular diseases such as heart attack, congestive heart failure, stroke, and peripheral vascular disease. Epidemiological studies demonstrated that the number of people with hypertension is increasing in both developed and developing countries [1, 2]. Moreover, there is a big problem that this increase is significant even in children. As mentioned by Taylor and coworkers [3], the percentage of children with prehypertension rose in USA (between 1988 and 2002) from 7.7% to 10%, while the percentage of children with hypertension increased from 2.7% to 3.7%. This means that more than 400,000 additional children are newly diagnosed with prehypertension or essential hypertension.

Hypertension is a complex trait resulting from the interactions of multiple genetic and environmental determinants. There is a growing evidence that the complex of these interactions plays an important role in determining an individual's risk of various common diseases including hypertension [4, 5]. Gibson [6] emphasized that gene–gene interactions and gene–environmental interactions must be ubiquitous, given the complexities of intermolecular interactions that are necessary to regulate gene expression and the hierarchical complexity of quantitative traits.

The interest in the genetic basis of human diseases has spanned centuries and discoveries of disease-related genes often suggest that tests to predict people at risk of future disease will soon be available. Progress in the battle against human diseases was accelerated by the availability of genomic information for humans, mice, and other organisms. The techniques of molecular biology and genetics as well as particular knowledge emerging from these genome projects have revolutionized the process of localizing and identifying genes involved in the disease. However, one should keep in mind that our knowledge could not always be translated into useful clinical applications. This is mainly true for common complex diseases. As our understanding of the role of genetics and the use of gene-based markers extend to complex multifactorial disease, physicians will have to learn how to recognize patients with increased risk.

It is true that not only genetic but also some environmental factors, for example, stress, dietary factors (salt, fat), ambient temperature, etc., could contribute to the development of a given disease [4, 5, 7], especially if they influence the organism in the "critical developmental periods" and/or "developmental windows." [4, 8].

The major goal of this chapter should be to integrate information on the relationships among the genetic determinants of high BP, environmental influences, and epigenetics. We are still in the situation that we can ask the following questions – *what should be the normal level of blood pressure in our population?, why we need higher BP?, what is the relationship between hypertension and other cardiovascular diseases?, is hypertension an adaptive trait?*, etc. Several hypotheses were proposed mainly for the last question [9]. These are the "slavery hypothesis" [10] and the "thrifty genotype theory" [11]. In both hypotheses, environmental factors play a very important role for selection of such genes that helped our ancestry to survive stressful conditions at the price of higher BP. However, both hypotheses have weak points, so that we still need more information in order to understand the complexity of hypertension.

Animal Models for Experimental Hypertension

As mentioned many times, hypertension is a polygenic trait with unknown etiology. There is no doubt that the study of such complicated disease is much easier in experimental animals than in humans, but a simple comparison of two strains, one normotensive and one hypertensive, could not answer the question about the primary causes of hypertension development and about the secondary consequences that could be involved in its maintenance. The use of special models and modern genetic approaches with gene manipulations are great advantages for the experimental approach that should help to understand the etiology of human hypertension and its effective prevention.

To understand how important animal models for the study of hypertension are, one should search any reference databases. It is impressive how the amount of such studies is increasing with time. Many different rat and mouse models of genetic hypertension have been developed with different etiology of hypertension [12–15]. These different genetic models provide the opportunity to investigate the genetic determinants of different types of hypertension, but one must be careful to transfer simply the results obtained in animal models to human essential hypertension. The advantages of having appropriate models are numerous. Due to many-sided interventions in animals (ethically impossible in humans), such models can substantially increase our understanding of the neural, renal, endocrine, or other variables triggering and/or maintaining hypertension. Due to the shorter life span of experimental animals, the role of various risk factors can be studied, alone or in combination, across the life span, to determine whether critical periods of sensitivity exist and to discover which physiological and biochemical events are associated with hypertension induction. Numerous environmental factors that may produce established hypertension can be manipulated, and thus animal models could help to answer our questions about the mechanisms responsible for hypertension development. Such models allow us to ask whether the mechanisms of salt-induced hypertension differ from those of stress-induced or renal hypertension and to look for some common mechanisms. In principle, such knowledge could enhance our understanding of this pathophysiological process and thus improve prevention and treatment of human essential hypertension [8]. Another great advantage of experimental models is that they are mostly inbred, for example, the individuals within the given strain are genetically identical. The

Table 1 Similarities between clinical and experimental forms of hypertension

Clinical forms	Experimental forms
Labile	Early phase of spontaneous hypertension
Essential	Spontaneous genetic hypertension (e.g., GH, SHR)
Neurogenic	Sinoaortal denervation, brainstem lesions
Pheochromocytoma	Norepinephrine infusion
Cushing syndrome	Glucocorticoid overproduction
Mineralocorticoid	Administration of mineralo-corticoids (e.g., DOCA)
Hyperaldosteronism	Adrenal regeneration
Renovascular	2K1C Goldblatt, ?1K1C Goldblatt
Aorta coarctation	Ligature of aorta, ?2K2C Goldblatt
High salt intake	Salt-sensitive strains (Dahl, Sabra)

GH genetically hypertensive rats, *SHR* spontaneously hypertensive rats, *DOCA* deoxycorticosterone acetate, *2K1C* two-kidney one-clip, *1K1C* one-kidney one-clip, *2K2C* two-kidney two-clip

same situation is known in monozygotic twins. The use of inbred strains is important for production of F_2 hybrids, recombinant inbred strains, backcross populations, etc., as a tool for the search for genetic determinants of hypertension and other cardiovascular diseases. In spite of the fact that any experimental model is inappropriate to human hypertension [16, 17], some similarities exist (Table 1).

The spontaneously hypertensive rat (SHR) has been widely studied as an animal model for essential hypertension. However, numerous other genetic or induced models of hypertension exist in the rat (Table 2). BP of SHR rises most rapidly between the ages of 4 and 13 weeks [8], and this elevation can be partially suppressed by kidney transplantation [18], ACE inhibitors [19, 20], or gene therapy [21, 22]. The SHR develops many features of hypertensive end-organ damage [23], but they have no tendency to develop atherosclerosis or vascular thrombosis. Several other substrains of SHR were developed to study a variety of clinical features of essential hypertension such as stroke, myocardial infarction, obesity, etc. [24]. In addition to rat models, mainly mice are

Table 2 The list of basic models of the rat

Genetic models

Genetically hypertensive rats – New Zealand (GH)

Spontaneously hypertensive rats (SHR)

Stroke-prone spontaneously hypertensive rats (SHRSP)

Lyon hypertensive rats (LH)

Münster spontaneously hypertensive rats (SHM)

Prague hypertriglyceridemic hypertensive rats (HTG)

Milan hypertensive strain (MHS)

Prague hypertensive rats (PHR)

Fawn-hooded hypertensive rats (FHR)

Dahl salt-sensitive rats (DS, SS/Jr)

Sabra hypertension-prone rats (SBH)

Induced models

Neurogenic hypertension

Hypertension from sino-aortic denervation

Renovascular (Goldblatt) hypertension – 1K1C, 2K1C, aorta coarctation, etc..

Hypertension from renal mass reduction – subtotal nephrectomy, etc.

Hypertension from dietary interventions –high-salt diet, high-fat diet, etc.

Mineralocorticoid hypertension – DOCA-salt

Insulin-resistant hypertension – high-fructose diet, etc.

NO-deficient hypertension – L-NAME treatment

DOCA deoxycorticosterone acetate, *NO* nitric oxide, *L-NAME* N^G-nitro-L-arginine methyl ester

often used irrespective of difficulties with the determination of particular phenotypes such as hemodynamic parameters, including BP. Their advantage is easier genetic manipulation, such as gene knockout, gene knock-in, etc.

Gene–Environment Interaction

There is no doubt that gene–environment interaction is not a static process, but it plays a very significant role throughout the whole life of a particular individual. This interaction is important not only for the modification of phenotypes but also for the expression of genetic information [4, 8]. As demonstrated earlier, gene–environment interaction is more pronounced in specific developmental periods, called "critical developmental periods" or "developmental windows," in which the organism is more sensitive to many environmental stimuli [8]. This is true even for humans

where the intrauterine period is very important for programming basic physiological functions. The association between low birth weight and raised blood pressure in later life has been studied [25–28]. According to this "programming hypothesis," an impairment of intrauterine environment modifies the fetus from its optimal development, leading to cardiovascular complications in later life. Although most clinical and experimental studies support this fetal programming hypothesis in relation to adult hypertension, there is still controversy regarding the cause and mechanisms underlying this phenomenon. Generally, the changes in maternal nutrition lead to abnormal fetal nutrition, which directly or indirectly influences growth and maturation of various organs. However, not all studies support this theory, suggesting that rather body size in early adolescence than birth weight is more important [29]. Eriksson et al. [28] have shown in a set of 2,003 people selected from the Helsinki birth cohort that two different paths of fetal, infant, and childhood growth precede the development of hypertension in adult life. In one path that was associated with more severe hypertension in people who tended to be obese, small body size at birth and during infancy was followed by rapid growth. In the other one, which was associated with a less severe hypertension, slow linear growth in utero and during infancy was followed by persisting small body size. More recently, animal and human studies support the hypothesis that congenital deficit in nephron number could be one of the possible common pathophysiological denominators between low birth weight and subsequent adult hypertension [30].

From the point of terminology one should keep in mind that the term *environment* means all stimuli that are not of genetic origin. This is important for understanding why there exists the variability of particular phenotypes in inbred strains or in monozygotic twins. Mainly monozygotic twins have been used to demonstrate the role of environmental factors in determining complex diseases and phenotypes but the true nature of the phenotypic discordance remains still poorly understood. It was demonstrated that the lighter twin has an elevated risk for adverse changes in body composition and risk for diabetes and hypertension later in life [31, 32], demonstrating that genetic factors do not fully account for the adult disease risk. One possibility could be that the uterine environment may not be the same for both individuals. For example, the possible effects of sharing different proportions of a common placenta on fetal growth and development are well recognized, as are the effects of placental anastomoses leading to partially shared circulations, which may also have long-term consequences [33]. In experimental twin research, Gärtner [34] has demonstrated that only 20–30% of the range of the body weight in inbred mice was directly estimated to be of environmental origin. He suggested the rest of the variability was due to a "third component" (in addition to the genetic and environmental factors), which is effective at or before fertilization and may originate from ooplasmic differences.

However, the link among changes in particular periods of life (e.g., between the intrauterine period and adulthood) can be explained only partially by time-dependent different expression of particular genes. There are also changes involved in epigenetic phenomena. Thus, environmental changes occurring in the intrauterine period or shortly after birth may ultimately lead to altered gene expression *via* epigenetic mechanisms, resulting in an increased susceptibility to chronic disease in adulthood [35]. This epigenetic process of imprinting is thought to particularly affect many of the genes regulating fetal and placental growth [36].

Epigenetic Phenomena – The Way How Environment Can Influence Genetic Information

Epigenetic inheritance is a complex process that depends on the participation of numerous components of epigenetic machinery. Four main types of epigenetic inheritance – DNA methylation, chromatin remodeling, genomic imprinting, and long-range control of chromatin structure – have been described [37]. It was even demonstrated that although the epigenetic pattern is not a part of DNA sequence, it is heritably transmitted during cell division [36, 38].

A typical example of epigenetic inheritance is the inheritance of the coat color gene *agouti* in the mouse [39, 40]. Several *agouti viable yellow* alleles (A^{hvy} or A^{IAP}) regulate the alternative production of black and yellow pigment in individual hair follicles. The coat color of mice with such an allele varies from yellow over mottled to wild-type agouti. Transcription of this gene occurs in the skin during a short period when the yellow subapical band is formed at the beginning of each hair growth cycle. When methylated, the *agouti* gene is expressed only in the hair follicles as in wild-type mice. On the other hand, unmethylated gene causes the yellow coat color. It was demonstrated that dietary supplementation of *a/a* dams with extra folic acid, vitamin B_{12}, choline, and betaine alters the phenotype of their A^{hvy}/a offspring through a different degree of methylation [41]. Thus, A^{hvy} expression, already known to be modulated by imprinting, maternal epigenetic inheritance, and strain-specific modifications, might also be modulated by the maternal diet. These results also suggested that through maternal epigenetic inheritance, the diet might positively affect health and longevity of the offspring [39] because yellow mice become obese and develop a tumor with age.

It was demonstrated that the epigenetic changes might be different in different developmental periods. Persistent epigenetic changes are more pronounced in early exposure to harsh conditions. This was demonstrated in the so-called "Dutch Hunger" study [42]. It was evident that individuals who were exposed to famine in utero had very different methylation patterns of genes involved in growth and metabolic disease compared to controls. Methylation of several genes (*IL-10, LEP, MEG3*, etc.) was higher, whereas methylation of *IGF2* was lower in these individuals [43]. This might be related to the fact that some mammalian genes are expressed preferentially from the paternal or maternal allele and are said to be genomically imprinted. Imprinted genes may regulate some of the crucial aspects of mammalian physiology connected with energy homeostasis, reproduction, growth, etc. Most imprinted genes are found in clusters and the best-characterized imprinted domain comprises the *insulin-like growth factor 2 (IGF2)* gene. The maternally imprinted *IGF2* gene on chromosome 11p15.5 is one of the best characterized epigenetically regulated loci. Recently, it has been demonstrated that substantial variation in DNA methylation of H19 and IGF2 region exists across individuals, suggesting that DNA methylation is a quantitative trait. Analysis of data in monozygotic and dizygotic twins revealed that a significant part of variation in DNA methylation could be attributed to heritable factors [44]. One of the most important findings of this study was the fact that the combined influence of environmental and stochastic factors did not increase from adolescence to middle age at the expense of heritability. On the contrary, Fraga et al. [45] observed age-related differences particularly in global DNA methylation, histone modification, and repetitive sequences. These authors speculated that the different results could be explained by heterogeneity in cell populations used for genomic DNA extraction. Moreover, we have demonstrated strong segregation of *IGF2* genotype with plasma triacylglycerols in the population of F_2 hybrids derived from Prague hypertriglyceridemic and Lewis progenitors [46]. There was also segregation between this genotype and blood pressure changes elicited by the blockade of either renin-angiotensin system or NO synthase. One could speculate that any epigenetic modification of the *IGF2* gene might be involved in these regulatory processes.

Perspectives and Concluding Remarks

There is no doubt that not only genetic but also environmental factors are very important for the regulation and maintenance of blood pressure. There is growing evidence that complex interactions between multiple genes and multiple environmental factors play an important role in determining an individual's risk of various common diseases including hypertension. Due to the complex trait it is still not simple to recognize individual genes, which should be the optimum target for genetic manipulation. Although some experimental results suggested certain possibilities, it is difficult to apply these techniques in humans. For example, gene therapy of 5-day-old SHR resulting in the long-term expression of AT_1 receptor antisense transcript successfully prevented the development of this type of genetic hypertension [21, 47], but the effect of such treatment was only transient in adult animals [48].

Conclusions

Increased understanding of the mechanisms by which environmental factors can modify the development of hypertension and other cardiovascular diseases may lead to the development of new strategies not only in the therapy but also in the prevention of these diseases. Some preclinical and clinical studies have demonstrated that exposure to factors such as diet, stress, smoking, air pollution, etc. are able to modify epigenetic markers. However, more investigations are needed to determine whether the accumulation of epigenetic alterations can increase the incidence of hypertension.

To decrease the incidence of important cardiovascular diseases we should pay more attention to epigenetic changes rather than to "gene hunting." This could be achieved by appropriate lifestyle modifications. At present, we can recommend the modification of lifestyle as a prevention of cardiovascular diseases including hypertension. Salt restriction to less than 6 g/day, maintenance of appropriate body weight, higher physical exercise, restriction of stress, augmented fruit and vegetable consumption, etc. should be a standard recommendation of physicians to their patients. Not only patients but the whole population must be motivated for lifestyle changes because most of the "civilization" diseases including hypertension have their roots in the earlier stages of ontogeny. Finally, it is evident that if a "sensitive" genome enters "toxic" environment during particular critical developmental period, there is a very high probability that disease will develop.

References

1. Reid CM, Thrift AG. Hypertension 2020: confronting tomorrow's problem today. Clin Exp Pharmacol Physiol. 2005;32:374–6.
2. Nugent R. Chronic diseases in developing countries: health and economic burdens. Ann NY Acad Sci. 2008;1136:70–9.
3. Taylor JY, Maddox R, Wu CY. Genetic and environmental risks for high blood pressure among African American mothers and daughters. Biol Res Nurs. 2009;11:53–65.
4. Kuneš J, Zicha J. Developmental windows and environment as important factors in the expression of genetic information: a cardiovascular physiologist's view. Clin Sci Lond. 2006;111:295–305.
5. Kuneš J, Zicha J. The interaction of genetic and environmental factors in the etiology of hypertension. Physiol Res. 2009;58(Suppl 2):S33–41.
6. Gibson G. Epistasis and pleiotropy as natural properties of transcriptional regulation. Theor Popul Biol. 1196;49:58–89.
7. Greenland S, Rothman KJ. Concepts of interaction. In: Rothman KJ, Greenland S, editors. Modern epidemiology. Philadelphia, PA: Lippincott-Raven; 1998. p. 329–42.
8. Zicha J, Kuneš J. Ontogenetic aspects of hypertension development: analysis in the rat. Physiol Rev. 1999; 79:1227–82.
9. Weder AB, Schork NJ. Adaptation, allometry, and hypertension. Hypertension. 1994;24:145–56.
10. Wilson TW, Grim CE. Biohistory of slavery and blood pressure differences in blacks today. A hypothesis. Hypertension. 1991;17(1 Suppl):I122–8.
11. Neel JV, Weder AB, Julius S. Type II diabetes, essential hypertension, and obesity as "syndromes of impaired genetic homeostasis": the "thrifty genotype" hypothesis enters the 21st century. Perspect Biol Med. 1998;42:44–74.
12. Rapp JP. Genetic analysis of inherited hypertension in the rat. Physiol Rev. 2000;8:135–72.
13. Cicila GT. Strategy for uncovering complex determinants of hypertension using animal models. Curr Hypertens Rep. 2000;2:1–10.
14. Glazier AM, Nadeu JH, Aitman TJ. Finding genes that underlie complex traits. Science. 2002;298:2345–9.
15. Svenson KL, Bogue MA, Peters LL. Identifying new mouse models of cardiovascular disease: a review of high-throughput screens of mutagenized and inbred strains. J Appl Physiol. 2003;94:1650–9.
16. Trippodo NC, Frohlich ED. Similarities of genetic (spontaneous) hypertension. Man and rat. Circ Res. 1981;48:309–19.
17. McGiff JC, Quilley CP. The rat with spontaneous genetic hypertension is not suitable model of human essential hypertension. Circ Res. 1981;48:455–63.
18. Rettig R, Folberth C, Stauss H, et al. Role of the kidney in primary hypertension: a renal transplantation study in rats. Am J Physiol. 1990;258:F606–11.
19. Campbell DJ, Duncan AM, Kladis A, et al. Converting enzyme inhibition and its withdrawal in spontaneously hypertensive rats. J Cardiovasc Pharmacol. 1995;26: 426–36.
20. de Souza Bomfim A, Mandarim-de-Lacerda CA. Effects of ACE inhibition during fetal development on cardiac microvasculature in adult spontaneously hypertensive rats. Int J Cardiol. 2005;101:237–42.
21. Iyer SN, Lu D, Katovich MJ, et al. Chronic control of high blood pressure in the spontaneously hypertensive rat by delivery of angiotensin type 1 receptor antisense. Proc Natl Acad Sci USA. 1996;93:9960–5.
22. Pachori AS, Huentelman MJ, Francis SC, et al. The future of hypertension therapy: sense, antisense, or nonsense? Hypertension. 2001;37:357–64.
23. Pinto YM, Paul M, Ganten D. Lessons from rat models of hypertension: from Goldblatt to genetic engineering. Cardiovasc Res. 1998;39:77–88.
24. Yamori Y. Implication of hypertensive rat models for primordial nutritional prevention of cardiovascular diseases. Clin Exp Pharmacol Physiol. 1999;26:568–72.
25. Barker DJP, Osmond C, Golding J, et al. Growth in utero, blood pressure in childhood and adult life, and mortality from cardiovascular disease. Br Med J. 1989;298:564–7.
26. Huxley RR, Shiel AW, Law CM. The role of size at birth and postnatal catch-up growth in determining systolic blood pressure: a systemic review of the literature. J Hypertens. 2000;18:815–31.
27. De Boo HA, Harding JE. The developmental origins of adult disease (Barker) hypothesis. Aust N Z J Obstet Gynaecol. 2006;46:4–14.
28. Eriksson JG, Forsón TJ, Kajantie E, et al. Childhood growth and hypertension in later life. Hypertension. 2007;49:1414–21.
29. Falkner B, Hulman S, Kushner H. Effect of birth weight on blood pressure and body size in early adolescence. Hypertension. 2004;43:203–7.
30. Zandi-Nejad K, Luyckx VA, Brenner BM. Adult hypertensuion and kidney disease. The role of fetal programming. Hypertension. 2006;47:502–8.
31. Bo S, Cavallo-Perin P, Scaglione L, et al. Low birthweight and metabolic abnormalities in twins with increased susceptibility to Type 2 diabetes mellitus. Diabet Med. 2000;17:365–70.
32. Iliadou A, Cnattingius S, Lichtenstein P. Low birthweight and Type 2 diabetes: a study on 11 162 Swedish twins. Int J Epidemiol. 2004;33:948–53.
33. Cheung YF, Taylor MJ, Fisk NM, et al. Fetal origins of reduced arterial distensibility in the donor twin in twin-twin transfusion syndrome. Lancet. 2000;355: 1157–8.
34. Gärtner K. A third component causing random variability beside environment and genotype. A reason for the limited success of a 30 year long effort to standardize laboratory animals? Lab Anim. 1990;24:71–7.
35. Waterland RA, Jirtle RL. Early nutrition, epigenetic changes at transposons and imprinted genes, and enhanced susceptibility to adult chronic diseases. Nutrition. 2004;20:63–8.

36. Reik W, Dean W, Walter J. Epigenetic reprogramming in mammalian development. Science. 2001;293:1089–93.

37. Nafee TM, Farrell WE, Carroll WD, et al. Epigenetic control of fetal gene expression. BJOG. 2008;115:158–68.

38. Surani MA. Reprogramming of genome function through epigenetic inheritance. Nature. 2001;414:122–8.

39. Wolff GL, Kodell RL, Moore SR, et al. Maternal epigenetics and methyl supplements affect agouti gene expression in Avy/a mice. FASEB J. 1998;12:949–57.

40. Morgan HD, Sutherland HG, Martin DI, et al. Epigenetic inheritance at the agouti locus in the mouse. Nat Genet. 1999;23:314–8.

41. Waterland RA, Jirtle RL. Transposable elements: targets for early nutritional effects on epigenetic gene regulation. Mol Cell Biol. 2003;23:5293–300.

42. Heijmans BT, Tobi EW, Stein AD, et al. Persistent epigenetic differences associated with prenatal exposure to famine in humans. Proc Natl Acad Sci USA. 2008;105:17046–9.

43. Tobi EW, Lumey LH, Talens RP, et al. DNA methylation differences after exposure to prenatal famine are common and timing- and sex-specific. Hum Mol Genet. 2009;18:4046–53.

44. Heijmans BT, Kremer D, Tobi EW, et al. Heritable rather than age-related environmental and stochastic factors dominate variation in DNA methylation of the human IGF2/H19 locus. Hum Mol Genet. 2007;16:547–54.

45. Fraga MF, Ballestar E, Paz MF, et al. Epigenetic differences arise during the lifetime of monozygotic twins. Proc Natl Acad Sci USA. 2005;102:10604–9.

46. Kadlecová M, Dobešová Z, Zicha J, et al. Abnormal Igf2 gene in Prague hereditary hypertriglyceridemic rats: its relation to blood pressure and plasma lipids. Mol Cell Biochem. 2008;314:37–43.

47. Martens JR, Reaves PY, Lu D, et al. Prevention of renovascular and cardiac pathophysiological changes in hypertension by angiotensin II type 1 receptor antisense gene therapy. Proc Natl Acad Sci USA. 1998;95:2664–9.

48. Katovich MJ, Gelband CH, Reaves P, et al. Reversal of hypertension by angiotensin II type 1 receptor antisense gene therapy in the adult SHR. Am J Physiol Heart Circ Physiol. 1999;277:H1260–4.

Phenotypic Overlap of Lethal Arrhythmias Associated with Cardiac Sodium Mutations: Individual-Specific or Mutation-Specific?

Naomasa Makita

Abstract

Mutations in cardiac sodium channel gene *SCN5A* are responsible for a spectrum of hereditary arrhythmias including type-3 long QT syndrome (LQT3), Brugada syndrome (BrS), conduction disturbance, and sinus node dysfunction. These syndromes were originally regarded as independent entities with distinct clinical manifestations and biophysical properties. However, recent evidence shows considerable clinical overlap among these disorders, implicating a new disease entity referred to as an overlap syndrome of cardiac sodium channelopathy. Class IC sodium channel blockers often induce BrS phenotype in some patients with LQT3. Furthermore, recent genetic studies have revealed that E1784K is the most prevalent *SCN5A* mutation responsible not only for LQT3 but BrS, confirming the clinical and genetic overlap of LQT3 and BrS. Here I show evidence that the clinical manifestations of *SCN5A* mutations are most probably determined by the biophysical and pharmacological properties of the mutations. I also provide an overview of current knowledge on the clinical features, prevalence, and molecular and biophysical mechanisms underlying the overlap syndrome to gain more insight into this complex issue and generate better therapeutic strategies for patient management.

Keywords

Brugada syndrome • Flecainide • Long QT syndrome • Overlap syndrome • *SCN5A*

N. Makita (✉)
Department of Molecular Physiology,
Nagasaki University Graduate School
of Biomedical Sciences, Nagasaki, Japan
e-mail: makitan@nagasaki-u.ac.jp

Introduction

Biochemistry and Biophysics of Cardiac Sodium Channels

Voltage-gated sodium channel is responsible for the rapid upstroke of the action potential in most excitable tissues and plays a pivotal role in the initiation, propagation, and maintenance of normal cardiac rhythm in the heart. Cardiac sodium channel consists of the most prevalent pore-forming α-subunit (Nav1.5) encoded by the gene *SCN5A* located on chromosome 3p21 and auxiliary β-subunits (Navβ1-Navβ4) encoded by the genes *SCN1B-SCN4B*, respectively. The α-subunits comprise a four-fold symmetry macromolecule consisting of structurally homologous domains (D1–D4), each containing six membrane-spanning segments (S1–S6) and a region (S5–S6 loop) controlling ion selectivity and permeation. The positively charged S4 segment of each domain functions as a voltage sensor [1, 2].

Na channels switch between three functional states (closed, open, inactivated), depending on the membrane potential. A membrane depolarization causes a rapid rise in local Na permeability due to the opening (activation) of Na channels from their resting closed state. Normally, activation of Na channels is transient owing to inactivation, another gating process mediated by structures located on the cytoplasmic face of the channel protein (mainly the D3–D4 linker). Na channels cannot reopen until the membrane is repolarized and they undergo recovery from inactivation. Membrane repolarization is achieved by fast inactivation of Na channels and is augmented by activation of voltage-gated K channels. Activation, inactivation, and recovery from inactivation occur within a few milliseconds. In addition to these rapid gating transitions, Na channels are also susceptible to slower inactivating processes (slow inactivation) if the membrane remains depolarized for a longer time. These slower events may contribute to determining the availability of active channels under various physiological conditions.

Table 1 Inherited cardiac sodium channelopathies

1. Cardiac Na channel α subunit (*SCN5A*)
    Congenital long QT syndrome (LQT3)
    Acquired long QT syndrome
    Brugada syndrome (BrS1)
    Cardiac conduction disturbance (CCD)
    Congenital sick sinus syndrome (SSS1)
    Atrial standstill
    AV block
    Sudden infant death syndrome (SIDS)
    Familial atrial fibrillation (FAF)
    Dilated cardiomyopathy (DCM)

2. Sodium channel β1 subunit (*SCN1B*)
    Brugada syndrome with CCD (BrS5)

3. Sodium channel β4 subunit (*SCN4B*)
    Congenital long QT syndrome (LQT10)

Genetics of Cardiac Sodium Channelopathies

Mutations of *SCN5A* are responsible for a spectrum of hereditary arrhythmias including type-3 congenial long QT syndrome (LQTS; LQT3) [3], acquired LQTS [4], Brugada syndrome (BrS; BrS1) [5], cardiac conduction disturbance (CCD) [6], congenital sick sinus syndrome (SSS) [7], atrial standstill [8–10], atrioventricular (AV) block [11], sudden infant death syndrome (SIDS) [12–14], and familial atrial fibrillation (FAF) [15–17] (Table 1). In addition to these primary electrical diseases which usually lack structural abnormalities, *SCN5A* mutations have also been reported in patients with dilated cardiomyopathy [15, 18]. Moreover, recent genetic studies have indicated that mutations in Na channel β-subunit genes, *SCN1B* and *SCN4B*, were associated with type-5 BrS complicated with CCD (BrS5) [19] and type-10 LQTS (LQT10), respectively.

Biophysical Properties of Cardiac Sodium Channel Channelopathies

Congenital LQTS is characterized by the prolongation of the QT interval on surface electrocardiograms (ECGs) and an increased risk of potentially fatal ventricular arrhythmias, especially torsade de pointes [20]. QT interval is

Table 2 Mutations in overlapped cardiac sodium channelopathies

Clinical manifestation	*SCN5A* and *SCN1B* ([a]) mutations	References
BrS + LQT3 (+/− CCD)	V411M, D1114N, W1191X, I1350T, ΔK1500, ΔKPQ, R1612P, P2006A	[21, 31–37]
BrS + LQT3 + SSS (+/− CCD)	G1262S, ΔF1617, E1784K, 1795insD	[7, 31, 38–43]
BrS + SSS	E161K, T187I, E1225K, ΔK1479, K1578fs. R1623X	[30, 44, 45]
BrS + AS	R367H	[10]
BrS + CCD	P336L, D356N, R376H, N406S, G752R, F861fs951X, E867X, G1319V	[45–49]
	G1406R, I1660V, S1710L, S1812X, E87Q[a], Y179X[a]	[19, 29, 45, 46, 50–52]
DCM (+/− CCD + SSS + AF)	T220I, R814W, F851fs, A1180V, D1275N, D1595H	[8, 15, 18]
CCD + SSS/AS	G1408R	[7]
AS + AF	L212P	[9]
LQT3 + CCD	P1332L, V1763M, M1766L, V1777M, P2005A	[53–60]

BrS Brugada syndrome, *LQT3* type-3 long QT syndrome, *CCD* cardiac conduction disturbance, *AS* atrial standstill, *AF* atrial fibrillation, *DCM* dilated cardiomyopathy, *SCN1B* mutations are shown with[a]

determined by the cardiac action potential which is orchestrated by a fine balance between inward and outward currents expressed in myocardial cells. After the first identification of the *SCN5A* mutation ΔKPQ, comprising a deletion of three conserved amino acids 1505–1507 in the cytoplasmic D3-D4 linker in 1995 [21], more than 100 distinct *SCN5A* mutations responsible for LQT3 have been reported. The common in vitro consequence of most of these mutations is a persistent Na current during the action potential plateau due to destabilized fast Na channel inactivation [3]. This failure of fast inactivation shifts the ionic balance during the plateau phase toward inward current (gain-of-function) and delays repolarization, thus increasing action potential duration and the corresponding QT interval. Na channel blockers, such as mexiletine (class IB) or flecainide (class IC), shorten QT in patients with LQT3 due to block of this persistent current [22–24], and therefore are theoretically useful in the management of affected patients.

BrS is another primary electrical disorder without underlying structural heart diseases characterized by the coved-type ST elevation in the right precordial leads [25, 26]. It predisposes affected individuals to ventricular fibrillation (VF). Mutations in *SCN5A* are identified in 20–30% patients with BrS, and most of the heterologously expressed mutant Na channels exhibit biophysical abnormalities resulting in reduced cardiac Na current (loss-of-function) [27]. Reduced Na current is thought to exaggerate differences in action potential duration between the inner (endocardium) and outer (epicardium) layers of ventricular muscle, thereby favoring substrate-promoting reentrant arrhythmias. Loss of function of cardiac Na channels is either owing to (a) haploinsufficiency due to nonfunctional mutations; (b) impaired altered channel gating properties including enhanced inactivation, disruption of activation, and impaired recovery from inactivation; or (c) impaired intracellular trafficking and decreased membrane surface expression of the channel molecules.

Clinical Overlap of Cardiac Sodium Channel Channelopathies

SCN5A mutations with loss-of-function properties have also been identified in patients with CCD [6, 28], SSS [7], and atrial standstill [8], and numbers of reports have shown that the mutation carriers tend to exhibit overlapping clinical properties of these syndromes [29, 30] (Table 2). Importantly, such loss-of-function properties are apparently opposite to those described in LQT3 (gain-of-function), and different *SCN5A* mutations were initially linked to separate arrhythmia syndromes. Surprisingly, some LQT3 patients display ECG findings characteristic of BrS, suggesting that a single mutation can be associated with a wide spectrum of disease phenotypes. Such phenotypic overlap between LQT3 and BrS was first reported in a large multigenerational Dutch family with an insertion mutation 1795insD, in which the mutation carriers showed ECG features of both LQT3 and BrS, and sinus node dysfunction (SND) [38, 39]. Importantly, sodium channel block in the overlap phenotype shortens QT but exacerbates the ST segment elevation BrS phenotype, and thus enhances arrhythmia risk [39]. Biophysical studies demonstrated that the mutant channels displayed enhancement of both closed-state inactivation and slow inactivation which was thought to sensitize carriers to the BrS phenotype during flecainide therapy [61], in addition to the persistent Na current, a hallmark Na channel property of LQT3.

The overlap between the LQT3 and BrS phenotypes was also reported in other *SCN5A* mutations, such as ΔKPQ [31, 62], E1784K [31], and ΔK1500 [32]. Priori et al. showed the additional evidence for the elusive link between these two clinical syndromes by the fact that the class IC sodium channel blocker flecainide induced ST-segment elevation in the right precordial leads not only in patients with BrS but also with LQT3 [31]. Out of 13 patients with 7 LQT3 families (*SCN5A* mutations of V411M, T1304M, ΔK1500, ΔKPQ, R1626P, E1784K, P2006A), six patients showed flecainide-induced ST elevation. However, they failed to identify the determinants of flecainide-induced ST elevation in patients with LQT3. In fact, they assumed that the clinical overlap appeared to be individual-specific, rather than gene-specific or mutation-specific, most likely because the number of their patients was rather small. Nonetheless, these observations raise a concern about the safety of class IC drug therapy in LQT3 patients and questions the underlying mechanisms.

Phenotypic variability in LQT3 has thus far been reported sporadically or only within a single kindred [38, 39]. Therefore, it is not clear whether development of the BrS phenotype in a patient with LQT3 is solely determined by the biophysical properties of the mutant channel, or by co-inherited genetic variations, gender, ethnicity, or other environmental factors. One approach to dissect such phenotypic variability is to perform a clinical assessment of individuals with multiple pedigrees from genetically heterogeneous populations with the same mutation. Recent multicenter large-scale genetic screening of *SCN5A* mutations revealed that E1784K is the most prevalent in both LQT3 (12%, 3/25) [63] and BrS (4.8%, 14/293) [64].

Clinical Phenotypes in 15 LQT3 Families with *SCN5A*-E1784K

We enrolled 44 genotyped LQT3 families with different ethnic backgrounds (Asian 20, Caucasian 24) ascertained in seven institutions of Japan, Italy, Germany, United Kingdom, and the United States. In 44 LQT3 families, E1784K was the most prevalent *SCN5A* mutation, identified in 15 families (34%). Two probands died suddenly, and 66 out of 93 surviving members underwent genetic testing. There were 41 mutation carriers and 25 noncarriers, and QTc was significantly prolonged in the carriers.

Spontaneous ST elevation in the right precordial leads was observed in 5/41 mutation carriers (shown with * in Fig. 1; coved-type: $n=1$, saddle-back type: $n=4$, Fig. 2a). Nine mutation carriers without diagnostic ST elevation at baseline underwent provocation with flecainide, ajmaline, or pilsicainide, and the test was positive (coved-type ST elevation, Fig. 2b) in five (shown with + in Fig. 1). Thus, the diagnosis of BrS was established in 9/41 mutation carriers (one individual, a; II:1, showed spontaneous saddle-back ST elevation which was converted to coved-type by ajmaline).

SND was common in the cohort, present in 16/41 mutation carriers (Fig. 2c), and 4 of these 16 carriers with SND also exhibited the BrS phenotype (Fig. 2b, d). Moreover, one carrier (a; III:5) showed SND without manifesting QT prolongation or ST elevation. Four patients received a permanent pacemaker and three received an implantable cardioverter defibrillator.

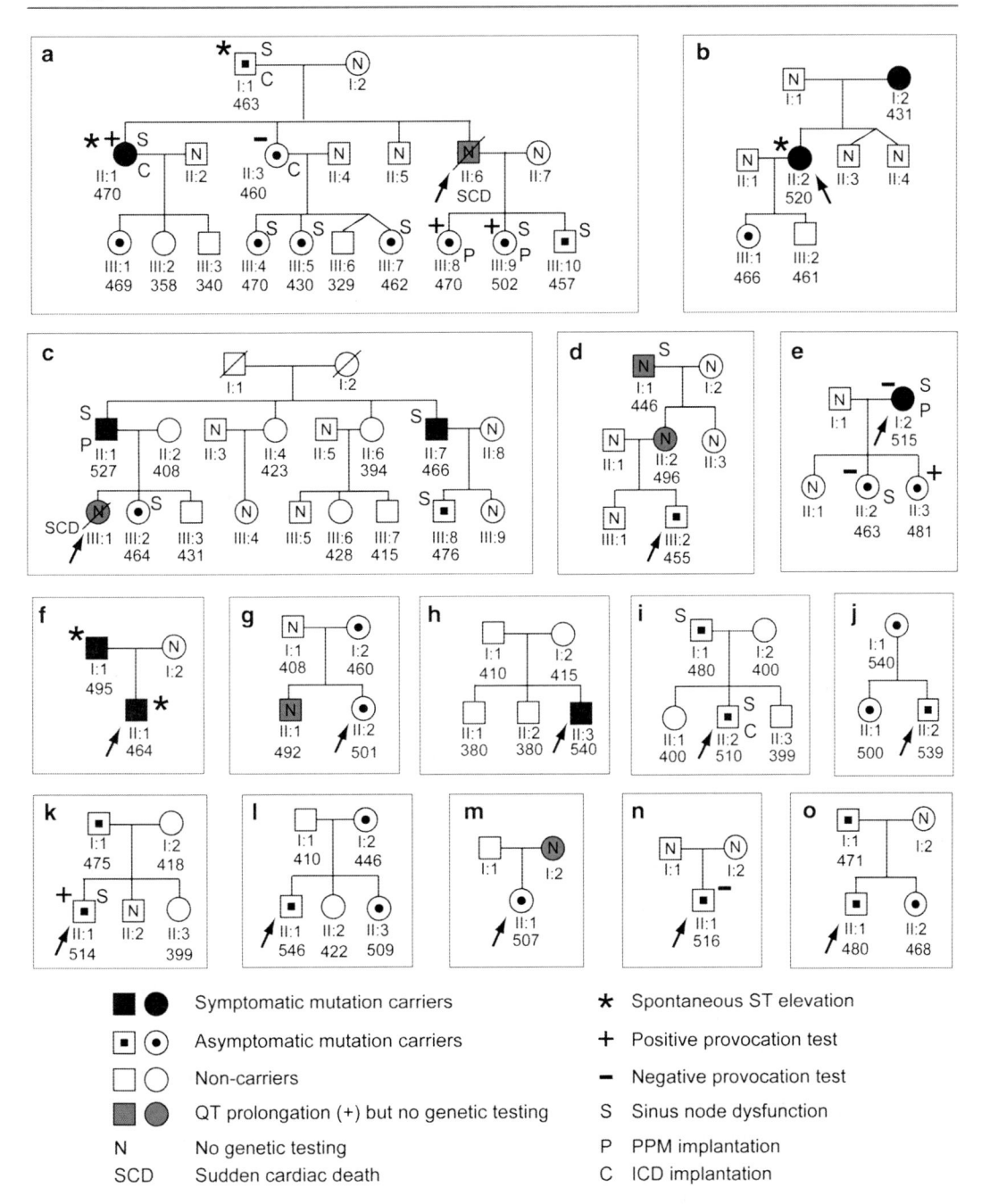

Fig. 1 Pedigrees of E1784K families. Pedigrees of 15 LQT3 families (**a–o**) carrying E1784K are shown. Probands are indicated by an *arrow*. Ten symptomatic mutation carriers, shown by the filled symbols, had episodes of syncope ($n=9$) and unexplained palpitations ($n=1$, **b**; II:2). Asymptomatic mutation carriers ($n=31$) are shown as symbols with a *dot*, and *shaded symbols* are the individuals with QT prolongation who declined genetic testing or sudden cardiac death victims (SCD; **a**;

II:6 and **c**; III:1). Individuals exhibiting ST elevation in the *right* precordial leads are depicted with an asterisk. Values for QTc intervals are given beneath each symbol. The Na-channel provocation test was positive in individuals with + (**a**; II:1, **a**; III:8, **a**; III:9, **e**; II:3, **k**; II:1), and negative in the individuals with − (**a**; II:3, **e**; I:2, **e**; II:2, **n**; II:1). Individuals with a positive and negative Na-channel blocker provocation test are shown with + and −, respectively (Modified with permission from [41])

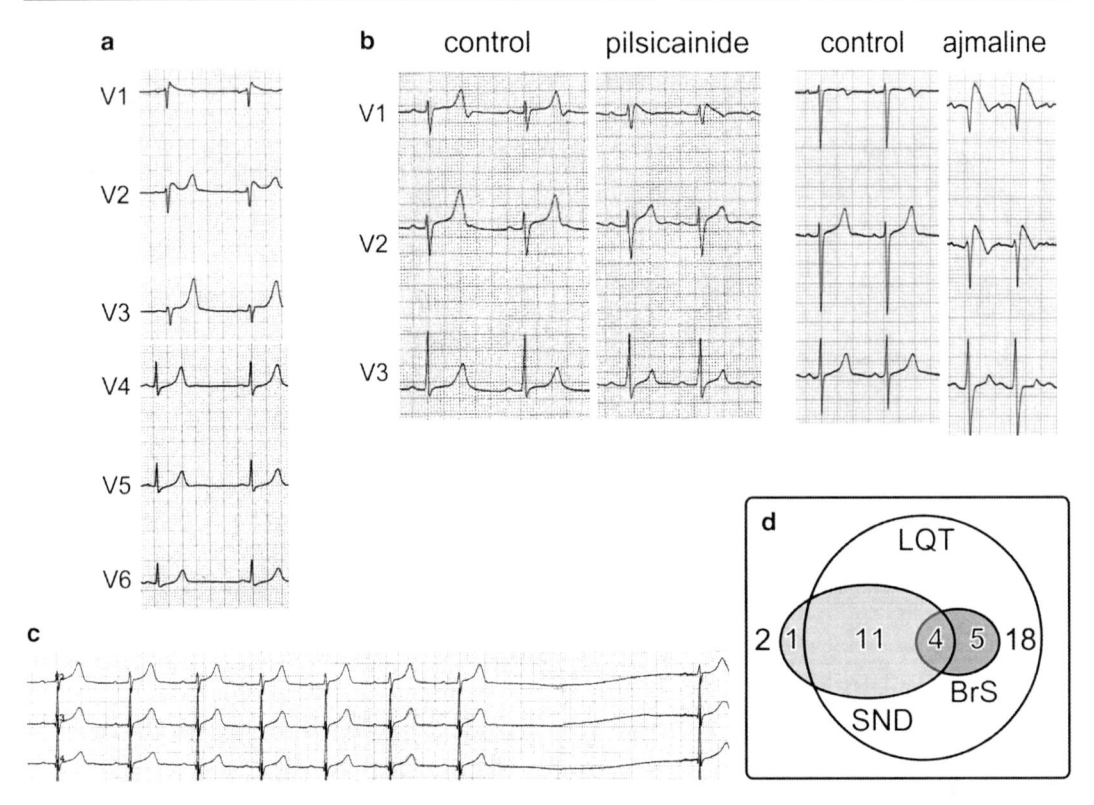

Fig. 2 ECG characteristics of E1784K mutation carriers. (a) QT prolongation (QTc=470 ms) and spontaneous saddle-back type ST elevation observed in the *right* precordial leads in a carrier, **a**; II:1. (b) ECG recordings before and after the Na-channel blocker provocation test. Pilsicainide (*left*, patient **k**; II:1) induced coved-type ST elevation in V1 and the QTc was concomitantly shortened (QTc: control 495 ms, pilsicainide 459 ms). Ajmaline (*right*, patient A; III:9) also induced coved-type ST elevation in V1 and V2 and QTc shortening (control 501 ms, ajmaline 490 ms). (c) SND demonstrated by a 3.9 s sinus arrest in a carrier, **a**; I:1. (d) A Venn diagram representing electrophysiological manifestation of 41 *SCN5A*-E1784K mutation carriers. Thirty eight carriers exhibited an abnormally long QTc; three individuals had a normal QTc, and one exhibited SND (SND) only. SND and BrS were observed in 15 and 9 individuals, respectively, with 4 displaying both phenotypes (Modified with permission from [41])

Biophysical Properties and Membrane Trafficking of E1784K

Whole-cell patch clamp recording showed that E1784K has the following biophysical abnormalities: (a) significantly smaller peak current density, (b) persistent Na current, (c) significantly faster macroscopic current decay, (d) hyperpolarizing shift of the steady-state inactivation, (e) significant depolarizing shift in the voltage-dependence of activation, and (f) normal recovery from inactivation. Furthermore, using Na channel plasmid construct with an extracellular FLAG epitope, membrane trafficking of E1784K determined by a confocal laser scanning microscopy was comparable to the wild type. These observations (Fig. 3) provide strong evidence that the loss-of-function properties displayed by E1784K are most likely attributable to the aforementioned changes in gating properties rather than a change in channel density.

Molecular Mechanisms of Enhanced Flecainide Sensitivity

Class IC drug challenge test was positive in 56% patients with E1784K. We therefore investigated tonic block and use-dependent block by flecainide in WT and E1784K channels, and compared

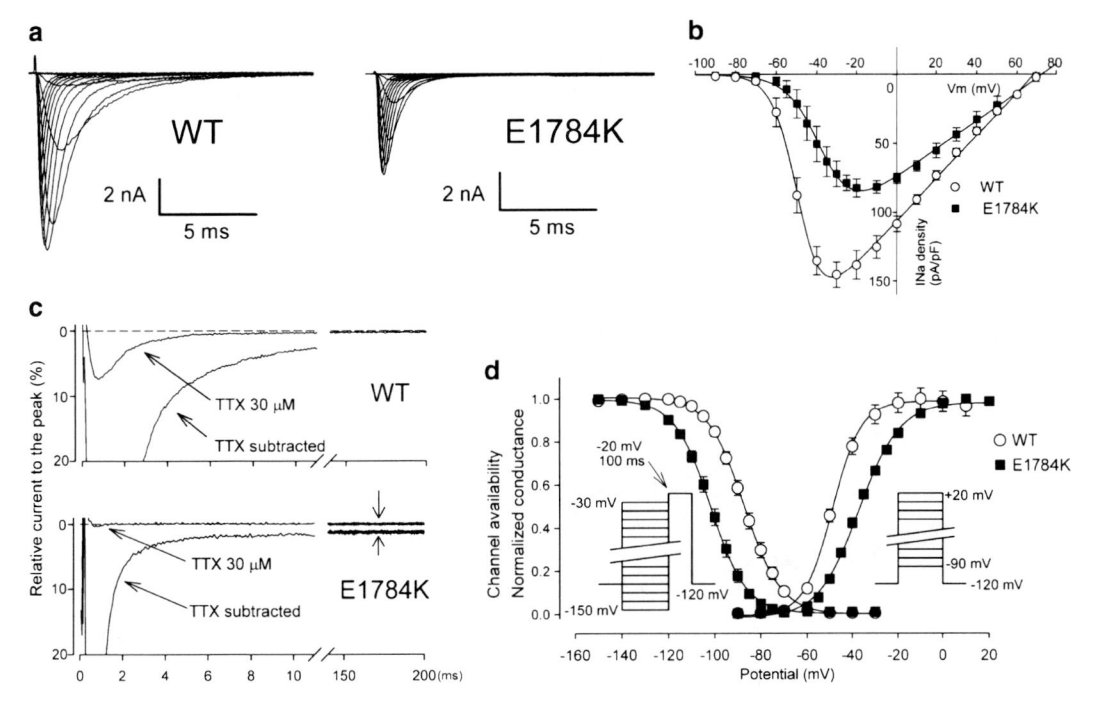

Fig. 3 Properties of E1784K whole-cell current. (**a**) Representative whole-cell current traces obtained from tsA-201 cells transfected with either WT or E1784K Na channels; all studies were conducted in cells co-transfected with human sodium channel β_1 subunits. Currents were recorded from a holding potential of −120 mV and stepped from −90 mV to +90 mV for 20 ms in 10 mV increments. (**b**) Current–voltage relationship. Current was normalized to cell capacitance to give a measure of Na current density. (**c**) Na currents were recorded with a test pulse potential of −20 mV from a holding potential of −120 mV and showed prominent tetrodotoxin (TTX)-sensitive late Na current (shown with *arrows*) and a faster decay in E1784K. (**d**) Steady-state availability for fast inactivation and the conductance-voltage relationship were measured with standard pulse protocols shown in the inset. *Curves* were fit with the Boltzmann equation. The voltage dependence of steady-state fast inactivation and activation was significantly shifted in the hyperpolarizing (−15.0 mV) and depolarizing (+12.5 mV) directions, respectively (Modified with permission from [41])

them with those of T1304M, a mutation that did not show ST elevation during the flecainide challenge test [31]. Cells transfected with WT, E1784K, or T1304M were depolarized by 2 Hz pulse trains in the absence or presence of 10 μM flecainide. During exposure to flecainide, peak currents normalized to predrug baseline were progressively reduced by the repetitive pulses (Fig. 4a, b). There was a remarkable difference in the extent of first pulse (tonic) block that was only 4.5 ± 4.0% for WT, and 7.1 ± 2.7% for T1304M, compared to substantial tonic block in E1784K (43.7 ± 8.0%, p < 0.001). Conversely, use-dependent block, determined by the difference in peak current values between the 1st and 100th test pulses relative to the first pulse, was slightly attenuated in E1784K. The net effect of flecainide after a train of 100 pulses was significantly greater in E1784K than WT but not in T1304M. Moreover, dose–response curves for flecainide block measured at a holding potential of −150 mV (thus representing drug affinity for the resting state) show that the E1784K channels were 7.5-fold more sensitive to resting-state block by flecainide than were the WT channels (IC$_{50}$: WT = 150.3 μM, E1784K = 20.4 μM) (Fig. 4c, d). These results indicate that the E1784K channels are much more sensitive to block by flecainide than are the WT and T1304M channels, and that this augmented sensitivity is attributable to enhanced tonic block rather than a change in use-dependent block.

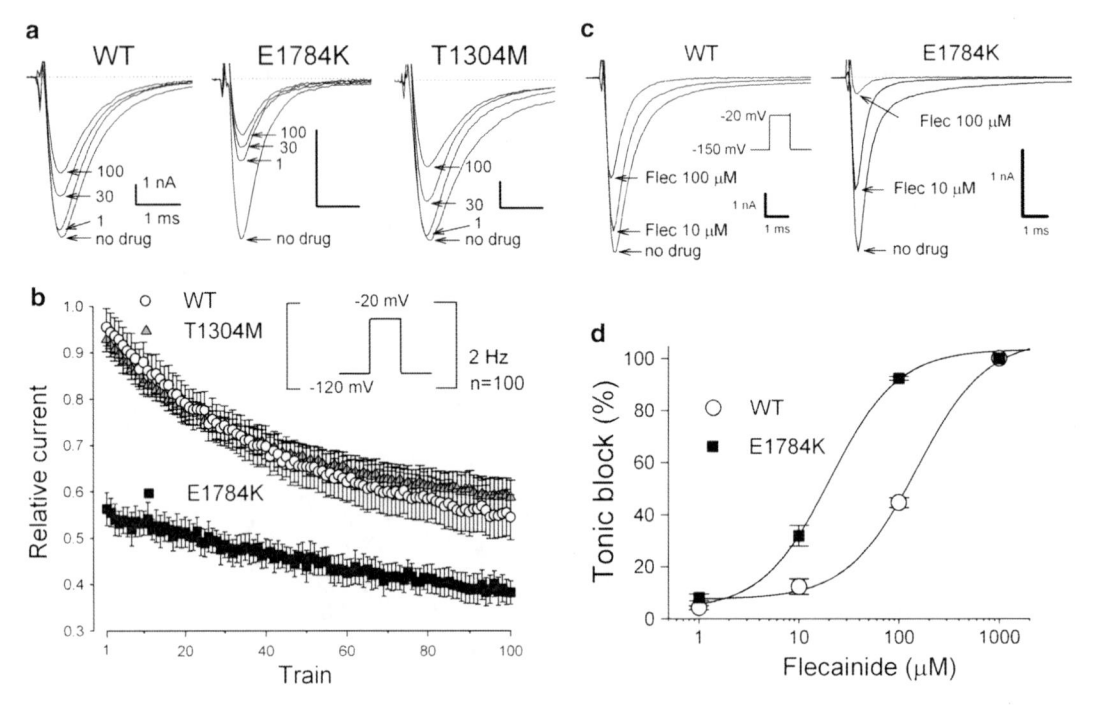

Fig. 4 Tonic block, use-dependent block, and the dose-dependence of flecainide. (**a**) Representative current traces of WT, E1784K, and T1304M before and after 10 μM flecainide. A train of 100 pulses (to −20 mV for 20 ms) was applied at 2 Hz from a holding potential of −120 mV. Numbers indicate the 1st (1), 30th (30), and 100th (100) pulse of the train. (**b**) Time course of the peak current levels after application of 10 μM flecainide. Peak current levels recorded with each pulse were normalized to the baseline prior to flecainide. (**c**) Representative steady-state current traces of WT and E1784K before and after flecainide (10 and 100 μM). Cells were depolarized by −20 mV from a holding potential of −150 mV. (**d**) Concentration-response curve for flecainide-induced tonic block in WT and E1784K. The normalized peak currents were fit to the Hill equation. The IC_{50} values, representing dissociation constants for resting state, were: WT, 150.3 μM; E1784K, 20.4 μM. Thus, the mutant channel was far more sensitive to tonic block by flecainide (Modified with permission from [41])

Functional Determinants of LQT3 Associated with BrS and SND

To explore the functional determinants for the phenotypic overlap of BrS in LQT3 patients, we compared the biophysical and pharmacological properties of reported LQT3 mutations, and sought features commonly and specifically observed in those manifesting the BrS phenotype (Table 3). The overlapping phenotype (LQT3 and BrS) has been previously reported for 1795insD [38, 39], ΔKPQ [31, 62], ΔK1500 [32], and E1784K [31]. In contrast, a carrier of T1304M did not show ST elevation during a flecainide test [31]. Similarly, SND has been reported in carriers of the same *SCN5A* mutations, 1795insD [65], ΔKPQ [68], ΔK1500 [32], E1784K [40], and

D1790G [23], but not in other *SCN5A* mutations, including T1304M. Thus, it is plausible to speculate that the biophysical characteristics common to these mutations but not found in T1304M are channel properties responsible for evoking mixed phenotypes of BrS and SND in patients with LQT3. To this end, Table 3 compares the functional properties of E1784K, and those reported for 1795insD, ΔKPQ, ΔK1500, E1784K, and T1304M [12]. Among the biophysical properties listed in Table 3, we found that both the negative shift in steady-state inactivation, and the enhanced tonic block by flecainide are common to 1795insD, ΔKPQ, ΔK1500, and E1784K, but not T1304M. This negative shift of inactivation will reduce the availability of the channels at the resting membrane potential, and increase the proportion

Table 3 Reported biophysical properties of LQT3 mutations

		SCN5A mutations				
		1795insD	ΔKPQ	ΔK1500	E1784K	T1304M
Clinical features	QT prolongation	+	+	+	+	+
	ST elevation[a]	+	+	+	+	−
	Sinus node dysfunction	+	+	+	+	−
Biophysical and pharmacological properties	Persistent Na current	+	+	+	+	+
	Shift of $V_{1/2}$ (inactivation)	Negative	Negative	Negative	Negative	Positive
	Shift of $V_{1/2}$ (activation)	Positive	Positive	Positive	Positive	Positive
	Current decay	Slower	Faster	↔	Faster	Faster
	Recovery from inactivation	Slower	Faster	ND	↔	Faster
	Slow inactivation	Enhanced	↔	ND	Enhanced	↔
	Tonic block by flecainide	Enhanced	Enhanced	Enhanced	Enhanced	↔
	UDB by flecainide	Enhanced	Enhanced	ND	Diminished	↔
References		[38, 39, 65, 66]	[3, 41, 67]	[32]	[40], [41]	[12], [41]

Modified with permission from [41]
ND not determined
[a]Spontaneous or Na-channel blocker-induced ST elevation; ↔: comparable to wild type

of inactivated channels in both the open and closed state, reducing Na current and increasing the sensitivity to Na-channel blockers. A positive shift in activation is another "loss-of-function" property evident in all the mutants including T1304M, making it less likely that this specific channel property underlies mixed clinical phenotypes in LQT3. Other channel properties such as current decay, recovery from inactivation, slow inactivation, or use-dependent block were not common among 1795insD, ΔKPQ, ΔK1500, and E1784K.

A negative shift in inactivation is observed in E1784K, 1795insD, ΔKPQ, and ΔK1500, and may play a role in the overlap of the LQT3 clinical phenotype with BrS and SND in the mutation carriers, although the number of LQT3 mutations that have been evaluated in this detail is still small, biophysical and pharmacological properties presented in a cultured cell line may not necessarily reflect the situation in vivo, and the effects of the mutation may be different in ventricular myocytes versus sinus node cells. Further studies that combine clinical and in vitro phenotyping in LQT3 mutations with and without overlapping clinical phenotypes will be required to confirm the findings of the present study. Nevertheless, a negative shift in inactivation and enhanced tonic block are common biophysical properties observed among *SCN5A* mutations with the LQT3/BrS overlapping phenotype. These findings suggest that prophylactic class IC drugs should be avoided in LQT3 mutations displaying these biophysical properties in vitro.

Conclusions

E1784K is the most common LQT3 mutation. In patients with this and other LQT3 mutations, overlap with BrS and SND is relatively common. In vitro studies with E1784K and previous reports in LQT3 mutations with and without this clinical overlap syndrome implicate a negative shift in inactivation and enhanced tonic block by drugs as underlying mechanisms. These data suggest that patients with LQT3 mutations displaying these characteristics in vitro should not receive class IC drugs. Furthermore, the present findings reinforce the general concept that in vitro characterization of the function of ion channel variants is a key component in generating specific therapeutic strategies for patient management.

Acknowledgments The author thanks the following investigators who were extensively involved in the international project "Functional characterization of the clinical overlap in cardiac sodium channelopathies" [41] for collecting clinical and genetic information on the LQT3 families, as well as the functional evaluation of the mutations: Elijah Behr (St George's University of London, London, UK), Wataru Shimizu (National Cardiovascular Center, Suita, Japan), Shigetomo Fukuhara and Naoki Mochizuki (National Cardiovascular Center Research Institute, Suita, Japan), Minoru Horie (Shiga University of Medical Science, Otsu, Japan), Akihiko Sunami (International University of Health and Welfare, Ohtawara, Japan), Lia Crotti and Peter J. Schwartz (University of Pavia, Pavia, Italy), Eric Schulze-Bahr (University of Muenster, Munster, Germany), and Alfred L. George Jr. and Dan M. Roden (Vanderbilt University, Nashville, USA). The author also thanks to Saori Mine and Atsuko Iida for technical assistance.

References

1. Catterall WA. From ionic currents to molecular mechanisms: the structure and function of voltage-gated sodium channels. Neuron. 2000;26:13–25.
2. George Jr AL. Inherited disorders of voltage-gated sodium channels. J Clin Invest. 2005;115:1990–9.
3. Bennett PB, Yazawa K, Makita N, et al. Molecular mechanism for an inherited cardiac arrhythmia. Nature. 1995;376:683–5.
4. Makita N, Horie M, Nakamura T, et al. Drug-induced long-QT syndrome associated with a subclinical SCN5A mutation. Circulation. 2002;106:1269–74.
5. Chen Q, Kirsch GE, Zhang D, et al. Genetic basis and molecular mechanism for idiopathic ventricular fibrillation. Nature. 1998;392:293–6.
6. Schott JJ, Alshinawi C, Kyndt F, et al. Cardiac conduction defects associate with mutations in SCN5A. Nat Genet. 1999;23:20–1.
7. Benson DW, Wang DW, Dyment M, et al. Congenital sick sinus syndrome caused by recessive mutations in the cardiac sodium channel gene (SCN5A). J Clin Invest. 2003;112:1019–28.
8. Groenewegen WA, Firouzi M, Bezzina CR, et al. A cardiac sodium channel mutation cosegregates with a rare connexin40 genotype in familial atrial standstill. Circ Res. 2003;92:14–22.
9. Makita N, Sasaki K, Groenewegen WA, et al. Congenital atrial standstill associated with coinheritance of a novel SCN5A mutation and connexin 40 polymorphisms. Heart Rhythm. 2005;2:1128–34.
10. Takehara N, Makita N, Kawabe J, et al. A cardiac sodium channel mutation identified in Brugada syndrome associated with atrial standstill. J Intern Med. 2004;255:137–42.
11. Wang DW, Viswanathan PC, Balser JR, et al. Clinical, genetic, and biophysical characterization of SCN5A mutations associated with atrioventricular conduction block. Circulation. 2002;105:341–6.
12. Wang DW, Desai RR, Crotti L, et al. Cardiac sodium channel dysfunction in sudden infant death syndrome. Circulation. 2007;115:368–76.
13. Otagiri T, Kijima K, Osawa M, et al. Cardiac ion channel gene mutations in sudden infant death syndrome. Pediatr Res. 2008;64:482–7.
14. Ackerman MJ, Siu BL, Sturner WQ, et al. Postmortem molecular analysis of SCN5A defects in sudden infant death syndrome. JAMA. 2001;286:2264–9.
15. Olson TM, Michels VV, Ballew JD, et al. Sodium channel mutations and susceptibility to heart failure and atrial fibrillation. JAMA. 2005;293:447–54.
16. Darbar D, Kannankeril PJ, Donahue BS, et al. Cardiac sodium channel (SCN5A) variants associated with atrial fibrillation. Circulation. 2008;117:1927–35.
17. Ge J, Sun A, Paajanen V, et al. Molecular and clinical characterization of a novel SCN5A mutation associated with atrioventricular block and dilated cardiomyopathy. Circ Arrhythm Electrophysiol. 2008;1:83–92.
18. McNair WP, Ku L, Taylor MRG, et al. SCN5A mutation associated with dilated cardiomyopathy, conduction disorder, and arrhythmia. Circulation. 2004;110:2163–7.
19. Watanabe H, Koopmann TT, Le Scouarnec S, et al. Sodium channel beta1 subunit mutations associated with Brugada syndrome and cardiac conduction disease in humans. J Clin Invest. 2008;118:2260–8.
20. Keating MT. The long QT syndrome. A review of recent molecular genetic and physiologic discoveries. Medicine. 1996;75:1–5.
21. Wang Q, Shen J, Splawski I, et al. SCN5A mutations associated with an inherited cardiac arrhythmia, long QT syndrome. Cell. 1995;80:805–11.
22. Schwartz PJ, Priori SG, Locati EH, et al. Long QT syndrome patients with mutations of the SCN5A and HERG genes have differential responses to Na+ channel blockade and to increases in heart rate. Implications for gene-specific therapy. Circulation. 1995;92:3381–6.
23. Benhorin J, Taub R, Goldmit M, et al. Effects of flecainide in patients with new SCN5A mutation: mutation-specific therapy for long-QT syndrome? Circulation. 2000;101:1698–706.
24. Schwartz PJ. The congenital long QT syndromes from genotype to phenotype: clinical implications. J Intern Med. 2006;259:39–47.
25. Brugada P, Brugada J. Right bundle branch block, persistent ST segment elevation and sudden cardiac death: a distinct clinical and electrocardiographic syndrome. A multicenter report. J Am Coll Cardiol. 1992;20:1391–6.
26. Wilde AA, Antzelevitch C, Borggrefe M, et al. Proposed diagnostic criteria for the Brugada syndrome. Eur Heart J. 2002;23:1648–54.
27. Antzelevitch C. The Brugada syndrome: ionic basis and arrhythmia mechanisms. J Cardiovasc Electrophysiol. 2001;12:268–72.
28. Tan HL, Bink-Boelkens MT, Bezzina CR, et al. A sodium-channel mutation causes isolated cardiac conduction disease. Nature. 2001;409:1043–7.
29. Shirai N, Makita N, Sasaki K, et al. A mutant cardiac sodium channel with multiple biophysical defects associated with overlapping clinical features of

Brugada syndrome and cardiac conduction disease. Cardiovasc Res. 2002;53:348–54.

30. Makiyama T, Akao M, Tsuji K, et al. High risk for bradyarrhythmic complications in patients with Brugada syndrome caused by *SCN5A* gene mutations. J Am Coll Cardiol. 2005;46:2100–6.

31. Priori SG, Napolitano C, Schwartz PJ, et al. The elusive link between LQT3 and Brugada syndrome: the role of flecainide challenge. Circulation. 2000;102:945–7.

32. Grant AO, Carboni MP, Neplioueva V, et al. Long QT syndrome, Brugada syndrome, and conduction system disease are linked to a single sodium channel mutation. J Clin Invest. 2002;110:1201–9.

33. Splawski I, Shen J, Timothy KW, et al. Spectrum of mutations in long-QT syndrome genes. KVLQT1, HERG, SCN5A, KCNE1, and KCNE2. Circulation. 2000;102:1178–85.

34. Priori SG, Napolitano C, Gasparini M, et al. Clinical and genetic heterogeneity of right bundle branch block and ST- segment elevation syndrome: a prospective evaluation of 52 families. Circulation. 2000;102:2509–15.

35. Shin DJ, Kim E, Park SB, et al. A novel mutation in the SCN5A gene is associated with Brugada syndrome. Life Sci. 2007;80:716–24.

36. Juang JM, Huang SK, Tsai CT, et al. Characteristics of Chinese patients with symptomatic Brugada syndrome in Taiwan. Cardiology. 2003;99:182–9.

37. Zareba W, Sattari MN, Rosero S, et al. Altered atrial, atrioventricular, and ventricular conduction in patients with the long QT syndrome caused by the ΔKPQ SCN5A sodium channel gene mutation. Am J Cardiol. 2001;88:1311–14.

38. Veldkamp MW, Viswanathan PC, Bezzina C, et al. Two distinct congenital arrhythmias evoked by a multidysfunctional Na+ channel. Circ Res. 2000;86:E91–977.

39. Bezzina C, Veldkamp MW, van Den Berg MP, et al. A single Na+ channel mutation causing both long-QT and Brugada syndromes. Circ Res. 1999;85:1206–13.

40. Wei J, Wang DW, Alings M, et al. Congenital long-QT syndrome caused by a novel mutation in a conserved acidic domain of the cardiac Na+ channel. Circulation. 1999;99:3165–71.

41. Makita N, Behr E, Shimizu W, et al. The E1784K mutation in SCN5A is associated with mixed clinical phenotype of type 3 long QT syndrome. J Clin Invest. 2008;118:2219–29.

42. Shin DJ, Jang Y, Park HY, et al. Genetic analysis of the cardiac sodium channel gene SCN5A in Koreans with Brugada syndrome. J Hum Genet. 2004;49:573–8.

43. Chen T, Inoue M, Sheets MF. Reduced voltage dependence of inactivation in the SCN5A sodium channel mutation delF1617. Am J Physiol Heart Circ Physiol. 2005;288:H2666–267676.

44. Smits JP, Koopmann TT, Wilders R, et al. A mutation in the human cardiac sodium channel (E161K) contributes to sick sinus syndrome, conduction disease and Brugada syndrome in two families. J Mol Cell Cardiol. 2005;38:969–81.

45. Schulze-Bahr E, Eckardt L, Breithardt G, et al. Sodium channel gene (SCN5A) mutations in 44 index patients with Brugada syndrome: different incidences in familial and sporadic disease. Hum Mutat. 2003;21:651–2.

46. Cordeiro JM, Barajas-Martinez H, Hong K, et al. Compound heterozygous mutations P336L and I1660V in the human cardiac sodium channel associated with the Brugada syndrome. Circulation. 2006;114: 2026–33.

47. Rossenbacker T, Carroll SJ, Liu H, et al. Novel pore mutation in SCN5A manifests as a spectrum of phenotypes ranging from atrial flutter, conduction disease, and Brugada syndrome to sudden cardiac death. Heart Rhythm. 2004;1:610–15.

48. Itoh H, Shimizu M, Tanaka S, et al. A novel missense mutation in the SCN5A gene associated with Brugada syndrome bidirectionally affecting blocking actions of antiarrhythmic drugs. J Cardiovasc Electrophysiol. 2005;16:486–93.

49. Potet F, Mabo P, Le Coq G, et al. Novel Brugada SCN5A mutation leading to ST segment elevation in the inferior or the right precordial leads. J Cardiovasc Electrophysiol. 2003;14:200–3.

50. Smits JP, Eckardt L, Probst V, et al. Genotype-phenotype relationship in Brugada syndrome: electrocardiographic features differentiate SCN5A-related patients from non-SCN5A-related patients. J Am Coll Cardiol. 2002;40:350–6.

51. Kyndt F, Probst V, Potet F, et al. Novel SCN5A mutation leading either to isolated cardiac conduction defect or Brugada syndrome in a large French family. Circulation. 2001;104:3081–6.

52. Tan BH, Valdivia CR, Song C, et al. Partial expression defect for the SCN5A missense mutation G1406R depends upon splice variant background Q1077 and rescue by mexiletine. Am J Physiol Heart Circ Physiol. 2006;291:H1822–8.

53. Kehl HG, Haverkamp W, Rellensmann G, et al. Images in cardiovascular medicine. Life-threatening neonatal arrhythmia: successful treatment and confirmation of clinically suspected extreme long QT-syndrome-3. Circulation. 2004;109:e205–2066.

54. Chang CC, Acharfi S, Wu MH, et al. A novel SCN5A mutation manifests as a malignant form of long QT syndrome with perinatal onset of tachycardia/bradycardia. Cardiovasc Res. 2004;64:268–78.

55. Tester DJ, Will ML, Haglund CM, et al. Compendium of cardiac channel mutations in 541 consecutive unrelated patients referred for long QT syndrome genetic testing. Heart Rhythm. 2005;2:507–17.

56. Valdivia CR, Ackerman MJ, Tester DJ, et al. A novel SCN5A arrhythmia mutation, M1766L, with expression defect rescued by mexiletine. Cardiovasc Res. 2002;55:279–89.

57. Ye B, Valdivia CR, Ackerman MJ, et al. A common human SCN5A polymorphism modifies expression of an arrhythmia causing mutation. Physiol Genomics. 2003;12:187–93.

58. Lupoglazoff JM, Cheav T, Baroudi G, et al. Homozygous SCN5A mutation in long-QT syndrome with functional two-to-one atrioventricular block. Circ Res. 2001;89:E16–2121.

59. Tester DJ, Ackerman MJ. Genetic testing for cardiac channelopathies: ten questions regarding clinical considerations for heart rhythm allied professionals. Heart Rhythm. 2005;2:675–7.

60. Shim SH, Ito M, Maher T, et al. Gene sequencing in neonates and infants with the long QT syndrome. Genet Test. 2005;9:281–4.

61. Viswanathan PC, Bezzina CR, George Jr AL, et al. Gating-dependent mechanisms for flecainide action in SCN5A-linked arrhythmia syndromes. Circulation. 2001;104:1200–5.

62. Moss AJ, Windle JR, Hall WJ, et al. Safety and efficacy of flecainide in subjects with long QT-3 syndrome (ΔKPQ mutation): a randomized, double-blind, placebo-controlled clinical trial. Ann Noninvasive Electrocardiol. 2005;10:59–66.

63. Kapa S, Tester DJ, Salisbury BA, et al. Genetic testing for long-QT syndrome: distinguishing pathogenic mutations from benign variants. Circulation. 2009;120:1752–60.

64. Kapplinger JD, Tester DJ, Alders M, et al. An international compendium of mutations in the SCN5A-encoded cardiac sodium channel in patients referred for Brugada syndrome genetic testing. Heart Rhythm. 2010;7:33–46.

65. Veldkamp MW, Wilders R, Baartscheer A, et al. Contribution of sodium channel mutations to bradycardia and sinus node dysfunction in LQT3 families. Circ Res. 2003;92:976–83.

66. Baroudi G, Chahine M. Biophysical phenotypes of SCN5A mutations causing long QT and Brugada syndromes. FEBS Lett. 2000;487:224–8.

67. Nagatomo T, January CT, Makielski JC. Preferential block of late sodium current in the LQT3 ΔKPQ mutant by the class IC antiarrhythmic flecainide. Mol Pharmacol. 2000;57:101–7.

68. Moss AJ, Zareba W, Benhorin J, et al. ECG T-wave patterns in genetically distinct forms of the hereditary long QT syndrome. Circulation. 1995;92:2929–34.

CLP-1-Mediated Transcriptional Control of Hypertrophic Gene Programs Underlying Cardiac Hypertrophy

M.A.Q. Siddiqui, Michael Wagner,
Jorge Espinoza-Derout, Facan Huang,
Daniel Beckles, and Eduardo Mascareno

Abstract

Cardiac hypertrophy is the heart's response to increased work, pressure, or volume overload. It begins with a compensatory phase that allows the heart to meet imposed demand through rapid expression of stress response genes. A decompensatory phase follows marked by additional adaptive stress response gene expression that with prolonged stress progressively turns maladaptive, leading the heart into failure. The transition from compensatory to decompensatory hypertrophy is likely to reflect changes in the transcription factors and regulatory molecules that control these programs in response to changes in stress stimuli and the status of cardiomyocytes throughout the hypertrophic process. Our laboratory has been studying the role of one such transcriptional regulatory molecule, CLP-1 (cardiac lineage protein-1), in the cellular response to hypertrophic stimuli. CLP-1, the mouse homolog of the human HEXIM1 gene, is an inhibitor of P-TEFb (transcription elongation factor b), a component of the transcriptional apparatus that controls RNA polymerase II activity and gene transcription. Knockout of the CLP-1 gene results in a severe form of hypertrophy in fetal mice suggesting that in the absence of the CLP-1 inhibitor, uninhibited P-TEFb activity may lead to unregulated expression of stress response genes and decompensatory hypertrophy. Because of its critical role in regulating the stress gene response to hypertrophic stimuli, we review our laboratory's work on CLP-1, its control of P-TEFb under various hypertrophic conditions, and how it may play an important role in a novel gene control mechanism, called promoter proximal pausing, that ensures the rapid expression of stress response genes in response to hypertrophic stimuli.

M.A.Q. Siddiqui (✉)
The Center for Cardiovascular and Muscle Research
and Department of Cell Biology, State University
of New York Downstate Medical Center,
Brooklyn, NY, USA
e-mail: MAQ.Siddiqui@downstate.edu

B. Ostadal et al. (eds.), *Genes and Cardiovascular Function*,
DOI 10.1007/978-1-4419-7207-1_19, © Springer Science+Business Media, LLC 2011

Keywords

AG490 • Cardiac hypertrophy • Cardiac lineage protein-1 • Compensatory hypertrophy • Cyclin T1 • Cyclin-dependent kinase 9 • Decompensatory hypertrophy • Jak2 kinase • Promoter proximal pausing • STAT transcription factors • Transcription elongation factor b

Introduction

The prevalence of hypertension, diabetes, and valvular diseases among an increasingly aged adult population is leading to an increase in one of the clinical consequences of these diseases – enlargement of the heart or cardiac hypertrophy. Hypertrophy is essentially a response to maintain normal cardiac output in the face of stress-inducing physiological imbalances that make the heart work harder, be they abnormally high blood pressure, compromised renal function, or decreased cardiac output from heart valve insufficiencies. When the heart is challenged with increased work, pressure, or volume overload, it mounts an adaptive response to normalize heart function by increasing contractility and ventricular wall thickness. This adaptive or compensatory phase, called physiological hypertrophy, initially meets imposed demand, but with prolonged load imposition, the compensatory response deteriorates into a maladaptive or decompensatory phase that is marked by depleted metabolic reserves [1, 2], fibrosis [3–6], apoptosis of myocardial cells [7, 8], and eventually heart failure. The decompensatory phase, called pathological hypertrophy, is essentially irreversible and has proven refractory to therapies designed to restore the myocardium to a functional state.

Our laboratory has been investigating the molecules involved in the signaling and transcriptional events that underlie the compensatory and decompensatory phases of cardiac hypertrophy. We have focused our studies on one such molecule, CLP-1 (cardiac lineage protein-1), that we have shown to be an important mediator by which hypertrophic signals evoke a genomic stress response. In this context, we discuss the interaction of the Jak/STAT (Janus kinase/signal transducer and activator of transcription) signal transduction pathway, a well-documented hypertrophic signaling pathway, with CLP-1. Given their central role in transmitting hypertrophic signals to the genome, CLP-1 and the Jak/STAT signaling pathway are likely to interact with a number of other pathways involved in transmitting the hypertrophic stimulus. Since several excellent reviews on these other potential CLP-1-interacting pathways have been published [9–12], our focus will be on the Jak/STAT pathway in this review.

Compensatory and Decompensatory Hypertrophy as Programs of Stress Response

Many, if not all of the events contributing to compensatory and decompensatory hypertrophy are driven by underlying gene programs. In the compensatory phase, gene programs direct heart cells to take adaptive measures to meet imposed demand, while in the decompensatory phase, similarly adaptive programs provide short-term relief but turn maladaptive with continued imposition of work, pressure, or volume overload. The adaptive gene programs include re-expression of the fetal program of contractile protein gene expression [13] and a program of increased protein synthesis [14] that results in increased cell size and thickened ventricular walls to normalize intramural pressure. The maladaptive gene programs include differentiation of fibroblasts into myofibroblasts producing collagen, expression of glycolytic enzymes for glucose metabolism, and eventually programmed cell death of irreversibly malfunctioning cardiomyocytes. The compensatory and decompensatory phases of hypertrophy can thus be viewed as genetic programs of stress response genes that direct cell behavior and ultimately heart function. Since the decompensatory phase leads to pathological hypertrophy, one way of controlling or managing cardiac hypertrophy clinically may be to prevent decompensatory hypertrophy by preventing expression of its underlying maladaptive gene programs.

As with hypertrophy, the maladaptive gene programs of decompensatory hypertrophy can be initially adaptive. For example, the cardiomyocyte adapts to increased energy demands by up-regulating the glycolytic program to make use of the more readily metabolized energy substrate, glucose [15]. While this works for a time, the continued demand for energy soon depletes the stores of glucose in adult heart cells, leaving the heart in metabolic distress and at risk of apoptosis. When the cells eventually die, a second compensatory program initiates to compensate for the loss of cardiomyocytes, which cannot be replaced by proliferation of healthy cardiomyocytes since these are post-mitotic. This compensatory program directs the expansion and differentiation of cardiac fibroblasts into myofibroblasts that produce and deposit increased amounts of extracellular collagen to compensate for the loss of cardiomyocytes, so-called replacement fibrosis [16]. As with glucose metabolism, this compensatory behavior is initially effective but soon turns maladaptive; continued collagen production leads to overproduction and increased stiffness of the myocardium or fibrosis, making contractility more labored and reducing, not increasing, heart function. From this it appears that the balance between glucose and fatty acid oxidation and fibroblast and myofibroblast differentiation and collagen deposition is critical to maintaining a compensatory versus decompensatory hypertrophy. Since these responses are driven by underlying gene programs, this balance is likely to be maintained by factors normally involved in the regulation of gene expression, in particular, regulatory molecules common to both processes and thus able to control the balance between compensatory and decompensatory

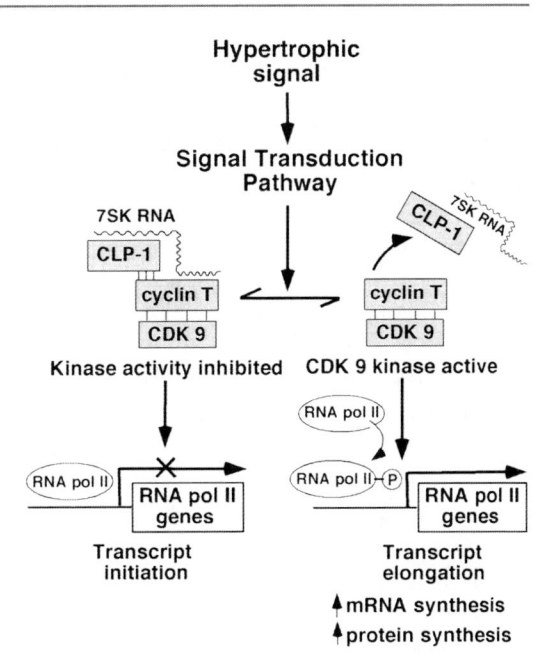

Fig. 1 The P-TEFb model of transcriptional regulation. The active form of P-TEFb is a complex of cyclin-dependent kinase (cdk) 9 and cyclin T1. The inactive form of P-TEFb comprises CLP-1 binding to cyclin T1 via a supporting scaffold of 7SK RNA. This binding inhibits cdk 9 and its phosphorylation activity. Dissociation of CLP-1 derepresses cdk9 kinase activity, allowing for phosphorylation of RNA polymerase (pol) II on its carboxy terminal. This causes RNA pol II to switch from its initiation state to elongation state and complete the synthesis of RNA transcript. In cardiac hypertrophy, we have proposed that this dissociation and the events controlling it may be critical to the up-regulation of RNA and protein synthesis that is a hallmark of cardiomyocyte hypertrophy

gene expression. Since these processes involve expression of stress response gene programs, this regulatory molecule is likely to be a transcription factor controlling these programs throughout the hypertrophic process. Our laboratory has been studying the role of one such regulatory molecule, CLP-1, in the cellular response to hypertrophic stimuli [17–22]. CLP-1, the mouse homolog of the human HEXIM1 gene [23–25], is an inhibitor of P-TEFb (transcription elongation factor b), a component of the transcriptional apparatus that controls RNA polymerase II activity and gene transcription (see Fig. 1) [24, 26].

CLP-1 is Central to the Hypertrophic Response Via its Ability to Control the Transcriptional Status of Stress Response Genes

Two properties of CLP-1 make this transcription cofactor an excellent candidate for regulating hypertrophic stress response gene programs. The first is that it is a general transcription cofactor regulating RNA polymerase (pol) II function and hence the expression of most if not all pol II, protein-encoding genes. It is therefore likely to be involved in the transcription of compensatory as well as decompensatory gene programs. Second, as a regulator of P-TEFb, CLP-1 could be instrumental in controlling the expression of stress response genes, many of which comprise the compensatory and decompensatory gene programs. Recent studies on the function of P-TEFb have provided new insights into how this complex, formed by the association of cyclin-dependent kinase (cdk) 9 and cyclin T1, controls stress response gene expression. A new control mechanism called "promoter-proximal pausing" in which P-TEFb plays a central role has emerged as a way of poising stress response genes to respond rapidly to stress and other stimuli [26–29]. Such a mechanism could allow the rapid expression of stress gene programs in response to hypertrophic stimuli. Because of its central role in regulating stress genes and the fact that stress gene expression is critical to the hypertrophic response, CLP-1 has continued to be the focus of our laboratory's research into the transcriptional mechanisms regulating the hypertrophic response. We review here our laboratory's initial discovery, characterization, and investigation into the properties of CLP-1 that place it at the center of the genomic response to hypertrophic stimuli.

A cDNA clone encoding CLP-1 was first isolated by our laboratory using expression screening of a stage 6 chicken embryo cDNA library designed to isolate transcription factors by their binding to a specific sequence within the myosin light chain-2 gene promoter [17]. This screen yielded a cDNA clone that upon in situ hybridization analysis and immunocytochemical analysis using an antibody made to a CLP-1 fusion protein showed enhanced expression in regions of the embryo specific for early cardiogenic progenitors, for example, the cardiac crescent, giving us our first indication of a cardiogenic function for CLP-1, from which it derived its name: cardiac lineage protein-1 or CLP-1. At this time, CLP-1 was a novel protein with no known homologues, but sequence analysis showed a nuclear localization sequence in the open reading frame that suggested a nuclear function that was later corroborated by immunofluorescent localization to cardiomyocyte nuclei [13]. Together, these data suggested that CLP-1 could be a nuclear factor important to the specification and/or development of early cardiac progenitors.

To facilitate further analysis of CLP-1, our laboratory then cloned the mouse CLP-1 gene from a genomic library and a mouse cDNA from an embryonic heart cDNA library [18]. As with the chicken studies, Northern blot analysis showed an early expression pattern in mouse embryos beginning at embryonic day (E) 7. During this time, other laboratories reported the isolation of human CLP-1, called HEXIM-1, and sequence comparison confirmed the homology between chicken, mouse, and human clones. A wider survey of tissues for CLP-1 expression showed a much wider array of tissues in which CLP-1 is expressed, suggesting that despite its early cardiogenic expression, it may perform a more generalized function in all tissues. This was also confirmed by promoter analysis showing the CLP-1 gene promoter to be active in both muscle cells and the 10T1/2 fibroblast cell line. Up until this point, our preliminary data, while not directly assessing CLP-1 function, nonetheless suggested a positive function related to transcription. When we examined CLP-1 functionally by determining if it could up-regulate the MLC2v gene promoter, we found that either no up-regulation occurred (unchanged promoter activity with increasing amounts of CLP-1 added) or promoter activity went down with added CLP-1 (see Fig. 2). This latter result was obtained in transfected rat primary cardiac cells, suggesting that on at least one cardiogenic promoter in cardiac cells, CLP-1 was acting to suppress transcription. Since the function

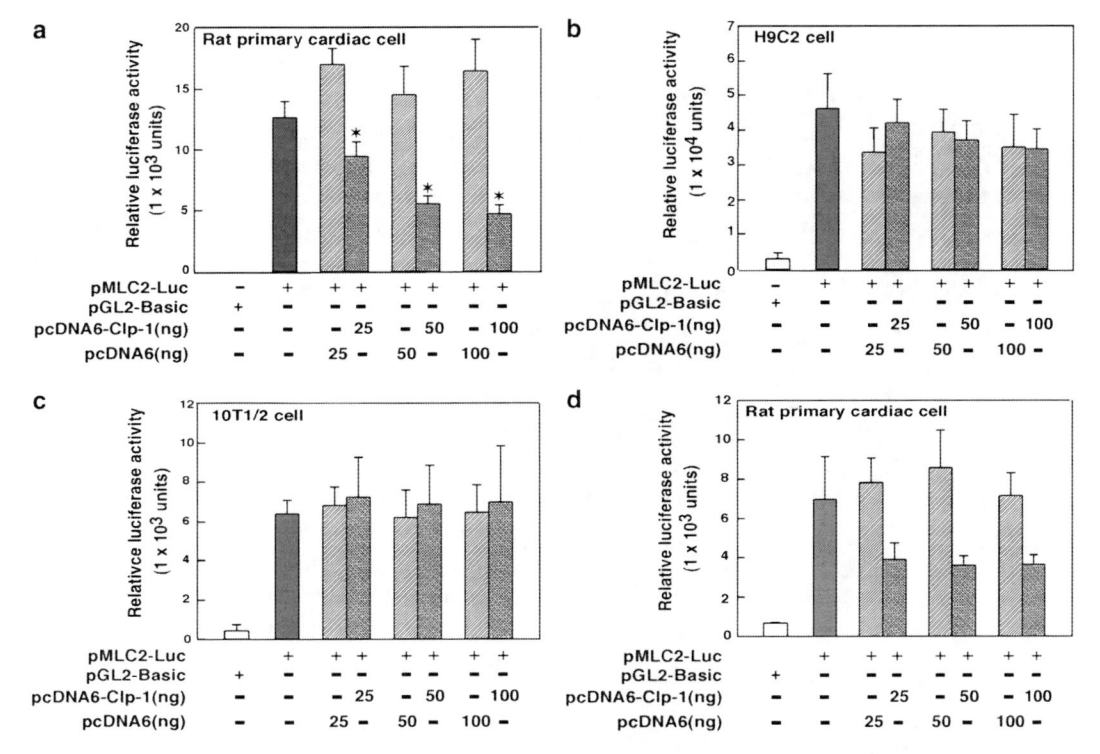

Fig. 2 Effect of CLP-1 expression on MLC-2V promoter activity. Cells were transfected with a cardiac MLC-2V promoter-luciferase reporter construct along with increasing amounts of CLP-expression vector or empty vector alone. Promoter activity is reported as luciferase activity relative to internal control (constitutive promoter construct). Transfected cell types: (**a**) Rat primary cardiac cells; (**b**) H9C2 cells; (**c**) 10T1/2 cells; (**d**) primary rat cardiac cells transfected with a truncated MLC2V promoter driving the luciferase reporter. In rat primary cardiac cells, increasing CLP-1 input leads to decreasing transcription suggesting that CLP-1 may be exerting a negative effect on transcription (Taken from [18] with permission)

of HEXIM1/CLP-1 as an inhibitor of P-TEFb activity and RNA transcription had yet to be described, these results were among the first to indicate a negative rather than a positive regulatory role for CLP-1 in transcription.

Ablation of the CLP-1 Gene Leads to a Fetal Form of Cardiac Hypertrophy

To delve further into the function of CLP-1 in vivo, we ablated the CLP-1 gene in mice [20]. The CLP-1 gene is a single copy gene that lacks introns. Knockout of one CLP-1 allele gave heterozygous mice that were phenotypically normal and viable. However, when these mice were crossed to generate the null CLP-1 phenotype,

genotype analysis of the first several litters showed no CLP-1−/− pups, indicating that the CLP-1 knockout was most likely embryonic lethal. When prenatal embryos and fetuses were genotyped, the expected 1:2:1 ratio for wild-type, heterozygote, and homozygote knockout genotype frequencies became skewed at E 17.5 resulting from a decrease in the number of knockout genotypes. This confirmed that the CLP-1 knockout was embryonic (or fetal) lethal beginning at approximately E17. Prior to E17, the overt appearance of embryos and fetuses showed all embryos to be similar in size and appearance; from E17 onward (until dead embryos were resorbed) the CLP-1 knockout fetuses began to exhibit decreased size and a much paler color than wild-type or heterozygous littermates (see Fig. 3). While an overall growth retardation phenotype

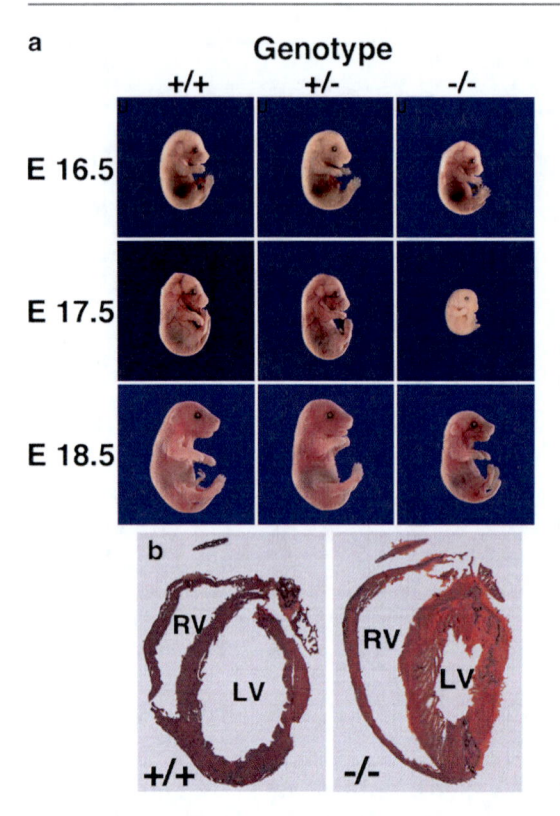

Fig. 3 (a) Overt appearance of wild-type, CLP-1 +/– and CLP-1 –/– fetuses. The CLP-1 phenotype of smaller body size and paler color becomes apparent starting at E16.5 and continues until the embryos are fully resorbed. Some variability is noted in the severity of the phenotype; this reflects slightly different ages from litter to litter and also an effect on phenotype due to litter size with knockout fetuses being affected more in larger litters. (b) Hematoxylin and eosin stained coronal sections of E17.5 wild-type and CLP-1 –/– hearts. E17.5 CLP-1 (–/–) fetal hearts show a thickened left ventricular wall and decreased left ventricular chamber size (Taken from [20] with permission)

could not be ruled out, analysis of internal organs, particularly the heart, showed that it was hypertrophic with a thickened left ventricular wall and decreased left ventricular chamber (see Fig. 3). To further test the possibility of hypertrophy, we examined CLP-1–/– hearts for molecular markers indicative of the hypertrophic state, that is, increased expression of atrial natriuretic factor, β (beta)-myosin heavy chain, and α-skeletal muscle actin, and found that these markers were uniformly elevated in E16 CLP-1–/– hearts relative to wild-type or heterozygous hearts. These results were consistent with the CLP-1–/– hearts being hypertrophic. Ultrastructural analysis using electron

microscopy showed cardiomyocytes from E15.5 to have normal nuclear morphology and sarcomeres with a normal banding pattern indicating a normal cell morphology and contractile apparatus. In contrast, E16.5 myocardium showed electron-dense chromatin masses coalesced near or abutting the nuclear envelope of cells and cytoplasmic mitochondria with far fewer cristae than in wild-type hearts. This morphology indicated that the E16.5 myocardium was undergoing apoptosis. In addition, the normal sarcomeric banding pattern seen in the myofibrils of E15.5 heart was completely destroyed in those of the E16.5 heart indicating a nonfunctioning contractile apparatus. Together, these data suggested that the E16.5 CLP-1 knockout hearts were hypertrophic and progressing to, if not already in, a stage of pathological hypertrophy and heart failure, the most likely cause of death for the CLP-1 knockout fetuses. In addition to its effect on heart function and hypertrophy, as a potential cardiogenic transcription factor or cofactor, we also wanted to examine how the absence of CLP-1 affected the expression of key cardiogenic genes such as Nkx2.5, eHAND, dHAND, and GATA4. Our results showed that dHAND was slightly decreased, but eHAND was completely absent in CLP-1–/– hearts as early as the E9.5 heart tube. Thattaliyath et al. have shown that in aorta-constricted mice with cardiac hypertrophy, eHAND expression is dramatically reduced [30]. In terms of eHAND expression in our CLP-1 knockout mice, this suggests that rather than being a transcription factor that is responsible for eHAND expression, a more likely explanation is that the absence of CLP-1 leads to cardiac hypertrophy, one consequence of which is a reduction in eHAND expression. Thus, this is another indication that the CLP-1 knockout leads to cardiac hypertrophy. Together, the results of our CLP-1 knockout studies indicate that eliminating CLP-1 results in a severe form of fetal cardiac hypertrophy. The developmental nature of the hypertrophy resulting from ablation of the CLP-1 gene could either indicate a requisite role for CLP-1 in critical developmental events or taken in a nondevelopmental context, a role in cardiac hypertrophy independent of developmental events and the developmental stage of the heart.

Hypertrophic Signals Lead to Dissociation of CLP-1 from the P-TEFb Complex, Suggesting that Transcriptional Deregulation is Key to Development of Hypertrophy

During this time, a number of reports were published that provided further support for the notion that CLP-1 was involved in hypertrophy and, perhaps equally important, that this role involved transcriptional regulation. Sano and colleagues were among the first to implicate P-TEFb and its regulation in the response of cardiomyocytes to hypertrophic stimuli [31]. At the time of their studies, it had been shown that P-TEFb was negatively regulated by a small RNA molecule, called 7SK, that bound to cyclin T1 to reversibly inhibit P-TEFb cdk9 kinase activity [32, 33]. The release of 7SK RNA from cyclin T1 derepressed the cyclinT1-cdk9 complex to activate cdk9 to phosphorylate and thus activate RNA pol II and transcriptional elongation. Sano et al. showed that 7SK RNA release from P-TEFb could be induced by hypertrophic stimuli, suggesting that this might be one way in which hypertrophic cardiomyocytes increased total RNA and protein levels, a classic hallmark of hypertrophic cardiac cells. It was not until subsequent studies by Yik et al. and Michels et al. that this model of P-TEFb regulation under stress conditions became further refined [23, 25]. These laboratories were the first to show that the actual cdk9 inhibitor was HEXIM1, the human homologue of mouse CLP-1. The key finding linking CLP-1/HEXIM1 to the findings of Sano et al. was the demonstration that 7SK RNA actually played a support role for CLP-1/HEXIM1 binding to the P-TEFb complex: CLP-1/HEXIM1 could only bind to cyclin T1 via a supporting bridge formed by 7SK RNA [34]. Release of 7SK RNA was important to activating P-TEFb kinase activity only insofar as it mediated the release of CLP-1/HEXIM1, the actual cdk9 inhibitor (see Fig. 1). The findings of these laboratories were extremely important for guiding our subsequent studies on CLP-1's role in cardiac hypertrophy.

With these insights into CLP-1's molecular function and how that function might be involved in controlling the stress gene response to hypertrophic stimuli, we turned our attention to linking the two observations by confirming the association of CLP-1 with components of the P-TEFb complex in cardiomyocytes and examining the behavior of this association under the stress conditions imposed by hypertrophic stimuli [21]. Our studies showed that CLP-1, cdk9, and cyclin T1 all are expressed in embryonic, fetal, and postnatal heart, as determined by Western blot analysis. Co-immunoprecipitation studies showed that CLP-1 and cdk9 can be co-immunoprecipitated using antibodies to cyclin T1, suggesting an association of CLP-1 with the P-TEFb complex. Co-localization of CLP-1 with cdk9 and cyclin T1 using immunohistochemical and immunocytochemical techniques further confirmed the co-localization of these proteins in the nucleus of cardiomyocytes (see Fig. 4). Based on the work of Sano et al. [31], we examined the status of CLP-1's association with the P-TEFb complex under normal versus hypertrophic conditions. Hypertrophy was induced in isolated cardiomyocytes using the well-documented technique of mechanically stretching cardiomyocytes by plating on expandable Flexcell 6-well plates and also by application of hypertrophic cytokines such as endothelin-1 and phenylephrine. Cell lysates were immunoprecipitated with antibodies to cyclin T1 and blotted with antibodies to either cdk9 or CLP-1. In all cases, hypertrophic cardiomyocytes showed P-TEFb complexes to be void of associated CLP-1 molecules indicating their release under hypertrophic conditions. We further tested this model by examining if CLP-1 can be released from P-TEFb complexes under conditions in which the hypertrophic response is abated by blocking a signal transduction pathway known to relay hypertrophic signals from membrane to nucleus, namely the Jak/STAT pathway (discussed in further detail below). Cardiomyocytes were treated with the Jak2 inhibitor AG490 prior to induction of hypertrophy by mechanical stretch. After 48 h of stretching, the cells were assayed by cyclin T1-CLP-1 co-immunoprecipitation assays. In cells treated with AG490, more CLP-1 was present in P-TEFb complexes than in cells left untreated, indicating that release of CLP-1 from P-TEFb occurs only under conditions in which

Fig. 4 Immuno-
cytochemical co-localization
of CLP-1, cyclin T1, and
cdk9 in isolated 2 day
postnatal rat cardiomyo-
cytes. (**A**) and (**B**). Confocal
microscopy shows CLP-1
and cdk9 to be co-localized
to the nucleus of MF20-
positive cardiomyocytes.
Panels i–k are magnified
images of nuclei showing
speckled-type nuclear
staining of cdk9 and
CLP-1. (**C**). Inhibition of
Jak2 kinase results in
decreased dissociation of
CLP-1 under hypertrophic
conditions. AG490 blocks
the dissociation of CLP-1
from the P-TEFb complex
(Taken from [21] with
permission of Oxford
University Press)

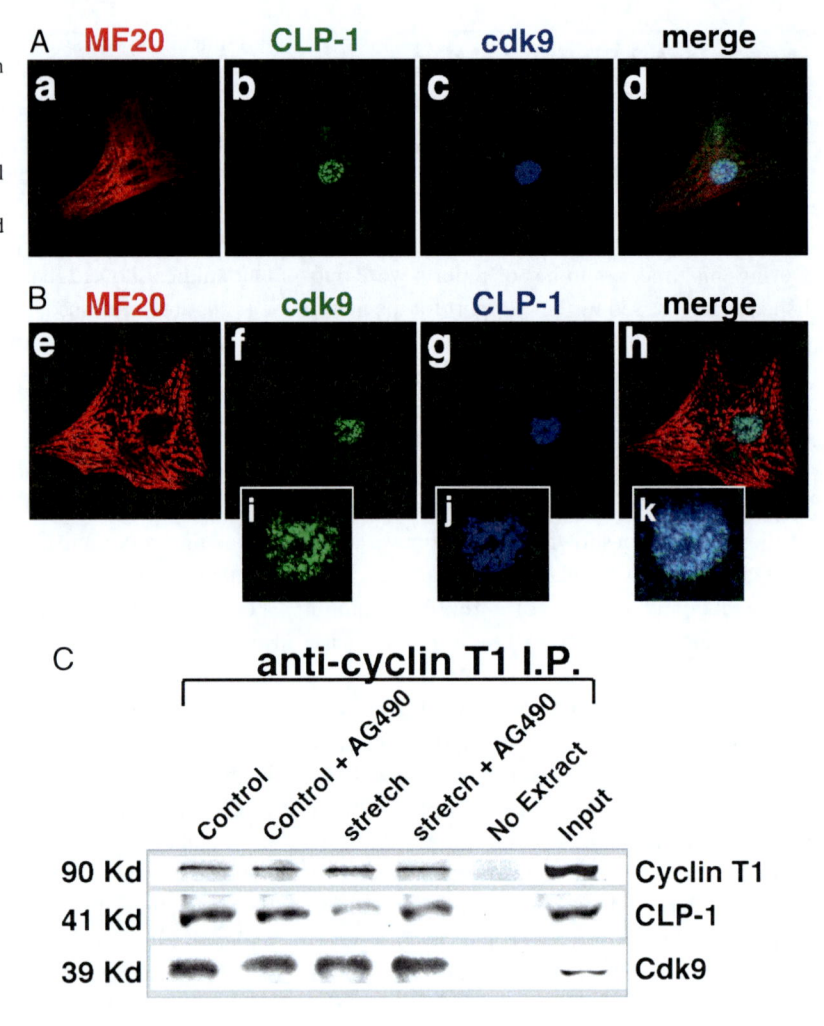

signal transduction pathways that transmit the hypertrophic signal are fully functional (see Fig. 4C). This suggests that the transduced Jak/STAT signal in some way controls the association and/or dissociation of CLP-1 with P-TEFb complexes, thereby controlling RNA pol II activity and transcriptional elongation. This work confirmed and extended the work of Sano et al. and placed CLP-1/HEXIM1 squarely in the center of the transcriptional response to hypertrophic stimuli. Despite the well-documented use of mechanical stretch and hypertrophic cytokines to induce hypertrophy, it still remained to be shown that CLP-1 regulation of P-TEFb activity is an integral part of the hypertrophic response in vivo in enlarged hearts.

Lowering CLP-1 Levels and Increasing P-TEFb Activity Exacerbates the Hypertrophy Seen in Transgenic Models of Cardiac Hypertrophy

To examine CLP-1 function in hypertrophic adult hearts, we resorted to the use of transgenic mice that develop hypertrophy from overexpression of specific genes in the heart [22]. We used two such mouse lines, a line of mice over-expressing calcineurin in the heart (MHC-CnA mice) [35] and a line of mice in which cyclin T1 is over-expressed in the heart (α-MHC-cyclin T1 mice) [31]. Calcineurin over-expressing mice exhibit compensatory hypertrophy during the first few postnatal months of life [36]. We determined CLP-1's association with P-TEFb and its effect on RNA pol II phosphorylation during this time and found that CLP-1 was associated with P-TEFb to a lesser degree than in age-matched wild-type hearts, and that RNA pol II was phosphorylated to a greater extent than in wild-type hearts. This indicates that CLP-1 is predominantly dissociated from P-TEFb complexes in hypertrophic hearts in vivo resulting in activation of P-TEFb kinase activity and RNA pol II, a finding in accord with our in vitro studies. We next sought to test our model of CLP-1 function in hypertrophic hearts by reversing the experimental design: rather than using hypertrophic hearts to determine if CLP-1 is dissociated from P-TEFb, we generated mice having elevated levels of cyclin T1 and decreased levels of CLP-1 and asked if under these conditions the hypertrophy normally seen in the cyclin T1 over-expressors is exacerbated by the lowered CLP-1 levels and the resulting increase in P-TEFb and RNA pol II activity. This is based on the model of CLP-1-P-TEFb interaction in which association of CLP-1 with cyclin T1 inhibits cdk9 kinase activity: by increasing the concentration of cdk9 activator (cyclin T1) and decreasing its inhibitor (CLP-1), we hypothesized that this would lead to increased cdk9 kinase activity, increased RNA pol II transcriptional elongation, and given our results with the CLP-1 knockout mice, an exacerbated hypertrophic response leading to enlarged hearts greater than that seen in MHC-cyclin T1 mice. The results of these experiments did in fact bear out this hypothesis. Alpha-MHC-cyclin T1/CLP-1+/− mice had much larger hearts than α (alpha)-MHC-cyclin T1 or CLP-1 +/− mice with the largest increase in heart-to-body weight ratio among these mice when compared to wild-type mice (see Fig. 5). Phosphorylation of serine 2 in the carboxy terminal domain of RNA pol II was increased by 50% in α (alpha)-MHC-cyclin T1/CLP-1 +/− hearts over that seen in α (alpha)-MHC-cyclin T1 hearts (Fig. 5). This particular phosphorylation is associated with the switch of RNA pol II from a transcriptional initiation state in which RNA synthesis is paused to one in which RNA pol II actively synthesizes the remaining

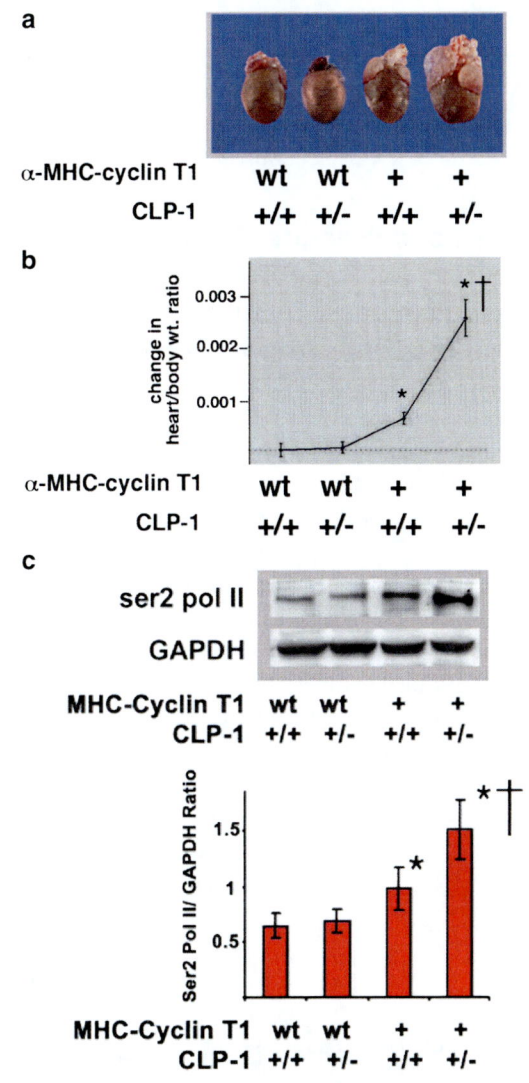

Fig. 5 Exacerbated hypertrophic response in α (alpha)-MHC-cyclin T1/CLP-1 +/− mice. (**a**) Photographs of adult mice hearts of the indicated genotypes. The α (alpha)-MHC-cyclin T1/CLP-1 +/− heart appears to be the most enlarged relative to all other genotypes. It also exhibited the largest change in heart/body weight ratio of all genotypes relative to wild-type mice. (**b**) Quantitation of the relative changes in heart to body weight ratios of the hearts pictured in (**a**). (**c**) The second serine in the domain targeted by cdk9 in the carboxy terminal end of RNA pol II exhibits 50% greater phosphorylation than the α (alpha)-MHC-cyclin T1 mouse heart. This suggests that decreased CLP-1 levels lead to increased cdk9 activity directed to RNA pol II (Taken from [22] with permission)

RNA transcript. Thus, in α (alpha)-MHC-cyclin T1/CLP-1 +/− hearts, RNA pol II's elongation activity is activated to a much greater extent than that in α (alpha)-MHC-cyclin T1 or CLP-1 +/– hearts. This most likely reflects an increase in P-TEFb cdk9 kinase activity, a finding that also bears out our hypothesis.

CLP-1 and Promoter Proximal Pausing Act to Control the Responsiveness of Stress Response Genes to Hypertrophic Stimuli

As our studies on CLP-1's control of P-TEFb in the hypertrophic response progressed, it became increasingly apparent from the work of other laboratories that P-TEFb and its regulatory molecules were at the center of a novel transcriptional control mechanism for the rapid up-regulation of stress response genes. These studies have provided new insights into gene transcription that have informed our understanding of how P-TEFb controls stress response gene expression, particularly as it relates to the hypertrophic stress response. A new control mechanism called "promoter-proximal pausing" has emerged as a way of poising stress response genes in a "ready state" to respond rapidly to stress and other stimuli

[26–29, 37]. In this mechanism, the basal or unstimulated state of stress response genes is one in which RNA pol II has assembled into an initiation complex that initiates RNA synthesis and synthesizes a small nascent but incomplete RNA transcript of very short length whose synthesis has been "paused." Stress signals act to "unpause" the RNA pol II to rapidly complete the transcript and allow for new RNA pol II enzymes to occupy the already assembled gene transcription apparatus and begin synthesizing more RNA (see Fig. 6). Controlling the paused state is P-TEFb. When CLP-1/HEXIM1 is bound to P-TEFb, its cdk9 kinase activity is repressed and its substrate, RNA pol II, is unphosphorylated and in a state of paused synthesis, having initiated synthesis of nascent transcripts. Upon receipt of the appropriate signals, CLP-1/HEXIM1 dissociates from P-TEFb derepressing cyclin T1 and activating cdk9 to phosphorylate the paused RNA pol II and its associated pause factors, NELF (negative elongation factor) [38] and DSIF (DRB sensitivity-inducing factor) [39]. Release of NELF allows RNA pol II to complete synthesis of nascent RNA transcripts into full-length mRNAs for translation into protein. By pre-assembling a transcriptional complex capable of immediately resuming

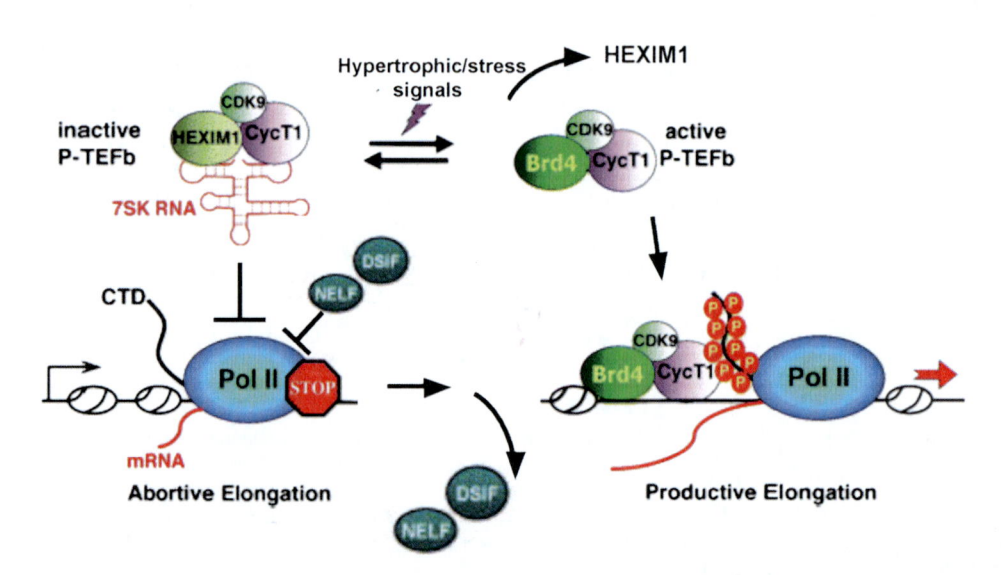

Fig. 6 Activation of P-TEFb by hypertrophic signals. CLP-1/HEXIM1 binds to the P-TEFb complex and inhibits cdk9 kinase activity, causing RNA pol II to remain in an abortive elongation stage (initiation complex) aided by presence of negative transcriptional elongation factors NELF and DSIF. Hypertrophic signals release CLP-1/ HEXIM1, NELF, and DSIF to promote RNA pol II activation by cdk9 and productive RNA chain elongation (Adapted from [47] with permission)

transcription upon receipt of stress signals, the genomic stress response can be launched much more quickly than if all the various components of the transcriptional apparatus had to be assembled de novo. Given our and others' observations on the behavior of P-TEFb and its regulatory components in the response of cardiomyocytes to hypertrophic stimuli, promoter-proximal pausing is likely to be an important transcriptional mechanism controlling the responsiveness of hypertrophic stress response genes to hypertrophic stimuli.

Transduction of Hypertrophic Signals Via the Jak/STAT Pathway Could Directly Affect CLP-1's Control of P-TEFb

While the transcriptional components involved in promoter-proximal pausing have been detailed, little is known about how these components interact with or respond to signals that promote "unpausing" of RNA synthesis and gene transcription. Since the hypertrophic genomic response is driven by hypertrophic signals, how these signals interact with P-TEFb to "unpause" hypertrophic stress response genes remains an essential aspect of this process that has yet to be fully elucidated. Some indication that signaling pathways can interact with P-TEFb has come from studies of stressed cells in which Ca^{2+}-based signaling, PI3K/Akt signaling, and MEK1 signaling pathways were shown to control P-TEFb activity [40–42]. None of these pathways, however, were examined in hypertrophic heart or cardiomyocytes. While such studies will no doubt prove informative, our laboratory has focused on the Jak/STAT signaling pathway as a potential regulator of CLP-1 dissociation from P-TEFb. Our laboratory has a long-standing interest in the Jak/STAT signal transduction pathway, which has been shown to be a major transducer of hypertrophic signals in hypertrophic hearts and cardiomyocytes (reviewed in [43]). The involvement of Jak/STAT in the stress gene response is also well documented with a number of studies showing STAT3 to be essential for inducing cardioprotective genes, a class of stress response genes promoting

cardiomyocyte survival in hypertrophic hearts and mechanically stretched cardiomyocytes (reviewed in [44]). Given that both Jak/STAT and P-TEFb are involved in up-regulating stress response genes, we asked if the STAT signaling pathway might be involved in regulating P-TEFb activity under hypertrophic conditions. Since CLP-1 appears to be fully or near fully dissociated from the P-TEFb complex during hypertrophy induced in cardiomyocytes and in our transgenic models of hypertrophy, we wanted to determine if blocking the Jak/STAT pathway under hypertrophic conditions would lead to CLP-1 being retained by P-TEFb complexes. To do this, we repeated studies in our laboratory in which cardiomyocytes pretreated with the Jak2 kinase inhibitor AG490 and then stimulated with hypertrophic agents failed to develop hypertrophy [45]. When we examined the interaction of CLP-1 with P-TEFb in these cells, we found that despite stimulation with hypertrophic agents, CLP-1 remained bound to P-TEFb [21] (see Fig. 4). Since inhibition of Jak2 prevents STAT activation and mobilization to the nucleus, these results suggested that activated STAT dimers may in some way interact with P-TEFb to prevent CLP-1 binding. For the Jak/STAT pathway to interact with P-TEFb during hypertrophy, Jak2 kinase must first phosphorylate and activate STAT dimers to translocate to the nucleus. Since STATs are not kinases, they most likely activate P-TEFb by competitively preventing or blocking CLP-1 binding. Hou et al. have shown in IL-6-treated HepG2 hepatocarcinoma cells that activated nuclear STAT3 binds to the cdk9/cyclin T complex prior to DNA interaction, suggesting that STAT3 may prevent CLP-1 binding and directly bring the active form of P-TEFb to STAT3-dependent genes to increase transcriptional elongation [46].

Our Jak2 inhibition experiments suggest that nuclear cdk9/cyclin T complexes may preferentially bind STAT3 dimers over CLP-1, thereby directing P-TEFb-cdk9 kinase activity to STAT3-responsive genes where they phosphorylate and switch RNA pol II from its "paused" to elongation state. Such a mechanism could up-regulate compensatory hypertrophic as well as cardioprotective genes in hypertrophic cardiomyocytes. Thus, in addition to promoter-based transcriptional activation, activated STAT dimers may also up-regulate gene transcription by promoting transcriptional elongation. The Jak/STAT pathway and its involvement in the hypertrophic response is an excellent example of how signaling transcription factors like the STATs might interact with P-TEFb to rapidly induce stress response genes. Because they bind specific promoter sequences, STATs could impart sequence specificity to the "unpausing" of stress response genes that P-TEFb would otherwise be unable to do. Documenting this will provide novel information on the role of STATs and CLP-1 in signal-dependent regulation of hypertrophic stress response genes.

Conclusions

In cardiac hypertrophy, work, volume, or pressure overload trigger signal transduction pathways to activate specific genetic programs that allow the heart to increase its output while maintaining normal hemodynamic function. Many of these genetic programs involve stress response genes that are poised to respond immediately to hypertrophic stress signals. This poised state is regulated by a mechanism known as promoter proximal pausing that in turn, is controlled by the transcriptional regulator CLP-1. To trigger the release of stress response genes from this paused state, hypertrophic stress signals must cause the release of CLP-1 from the promoter proximal pausing complex to allow for transcription of response genes. By acting as a signal-dependent switch regulating the transition from poised to active transcription, CLP-1 can control the expression of genes that comprise the genomic compensatory stress response to hypertrophic stimuli.

References

1. Luptak I, Balschi JA, Xing Y, et al. Decreased contractile and metabolic reserve in peroxisome proliferator-activated receptor-alpha-null hearts can be rescued by increasing glucose transport and utilization. Circulation. 2005;112:2339–46.
2. Ingwall JS. Energy metabolism in heart failure and remodeling. Cardiovasc Res. 2009;81:412–9.
3. Eghbali M, Weber KT. Collagen and the myocardium: fibrillar structure, biosynthesis and degradation in relation to hypertrophy and its regression. Mol Cell Biochem. 1990;96:1–14.
4. Boluyt MO, O'Neill L, Meredith AL, et al. Alterations in cardiac gene expression during the transition from stable hypertrophy to heart failure. Marked upregulation of genes encoding extracellular matrix components. Circ Res. 1994;75:23–32.
5. Mujumdar VS, Tyagi SC. Temporal regulation of extracellular matrix components in transition from compensatory hypertrophy to decompensatory heart failure. J Hypertens. 1999;17:261–70.
6. Ho CY, Lopez B, Coelho-Filho OR, et al. Myocardial fibrosis as an early manifestation of hypertrophic cardiomyopathy. N Engl J Med. 2010;363:552–63.
7. Dorn 2nd GW. Apoptotic and non-apoptotic programmed cardiomyocyte death in ventricular remodeling. Cardiovasc Res. 2009;81:465–73.
8. van Empel VP, Bertrand AT, Hofstra L, et al. Myocyte apoptosis in heart failure. Cardiovasc Res. 2005;67:21–9.
9. Heineke J, Molkentin JD. Regulation of cardiac hypertrophy by intracellular signaling pathways. Nat Rev Mol Cell Biol. 2006;7:589–600.
10. Rose BA, Force T, Wang Y. Mitogen-activated protein kinase signaling in the heart: angels versus demons in a heart-breaking tale. Physiol Rev. 2010;90:1507–46.
11. Clerk A, Cullingford TE, Fuller SJ, et al. Signaling pathways mediating cardiac myocyte gene expression in physiological and stress responses. J Cell Physiol. 2007;212:311–22.
12. Kehat I, Molkentin JD. Extracellular signal-regulated kinase 1/2 (ERK1/2) signaling in cardiac hypertrophy. Ann NY Acad Sci. 2010;1188:96–102.
13. Black FM, Packer SE, Parker TG, et al. The vascular smooth muscle alpha-actin gene is reactivated during cardiac hypertrophy provoked by load. J Clin Invest. 1991;88:1581–8.
14. Bernardo BC, Weeks KL, Pretorius L, et al. Molecular distinction between physiological and pathological cardiac hypertrophy: experimental findings and therapeutic strategies. Pharmacol Ther. 2010;128:191–227.
15. Lehman JJ, Kelly DP. Gene regulatory mechanisms governing energy metabolism during cardiac hypertrophic growth. Heart Fail Rev. 2002;7:175–85.
16. Mann DL. Mechanisms and models in heart failure: a combinatorial approach. Circulation. 1999;100:999–1008.
17. Ghatpande S, Goswami S, Mathew S, et al. Identification of a novel cardiac lineage-associated protein(cCLP-1): a candidate regulator of cardiogenesis. Dev Biol. 1999;208:210–21.
18. Huang F, Wagner M, Siddiqui MA. Structure, expression, and functional characterization of the mouse CLP-1 gene. Gene. 2002;292:245–59.
19. Rice AP. Dysregulation of positive transcription elongation factor B and myocardial hypertrophy. Circ Res. 2009;104:1327–9.

20. Huang F, Wagner M, Siddiqui MA. Ablation of the CLP-1 gene leads to down-regulation of the HAND1 gene and abnormality of the left ventricle of the heart and fetal death. Mech Dev. 2004;121:559–72.

21. Espinoza-Derout J, Wagner M, Shahmiri K, et al. Pivotal role of cardiac lineage protein-1 (CLP-1) in transcriptional elongation factor P-TEFb complex formation in cardiac hypertrophy. Cardiovasc Res. 2007;75:129–38.

22. Espinoza-Derout J, Wagner M, Salciccioli L, et al. Positive transcription elongation factor b activity in compensatory myocardial hypertrophy is regulated by cardiac lineage protein-1. Circ Res. 2009;104: 1347–54.

23. Yik JH, Chen R, Nishimura R, et al. Inhibition of P-TEFb (CDK9/Cyclin T) kinase and RNA polymerase II transcription by the coordinated actions of HEXIM1 and 7SK snRNA. Mol Cell. 2003;12:971–82.

24. Dey A, Chao SH, Lane DP. HEXIM1 and the control of transcription elongation: from cancer and inflammation to AIDS and cardiac hypertrophy. Cell Cycle. 2007;6:1856–63.

25. Michels AA, Nguyen VT, Fraldi A, et al. MAQ1 and 7SK RNA interact with CDK9/cyclin T complexes in a transcription-dependent manner. Mol Cell Biol. 2003;23:4859–69.

26. Peterlin BM, Price DH. Controlling the elongation phase of transcription with P-TEFb. Mol Cell. 2006;23:297–305.

27. Price DH. Poised polymerases: on your mark…get set…go! Mol Cell. 2008;30(1):7–10.

28. Kohoutek J. P-TEFb- the final frontier. Cell Div. 2009;4:19.

29. Core LJ, Lis JT. Transcription regulation through promoter-proximal pausing of RNA polymerase II. Science. 2008;319:1791–2.

30. Thattaliyath BD, Livi CB, Steinhelper ME, et al. HAND1 and HAND2 are expressed in the adult-rodent heart and are modulated during cardiac hypertrophy. Biochem Biophys Res Commun. 2002;297:870–5.

31. Sano M, Abdellatif M, Oh H, et al. Activation and function of cyclin T-Cdk9 (positive transcription elongation factor-b) in cardiac muscle-cell hypertrophy. Nat Med. 2002;8:1310–7.

32. Yang Z, Zhu Q, Luo K, et al. The 7SK small nuclear RNA inhibits the CDK9/cyclin T1 kinase to control transcription. Nature. 2001;414:317–22.

33. Nguyen VT, Kiss T, Michels AA, et al. 7SK small nuclear RNA binds to and inhibits the activity of CDK9/cyclin T complexes. Nature. 2001;414:322–5.

34. Michels AA, Fraldi A, Li Q, et al. Binding of the 7SK snRNA turns the HEXIM1 protein into a P-TEFb (CDK9/cyclin T) inhibitor. EMBO J. 2004;23: 2608–19.

35. Molkentin JD, Lu JR, Antos CL, et al. A calcineurin-dependent transcriptional pathway for cardiac hypertrophy. Cell. 1998;93:215–28.

36. Semeniuk LM, Severson DL, Kryski AJ, Swirp SL, Molkentin JD, Duff HJ. Time-dependent systolic and diastolic function in mice overexpressing calcineurin. Am J Physiol Heart Circ Physiol. 2003;284:H425–30.

37. Zeitlinger J, Stark A, Kellis M, et al. RNA polymerase stalling at developmental control genes in the Drosophila melanogaster embryo. Nat Genet. 2007; 39:1512–6.

38. Fujinaga K, Irwin D, Huang Y, et al. Dynamics of human immunodeficiency virus transcription: P-TEFb phosphorylates RD and dissociates negative effectors from the transactivation response element. Mol Cell Biol. 2004;24:787–95.

39. Yamada T, Yamaguchi Y, Inukai N, et al. P-TEFb-mediated phosphorylation of hSpt5 C-terminal repeats is critical for processive transcription elongation. Mol Cell. 2006;21:227–37.

40. Chen R, Liu M, Li H, et al. PP2B and PP1alpha cooperatively disrupt 7SK snRNP to release P-TEFb for transcription in response to Ca2+ signaling. Genes Dev. 2008;22:1356–68.

41. Contreras X, Barboric M, Lenasi T, et al. HMBA releases P-TEFb from HEXIM1 and 7SK snRNA via PI3K/Akt and activates HIV transcription. PLoS Pathog. 2007;3:1459–69.

42. Fujita T, Ryser S, Piuz I, et al. Up-regulation of P-TEFb by the MEK1-extracellular signal-regulated kinase signaling pathway contributes to stimulated transcription elongation of immediate early genes in neuroendocrine cells. Mol Cell Biol. 2008;28:1630–43.

43. Yamauchi-Takihara K. gp130-mediated pathway and heart failure. Future Cardiol. 2008;4(4):427–37.

44. Wagner M, Siddiqui MA. Signaling networks regulating cardiac myocyte survival and death. Curr Opin Investig Drugs. 2009;10:928–37.

45. Beckles DL, Mascareno E, Siddiqui MA. Inhibition of Jak2 phosphorylation attenuates pressure overload cardiac hypertrophy. Vascul Pharmacol. 2006;45:350–7.

46. Hou T, Ray S, Brasier AR. The functional role of an interleukin 6-inducible CDK9.STAT3 complex in human gamma-fibrinogen gene expression. J Biol Chem. 2007;282:37091–102.

47. Zhou Q, Yik JH. The Yin and Yang of P-TEFb regulation: implications for human immunodeficiency virus gene expression and global control of cell growth and differentiation. Microbiol Mol Biol Rev. 2006;70: 646–59.

Molecular Mechanisms of Subcellular Remodeling in Congestive Heart Failure

Andrea P. Babick, Alison L. Müller, and Naranjan S. Dhalla

Abstract

Cardiac dysfunction in congestive heart failure (CHF) is generally associated with changes in the biochemical activity of different subcellular organelles including the sarcolemma (SL), sarcoplasmic reticulum (SR), and myofibrils (MF). Extensive research has been carried out by employing a wide variety of experimental models as well as myocardial tissue from patients with CHF to examine if changes in the activities of subcellular organelles are due to corresponding changes in cardiac protein content and gene expression. Varying degrees of alterations in mRNA levels and protein content for SL, SR, and MF have been observed in the failing heart. Furthermore, improvement in cardiac function in CHF by different pharmacologic interventions has been associated with attenuation of changes in gene and protein expression for SL, SR, and MF. These observations are consistent with the view that subcellular remodeling and subsequent cardiac dysfunction in CHF may be a consequence of alterations in cardiac gene expression.

Keywords

Ca^{2+} transport • Ca^{2+}-pump ATPase • Cardiac dysfunction • Cardiac remodeling • Congestive heart failure • Myofibrillar ATPase • Myofibrils • Na^+-Ca^{2+} exchange • Na^+-K^+ ATPase • Sarcolemma • Sarcoplasmic reticulum • Subcellular remodeling

Introduction

It is generally accepted that cardiac dysfunction in congestive heart failure (CHF) is due to changes in the size and shape of the heart (cardiac remodeling) [1–4]. However, there are several experimental and clinical situations where cardiac dysfunction has been observed without any

N.S. Dhalla (✉)
Institute of Cardiovascular Sciences, St. Boniface General Hospital Research Centre, Winnipeg, Canada

Department of Physiology, University of Manitoba, Winnipeg, Canada
e-mail: nsdhalla@sbrc.ca

evidence of cardiac remodeling and vice versa [5–8]. In fact, cardiac remodeling at initial stages of myocardial hypertrophy is accompanied by no changes or hyperfunction of the heart [9]. Accordingly, it has been proposed that cardiac dysfunction in CHF is associated with remodeling of subcellular organelles including sarcolemma (SL), sarcoplasmic reticulum (SR), myofibrils (MF), and mitochondria (MIT), as well as extracellular matrix (ECM) [5–8]. It should be noted that subcellular remodeling refers to changes in molecular and physical structure as well as the chemical composition of different organelles in the myocardium. Such defects may occur in one or more organelles depending upon the stage of CHF development as well as the type of pathophysiologic stimulus for heart disease. Although different mechanisms concerned with the synthesis and degradation of subcellular organelles are considered to result in subcellular remodeling [5–8], the present article is intended to focus on changes in some of the gene and protein expressions which have been reported to induce subcellular defects for the occurrence of cardiac dysfunction in CHF. In particular, it is planned to highlight the significance of alterations in the expression of some proteins for the remodeling of SL, SR, and MF, which are known to play a major role in determining the subcellular activities and thereby the status of heart function. It is pointed out that it is not our intention to undermine the importance of MIT or ECM remodeling in inducing cardiac dysfunction during the development of CHF as these mechanisms of heart disease are known to play a major role in energy production and maintenance of the shape and size of the heart, respectively.

Remodeling of SL Membrane in CHF

Although SL membrane contains several receptors, exchangers, transporters, and enzymes that play an important role in the regulation and maintenance of cardiac function, it is planned to limit the discussion to the Na^+-K^+ ATPase and Na^+-Ca^{2+} exchanger to illustrate their remodeling and modification of their function in CHF. The Na^+-K^+

ATPase is a prominent member of the SL protein family [10], which exists in virtually all animal tissues, as well as the human myocardium [11]. This enzyme is responsible for the active transport of Na^+ ions out of the cell, while simultaneously importing K^+ ions [10], and hence functions to maintain cell volume, establish ionic gradients, and preserve membrane potential of the cardiomyocyte [12]. Consequently, a defect in the function of this enzyme was found to be related to abnormalities in cardiac performance and has been outlined as a salient feature of the subcellular basis of CHF [11–15]. A wide variety of changes in the mRNA level, protein content, and activities of Na^+-K^+ ATPase as well as Na^+-Ca^{2+} exchanger were observed in different studies, as shown in Table 1 [16–22].

It is noteworthy that Na^+-K^+ ATPase is composed of different subunits such as α_1, α_2, α_3, β_1, β_2, and β_3, and several investigators have examined alterations in these subunits in heart disease. Charlemagne et al. [13] reported that there was a reduction in the α_2 mRNA and protein levels in mild and severe stages of hypertrophy, while the compensated stage of hypertrophy revealed no alterations in the α_1 and β_1 mRNA and protein levels. Furthermore, the α_3 mRNA and protein levels were increased at 5 days and 30–50 post-stenosis of the abdominal aorta, respectively. In another study, Semb et al. [15] observed that 6 wks post-MI showed a reduction in α_2 mRNA and protein levels, with no alterations in the expression of the α_1 and β_1 subunits; however an increase in the α_3 subunit at the transcriptional level was noted. This was supported by Book et al. [23], who indicated that at 8 wks post-stenosis of the left renal artery, there was a decrease in the α_2 mRNA and protein levels with unchanged α_1 expression, and a reduction in the β_1 protein levels. A unique experimental animal model of heart failure, UM-X7.1 cardiomyopathic hamsters, was studied by Kato et al. [14], who reported a decrease in the α_2 mRNA, protein and α_3 protein levels with enhanced α_1 and β_1 mRNA and protein levels, with contrasting undetected levels of α_3 mRNA.

In terms of the functional alterations in the Na^+-K^+ ATPase, Dixon et al. [24] monitored its

Table 1 Modifications in SL membrane protein and gene expressions post myocardial infarction

Animal model/time point	Genes of interest	Findings	Reference
Male SD rat, CL/8 wks	Na⁺/K⁺ ATPase	↓ Na⁺/K⁺ α_2 *mRNA* and *protein* ↑ Na⁺/K⁺ α_3 *mRNA* and *protein* NC Na⁺/K⁺ α_1 and β_1	Guo et al. [16]
Male SD rat, CL/7 wks	NCX, Na⁺/K⁺ ATPase	↓ NCX *mRNA* and *protein* levels ↓ Na⁺/K⁺ $\alpha_{1,2}$ and β_1 *protein* levels ↑ Na⁺/K⁺ α_3 *protein* levels	Shao et al. [17]
Male SD rat, CL/37 wks	NCX, Na⁺/K⁺ ATPase	↓ Na⁺/K⁺ α_2 *mRNA* levels ↑ Na⁺/K⁺ $\alpha_{1,2}$ *mRNA* levels ↑ NCX *mRNA* levels	Ren et al. [18]
Human end stage heart failure	NCX	↑ NCX *protein* levels	Schillinger et al. [19]
Male Wistar rat, CL/110 days	NCX	↑ NCX *mRNA* and *protein* levels	Sjaastad et al. [20]
Male Wistar rat, CL/4 and 12 wks	NCX	↑ NCX *mRNA* at 4 and 12 wks	Hanatani et al. [21]
Male Wistar rat, CL/1 wk, 3 wks, 3 months	NCX	↑ NCX *mRNA* at 1 and 3 wks ↓ NCX *mRNA* at 3 months	Yoshiyama et al. [22]

SD Sprague Dawley, *CL* coronary ligation, *SHR* spontaneously hypertensive rats, *NCX* Na⁺/Ca²⁺ exchanger, *Na⁺/K⁺* Na⁺/K⁺ ATPase, *wks* weeks, *NC* no change observed

activity at 4, 8, and 16 wks post-MI, and discovered that at 4 wks, the activity was unchanged, but at 8 and 16 wks the activity was significantly decreased. This finding suggested that the activity of the Na⁺-K⁺ ATPase may conceivably play a part in the adaptive mechanism of the heart that occurs during the development of CHF. Auxiliary investigations by Shao et al. [17] demonstrated that reduced activity of this SL enzyme was coupled with the reduction in the expression of the α_1, α_2, and β_1 mRNA and protein levels, in addition to an elevation in the expression of the α_3 subunit. Shao et al. [17] further demonstrated that when imidapril (an angiotensin converting enzyme inhibitor (ACE)) was administered in animals with CHF, the Na⁺-K⁺ ATPase activity improved and the changes in the gene expression of the SL proteins were attenuated as a consequence of the blockade of the renin-angiotensin system (RAS). Further studies by Ren et al. [18] revealed that after 37 wks of treatment of 3 wks post-MI with imidapril attenuated the reduction in the activity of the Na⁺-K⁺ ATPase, with paralleled trends in the expression of both the mRNA and protein content.

The Na⁺-Ca²⁺ exchange protein, which uses the influx of Na⁺ to extrude intracellular Ca²⁺, is a prominent member of the SL proteins and is situated in the T-tubules closest to the sites of Ca²⁺ release from the SR [25]. The fully mature form of the Na⁺-Ca²⁺ exchanger exists as 120 kDa and is responsible for maintaining Ca²⁺ homeostasis in the cell [26]. Since its discovery, the kinetic parameters of this enzyme suggest that this system can encompass rapid Ca²⁺ transport in and out of the myocardial cell during the cardiac contractile cycle [27]. Though its significance in cardiac excitation-contraction coupling in the normal heart has been well established, its role in the failing myocardium has yet to be fully characterized. Some of the studies [17–22] indicating alterations in SL Na⁺-Ca²⁺ exchanger activity, as well as gene and protein expressions, are shown in Table 1. In a clinical study on dilated cardiomyopathy (DCM) and coronary artery disease (CAD), Studer et al. [28] evaluated the expression of the Na⁺-Ca²⁺ exchanger together with the SR Ca²⁺-pump ATPase (SERCA). Among the two patient groups employed, the mRNA and protein levels of the Na⁺-Ca²⁺ exchanger were elevated in contrast to the reduction in the mRNA and protein levels of SERCA [28]; this observation gave rise to the idea that the increased expression of the Na⁺-Ca²⁺ exchanger somewhat compensated for the diminished function of the SR to remove Ca^{2+} from the cytosol during relaxation. Furthermore, these findings were supplemented by Hasenfuss et al. [29] who affirmed that the decreased levels of SERCA in concert with unaltered levels of the Na^+-Ca^{2+}exchange, accounted for the disorder in diastolic dysfunction. On the other hand, early stages of CHF due to MI have shown a reduction in the activity, mRNA, and protein expression of Na^+-Ca^{2+} exchange [17, 30]. Schillinger et al. [19] illustrated, in the hours preceding cardiac transplantation, that the increase in the Na^+-Ca^{2+} exchanger, collectively with the reduction in SERCA, provided a substantial association amongst changes in neurohormonal levels of epinephrine and SL activity of Na^+-Ca^{2+} exchange. They further projected that during CHF, the activation of the sympathetic nervous system conceivably amplified the expression of the Na^+-Ca^{2+} exchanger, which may potentially have a role in the onset of malignant ventricular arrhythmias. The intensifying concern of progressing arrhythmias in CHF was previously examined by Reinecke et al. [31]. It was indicated that the enhanced activity of the Na^+-Ca^{2+} exchange in end-stage HF was a result of its increased protein levels, and that this increase provided an augmented influx of Na^+, which was further associated with potential membrane depolarizations to create amplified arrhythmogenesis. Nonetheless, alterations in the activation as well as mRNA and protein levels for both Na^+-Ca^{2+} exchanger and Na^+-K^+ ATPase suggest the occurrence of SL remodeling during the development of CHF.

Remodeling of SR Membrane in CHF

During cardiac relaxation, Ca^{2+} is pumped from the cytosol into the SR through the 105 kDa SR Ca^{2+}-pump ATPase [32, 33]. As this enzyme is responsible for the diastolic phase of the cardiac cycle, any impairments in this process of Ca^{2+} sequestration could possibly contribute to the pathophysiology of CHF. Supporting evidence for this postulation regarding cardiac contractile dysfunction in the failing heart include (a) an increased abundance of SERCA with contrasting decreased levels of PLB in response to prolonged exposure to thyroxine [34, 35]; (b) an abnormal force–frequency relationship, whereby increased frequency of stimulation gives a decreased developed tension [36]; and (c) a down-regulated β-adrenergic receptor to give rise to reduced levels of cAMP, which further affects the regulation of PLB and, in turn, disrupts its negative inhibitory regulation of SERCA2a [37, 38]. Extensive research has been focused on elucidating the mechanisms involved in the development of CHF in various experimental models. Clinical studies performed on the isolated human myocardium have shown an overall decrease in SERCA mRNA [39–41] and protein levels, in addition to a reduction in the abnormal handling of Ca^{2+} by SERCA itself [42, 43]. To assess the validity of these applications, different investigators have attempted to compare the findings in animal models of CHF with the failing human myocardium. In a report by Movsesian et al. [44], findings showed a reduction in the Ca^{2+} sequestration of the failing human myocardium, consistent with those of the animal models, and can be attributed to decreased levels of SERCA mRNA produced during gene transcription. Further studies supporting this decrease in SERCA expression and function in the failing heart include models of the pressure-overloaded rat [33], the tachycardia-induced mongrel dog [45], the volume-overloaded rat [46], and the transgenically engineered hypertensive rat [47]. Though this offers insight into the molecular pathogenesis of CHF, the data accumulated thus far raises more questions than have been answered. If in fact the protein level of SERCA remains unchanged in the failing heart, the answer may possibly lie in the complex mechanisms concerning transcription, translation, and protein degradation of the SR membrane [44]. Varying degrees of alterations in different SR protein content and gene expressions indicating remodeling SR membrane in CHF due to MI are shown in Table 2 [17–19, 21, 28, 29, 48–60].

The Ca^{2+} uptake process of SERCA is intimately modulated through another SR protein, PLB, which is composed of five equal monomers. This 30 kDa protein [61] inhibits SERCA through

Table 2 Modifications in SR protein and gene expressions post myocardial infarction

Animal model/time point	Genes of interest	Findings	Reference
Male SD rat, CL/5 wks	SERCA2a/PLB/RyR	↓ SERCA2a/PLB/RyR *mRNA* ↓ SERCA2a/PLB/RyR *protein*	Sanganalmath et al. [48]
Male SD rat, CL/1 day, 2 wks, 4 wks	SERCA2a	↓ SERCA2a *mRNA* day 1 ↓ SERCA2a *protein* at 4 wks	Sallinen et al. [49]
Male Wistar rat, CL/12 wks	SERCA2a	↓ SERCA2a *mRNA* levels	Prunier et al. [50]
Male SD rat, CL/7 wks	SERCA2a/PLB/RyR	↓ SERCA2a/PLB/RyR *mRNA* levels	Shao et al. [17]
Male SD rat, CL/37 wks	SERCA2a/PLB/ RyR/CQS	*NC* SERCA2a/RyR/CQS *mRNA* ↓ PLB *mRNA* levels	Ren et al. [18]
Male SD rat, CL/16 wks	SERCA2a/PLB/RyR	↓ SERCA2a, PLB *mRNA* levels ↑ RyR *mRNA* levels	Xu et al. [51]
Male SD rat, CL/7 wks	SERCA2a/PLB/ RYR/CQS	↓ SERCA2a/PLB/RyR/CQS *mRNA* ↓ SERCA2a/PLB/RyR/CQS *protein*	Guo et al. [52]
Human end stage heart failure	SERCA2a	↓ SERCA2a *protein*	Schillinger et al. [19]
Male SD rat, CL/12 wks	SERCA2a/RyR	↓ SERCA2a/RyR *mRNA* levels	Sakai et al. [53]
Male SD rat, CL/6 wks	SERCA2a/PLB	*NC*	Ambrose et al. [54]
Human heart DCM, ICM	SERCA2a	↓ SERCA2a *protein* levels	Hasenfuss et al. [29]
Male SD rat, CL/8 wks	SERCA2a/PLB	↓ SERCA2a/PLB *mRNA* & *protein*	Shao et al. [55]
Male SD rat, CL/3 wks	SERCA2a	↓ SERCA2a *protein* levels	Zhang et al. [56]
Male SD rat, CL/4, 12 wks	SERCA2a	↓ SERCA2a *mRNA* 12 wks	Hanatani et al. [21]
Male SD rat, CL/4 wks	SERCA2a	↓ SERCA2a *mRNA* levels	Iijima et al. [57]
Human idiopathic DCM	SERCA2a/PLB	*NC*	Munch et al. [58]
Male SD rat CL/1 day, 1 wk and 6 wks	SERCA2a/PLB	*NC* in SERCA2a *mRNA* or *protein* ↓ PLB *mRNA* transiently on day1	Yue et al. [59]
Male SD rat, CL/4, 8 and 16 wks	SERCA2a	↓ SERCA2a *mRNA* at 4, 8, 16 wks ↓ SERCA2a *protein* at 8 and 16 wks	Zarain-Herzberg et al. [60]
Human DCM, CAD	SERCA2a	↓ SERCA2a *mRNA* and *protein*	Studer et al. [28]

SD Sprague Dawley, *CL* coronary ligation, *SERCA2a* sarco(endo)plasmic reticulum Ca²⁺ ATPase, *PLB* phospholamban, *RyR* ryanodine receptor, *CQS* calsequestrin, *DCM* dilated cardiomyopathy, *ICM* idiopathic cardiomyopathy, *CAD* coronary artery disease, *NC* no change observed, *wks* weeks

direct interaction, which depresses the transport of Ca^{2+} into the SR [62]. As phosphorylation of PLB relieves this inhibition and allows for Ca^{2+} uptake to occur, it is thought that this resulting de-inhibition through kinase activity is the principal molecular mechanism responsible for the inotropic effects involved in the β-adrenergic receptor system [44]. Compelling evidence to substantiate this phenomenon was seen in a study involving the isoproterenol myocardial response in mice deficient in the PLB gene in comparison to their control [63]. This investigation has demonstrated that the PLB-deficient mice exhibited high rates of contraction and relaxation in the absence of isoproterenol with no increase in response in its presence, which correlated well with the observation that the control mice had

low rates of contraction and relaxation in the absence of isoproterenol, but showed increased rates with progressive exposure to isoproterenol. In accordance, these results reflect the mechanism by which the phosphorylation of PLB removes the inhibitory effect on SERCA to permit the transport of Ca^{2+} into the SR.

Ca^{2+} release from the SR is achieved through the RyR, which is composed of four monomers of ~560,000 kDa [64, 65]. Evidently, the cardiac RyR mRNA is unique to the myocardium and is not expressed in fast- or slow-twitch skeletal muscle [66, 67]. Although the status of Ca^{2+} pumping into the SR has been extensively studied in CHF of humans and animal models, relatively fewer studies are available on the Ca^{2+} release process in the failing heart. When SR membrane vesicles were incorporated into artificial planar phospholipid bilayers with the activity of single channels subsequently recorded using voltage clamp conditions, unaltered characteristic behavior of these channels was observed in CHF from ischemic cardiomyopathy, DCM, congenital disease, or valvular disease as compared to normal hearts [68, 69]. Yet contradictory to these results, another study revealed that the threshold of Ca^{2+} release, as induced by caffeine, was remarkably increased in the hearts of patients with DCM as opposed to normal hearts, thus suggesting an impaired gating mechanism in the Ca^{2+}-release channel [70]. While comparing the Ca^{2+}-release activity in both pressure-overloaded and volume-overloaded rats, Hisamatsu et al. [46] have documented enhanced Ca^{2+} release in the compensated left ventricular hypertrophy stage of the pressure-overloaded model, with a contrasting decrease in Ca^{2+}-release activity and number of RyR in the volume-overloaded model. Cory et al. [71] have observed that both the density of the SR terminal cisternae and the activity of RyR were reduced in the Doberman Pinscher dog CHF model, as well as during rapid ventricular pacing in mongrel dogs. Additionally, Arai et al. [41] documented a reduction in RyR mRNA in patients suffering from end-stage CHF from primary pulmonary hypertension, DCM, or ischemic heart disease. Furthermore, Pennock et al. [72] described that after ligation of the circumflex artery in New Zealand white rabbits, the administration of 3,5-diiodothyropropionic acid (DITPA) prevented the reduction in the protein density of RyR, with no measurable changes at the gene mRNA level, thereby improving SR function in the infarcted rabbit heart. In view of these studies, it offers that changes in the expression of mRNA and protein content for RyR may depend upon the stage of SR remodeling during the development of CHF.

Remodeling of MF in CHF

The structural contractile unit of the myocardium controls the transition of the diastolic state to the systolic state through various intricate steric,

allosteric, and cooperative mechanisms of the MF thick and thin filaments [73]. Upon cardiac distress, the MF, which represent more than 50% of the cell volume, are considered to adapt by increasing in size, number, and overall expression [74]. One of the major components of the cardiac contractile apparatus is the myosin motor of the thick filament protein system, which acts as the cross-bridge for interacting with the thin filament system to produce force via ATP hydrolysis [75]. As shown in Table 3 [76–83], various studies have revealed a significant reduction in MF ATPase activity in the failing heart [84], including CHF due to mitral valve insufficiency, pressure overload, idiopathic cardiomyopathy, and CAD [85–89]. Composed of two heavy chains, each associated with two different light chains [90, 91], myosin is involved in the imperative process that influences cardiac systolic and diastolic functions. The myosin light chains (MLC) are categorized into special groups and are called essential MLC (MLC-1) and regulatory MLC (MLC-2). In contrast to the thick filament family, the troponin network is a collection of proteins that encompasses the thin filament regulatory elements [92] and plays a crucial role in Ca^{2+} sensitivity on the MF and regulating MF ATPase activity [93]. Currently, it is believed that the binding and removal of Ca^{2+} from troponin transmits conformational changes to tropomyosin, which, in due course, activates the contractile elements for triggering the cross-bridge interaction between the actin and myosin [94–98]. Since the MF are considered as the contractile machinery in the cell, any structural or functional modifications to myosin, actin, troponin, and tropomyosin may contribute to MF remodeling in heart disease.

There are two genes of particular interest located in tandem on chromosome 14 that encode the cardiac myosin heavy chain (MHC), and are termed α-MHC and β-MHC [99, 100]. Given that the α-MHC isoform results in a high-power, low economy ATPase activity, whereas the β-MHC isoform gives rise to a low-power, high economy ATPase myofilament activity, the events associated with cardiac stress promote a shift in expression toward the β-MHC for a more efficient performance [101–106]. In a study by

Table 3 Modifications in MF protein and gene expressions post myocardial infarction

Animal model/time point	Genes of interest	Findings	Reference
Male SD rat, CL/4 wks	α- and β-MHC	↓ α-MHC *mRNA*; ↑ β-MHC *mRNA*	Hart et al. [76]
Male SD rat, AB (PO)/15 wks	α- and β-MHC	↓ α-MHC *mRNA*; ↑ β-MHC *mRNA*	Schwarzer et al. [77]
Male SD rat, CL/5 wks	α- and β-MHC	↓ α-MHC *mRNA*; ↑ β-MHC *mRNA* ↓ α-MHC *protein*; ↑ β-MHC *protein*	Sanganalmath et al. [48]
Male SD rat, ACS (VO)/4,10 wks	α-/β-MHC/α-cardiac/α-SK	↑ β-MHC *mRNA* at 4 and 10 wks NC α-MHC/α-cardiac/α-SK 4 wks ↓ α-MHC *mRNA* at 10 wks NC α-cardiac/α-SK at 10 wks	Freire et al. [78]
Male SD rat, CL/8 wks	α- and β-MHC	↓ α-MHC *mRNA*; ↑ β-MHC *mRNA*	Wang et al. [79]
Male SD rat, CL/7 wks	α- and β-MHC	↓ α-MHC *mRNA*; ↑ β-MHC *mRNA*	Wang et al. [80]
Male Wistar rat, AB (PO)/18 wks	α- and β-MHC	↓ α-MHC *mRNA*; ↑ β-MHC *mRNA*	Huang et al. [81]
Male SD rat/1 day, 1 wk, 6 wks	β-MHC/α-SK	↑ β-MHC *mRNA* 1 day/1 wk/6 wks ↑ α-SK *mRNA* 1 day/1 wk/6 wks	Yue et al. [59]
Male SD rat, AB (PO)/22 wks	α- and β-MHC	↓ α-MHC *protein*; ↑ β-MHC *protein*	Chang et al. [82]
Male Wistar rat, CL/1 wk, 3 wks and 3 months	α-/β- MHC/α-cardiac/α-SK	↓ α-MHC *mRNA* levels ↑ β-MHC/α-SK *mRNA* levels NC α-cardiac *mRNA* levels	Yoshiyama et al. [22]
Male SD rat, CL/20 wks	α-SK	↓ α-SK *mRNA* levels	Simonini et al. [83]

SD Sprague Dawley, *CL* coronary ligation, *MHC* myosin heavy chain, *a-cardiac* α-actin cardiac, *a-SK* α actin skeleton, *ACS* aortocaval shunt, *AB* aortic banding, *PO* pressure overload, *SHR* spontaneously hypertensive rat, *VO* volume overload, *NC* no change observed, *wks* weeks

Swoap et al. [107], both systemic hypertension and caloric restriction resulted in the enhanced expression of β-MHC protein and mRNA levels due to increased transcription activity, in concert with a reduction in the expression of α-MHC protein and mRNA levels. Eble et al. [108] conducted another molecular study in the failing hearts of rabbits, and reported an increase in the MHC synthesis in left ventricular dysfunction due to chronic ventricular tachycardia that could be explained by an increased MHC translational efficiency. Such a change was further supported by Imamura et al. [109], who reported an elevated synthesis in MHC in dogs subjected to pressure overload. Furthermore, in the rat model of pressure-overload hypertrophy, Toffolo et al. [110] described an augmentation in cell size followed by a change in the expression of myosin, to produce the slow migrating, economic V_3 isoform, while exhibiting an increased number of myofibril units during the adaptive process of the myocardium. These observations are consistent with the view that remodeling of MF occurs with respect to its protein content in CHF and such a defect seems to be due to alterations in the expression of genes for different MF proteins.

Conclusions

From the foregoing discussion, it is evident that cardiac dysfunction in CHF is associated with a wide variety of alterations in the activities as well as the expressions of genes and proteins for SL, SR, and MF. It should be noted that changes in cardiac gene expressions can be seen to result in alterations in the content of SL, SR, and MF proteins and thus may form the molecular basis for changes in the chemical composition of the subcellular organelles in the failing heart. Such a mechanism based on changes in cardiac gene expression does not rule out the participation of other mechanisms such as depression in the activity of different subcellular proteins due to changes in myocardial metabolisms or cation homeostasis in the cell. In addition, proteolysis of SL, SR, and MF proteins by the activation of various proteolytic enzymes has also been indicated to account for subcellular remodeling and cardiac dysfunction during the development of CHF [5–8]. Furthermore, remodeling of one or more subcellular organelles may depend on the type and stage of CHF and some of the subcellular changes at any given time-point may be adaptive or pathogenetic in nature. Various signal transduction mechanisms, which are altered during the development of CHF, may also affect cardiac gene and protein expressions, as well as the subcellular activities in the myocardium. Thus, a great deal of caution should be exercised while interpreting the data on subcellular remodeling and its consequence in the development of cardiac dysfunction in CHF. Nonetheless, prevention of subcellular remodeling in the failing heart represents a real challenge for the development of novel therapies and the improvement of cardiac function in CHF.

Acknowledgments The work in this article was supported by a grant from the Canadian Institutes of Health Research. The infrastructure support for this project was provided by the St. Boniface Hospital Research Foundation.

References

1. Cohn JN, Ferrari R, Sharpe N. Cardiac remodeling – concepts and clinical implications: a consensus paper from an international forum on cardiac remodeling. J Am Coll Cardiol. 2000;35:569–82.
2. Dhalla NS, Afzal N, Beamish RE, et al. Pathophysiology of cardiac dysfunction in congestive heart failure. Can J Cardiol. 1993;9:873–87.
3. Swynghedauw B. Molecular mechanisms of myocardial remodeling. Physiol Rev. 1999;79:215–62.
4. Pfeffer MA, Braunwald E. Ventricular remodeling after myocardial infarction: experimental observations and clinical implications. Circulation. 1990;81: 1161–72.
5. Dhalla NS, Shao Q, Panagia V. Remodeling of cardiac membranes during the development of congestive heart failure. Heart Fail Rev. 1998;2:261–72.
6. Dhalla NS, Saini-Chohan HK, Rodriguez-Leyva D, et al. Subcellular remodeling may induce cardiac dysfunction in congestive heart failure. Cardiovasc Res. 2009;81:429–38.
7. Dhalla NS, Dent MR, Tappia PS, et al. Subcellular remodeling as a viable target for the treatment of congestive heart failure. J Cardiovasc Pharmacol Ther. 2006;11:31–45.
8. Babick AP, Dhalla NS. Role of subcellular remodeling in cardiac dysfunction due to congestive heart failure. Med Princ Pract. 2007;16:81–9.
9. Dhalla NS, Heyliger CE, Beamish RE, et al. Pathophysiological aspects of myocardial hypertrophy. Can J Cardiol. 1987;4:183–96.
10. Skou JC. Enzymatic basis for the active transport of Na$^+$ and K$^+$ across cell membrane. Physiol Rev. 1965;45:596–617.
11. Schwinger RHG, Bundgaard H, Muller-Ehmsen J, et al. The Na, K-ATPase in the failing human heart. Cardiovasc Res. 2003;57:913–20.
12. Horisberger JD, Lemas V, Kraehenbuhl JP, et al. Structure-function relationship of Na, K-ATPase. Annu Rev Physiol. 1991;53:565–84.
13. Charlemagne D, Orlowski J, Oliviero P, et al. Alteration of Na, K-ATPase subunit mRNA and protein levels in hypertrophied rat heart. J Biol Chem. 1994;269:1541–7.
14. Kato K, Lukas A, Chapman D, et al. Changes in the expression of cardiac Na$^+$-K$^+$ATPase subunits in the UM-X7.1 cardiomyopathic hamster. Life Sci. 2000; 67:1175–83.
15. Semb SO, Lunde PK, Holt E, et al. Reduced myocardial Na$^+$, K$^+$-pump capacity in congestive heart failure following myocardial infarction in rats. J Mol Cell Cardiol. 1998;30:1311–28.
16. Guo X, Wang J, Elimban V, et al. Both enalapril and losartan attenuate sarcolemmal Na$^+$-K$^+$-ATPase remodeling in failing rat heart due to myocardial infarction. Can J Physiol Pharmacol. 2008;86:139–47.
17. Shao Q, Ren B, Elimban V, et al. Modification of sarcolemmal Na$^+$-K$^+$ ATPase and Na$^+$/Ca^{2+} exchanger expression in heart failure by blockade of renin-angiotensin system. Am J Physiol Heart Circ Physiol. 2005;288:H2637–46.
18. Ren B, Shao Q, Ganguly PK, et al. Influence of long-term treatment of imidapril on mortality, cardiac function, and gene expression in congestive heart failure due to myocardial infarction. Can J Physiol Pharmacol. 2004;82:1118–27.
19. Schillinger W, Schneider H, Minami K, et al. Importance of sympathetic activation for the expression of Na$^+$-Ca^{2+} exchanger in end-stage failing human myocardium. Eur Heart J. 2002;23:1118–24.
20. Sjaastad I, Sejersted OM, Ilebekk A, et al. Echocardiographic criteria for detection of postinfarction congestive heart failure in rats. J Appl Physiol. 2000;89:1445–54.
21. Hanatani A, Yoshiyama M, Takeuchi K, et al. Angiotensin II type 1-receptor antagonist candesartan cilexitil prevents left ventricular dysfunction in myocardial infarcted rats. Jpn J Pharmacol. 1998;78:45–54.
22. Yoshiyama M, Takeuchi K, Hanatani A, et al. Effect of cilazapril on ventricular remodeling assessed by Doppler-echocardiographic assessment and cardiac gene expression. Cardiovasc Drugs Ther. 1998;12: 57–70.
23. Book CB, Moore RL, Semanchik A, et al. Cardiac hypertrophy alters expression of Na$^+$, K$^+$-ATPase

subunit isoforms at mRNA and protein levels in rat myocardium. J Mol Cell Cardiol. 1994;26:591–600.

24. Dixon IM, Hata T, Dhalla NS. Sarcolemmal Na⁺-K⁺-ATPase activity in congestive heart failure due to myocardial infarction. Am J Physiol. 1992;262:C664–71.

25. Frank JS, Mottino G, Reid D, et al. Distribution of the Na⁺-Ca²⁺ exchange protein in mammalian cardiac myocytes: an immunofluorescence and immunocolloidial gold-labeling study. J Cell Biol. 1992;117:337–45.

26. Nicoll DA, Longory S, Philipson KD. Molecular cloning and functional expression of the cardiac sarcolemmal Na⁺-Ca²⁺ exchanger. Science. 1990;250: 562–5.

27. Reuter H. Exchange of calcium ions in the mammalian myocardium: mechanisms and physiological significance. Circ Res. 1974;34:599–605.

28. Studer R, Reinecke H, Bilger J, et al. Gene expression of the cardiac Na⁺-Ca²⁺ exchanger in end-stage human heart failure. Circ Res. 1994;75:443–53.

29. Hasenfuss G, Schillinger W, Lenhart SE, et al. Relationship between Na⁺-Ca²⁺ -exchanger protein levels and diastolic function of failing human myocardium. Circulation. 1999;99:641–8.

30. Dixon IMC, Hata T, Dhalla NS. Sarcolemmal calcium transport in congestive heart failure due to myocardial infarction in rats. Am J Physiol Heart Circ Physiol. 1992;31:H1387–94.

31. Reinecke H, Studer R, Vetter R, et al. Cardiac Na⁺/Ca²⁺ exchange activity in patients with end-stage heart failure. Cardiovasc Res. 1996;31:48–54.

32. Brandl CJ, de Leon S, Martin DR, et al. Adult forms of the Ca²⁺ATPase of sarcoplasmic reticulum. Expression in developing skeletal muscle. J Biol Chem. 1987;262:3768–74.

33. Komuro I, Kurabayashi M, Shibazaki Y, et al. Molecular cloning and characterization of a Ca²⁺ + Mg²⁺ -dependent adenosine triphosphatase from rat cardiac sarcoplasmic reticulum. J Clin Invest. 1989; 83:1102–8.

34. Beekman RE, van Hardeveld C, Simonides WS. On the mechanism of the reduction by thyroid hormone of β-adrenergic relaxation rate stimulation in rat heart. Biochem J. 1989;259:229–36.

35. Fisher DJ, Phillips S, McQuinn T. Regulation of SERCA2 expression by thyroid hormone in cultured chick embryo cardiomyocytes. Am J Physiol Heart Circ Physiol. 1996;270:H638–44.

36. Muliere LA, Hasenfuss G, Leavitt B, et al. Altered myocardial force-frequency relation in human heart failure. Circulation. 1992;85:1743–50.

37. Bristow MR, Ginsburg R, Minobe W, et al. Decreased catecholamine sensitivity and β-adrenergic receptor density in failing human hearts. N Engl J Med. 1982;307:205–11.

38. Bristow MR, Ginsberg R, Umans V, et al. β₁- and β₂-adrenergic-receptor subpopulations in nonfailing and failing human ventricular myocardium: coupling of both receptor subtypes to muscle contraction and selective β₁-receptor down-regulation in heart failure. Circ Res. 1986;59:297–309.

39. Mercadier JJ, Lompre AM, Duc P, et al. Altered sarcoplasmic reticulum Ca²⁺-ATPase gene expression in the human ventricle during end-stage heart failure. J Clin Invest. 1990;85:305–9.

40. Brillantes AM, Allen P, Takahashi T, et al. Differences in cardiac calcium release channel (ryanodine receptor) expression in myocardium from patients with end-stage heart failure caused by ischemic versus dilated cardiomyopathy. Circ Res. 1992;71:18–26.

41. Arai M, Alpert NR, MacLennan DH, et al. Alterations in sarcoplasmic reticulum gene expression in human heart failure. A possible mechanism for alterations in systolic and diastolic properties of the failing myocardium. Circ Res. 1993;72:463–9.

42. Schwinger RHG, Bohm M, Schmidt U, et al. Unchanged protein levels of SERCA II and phospholamban but reduced Ca²⁺ uptake and Ca²⁺ ATPase activity of cardiac sarcoplasmic reticulum from dilated cardiomyopathy patients compared with patients with nonfailing hearts. Circulation. 1995;92:3220–8.

43. Meyer M, Schilinger W, Pieske B, et al. Alterations of sarcoplasmic reticulum proteins in failing human dilated cardiomyopathy. Circulation. 1995;92:778–84.

44. Movsesian MA, Schwinger RHG. Calcium sequestration by the sarcoplasmic reticulum in heart failure. Cardiovasc Res. 1998;37:352–9.

45. Igarashi-Saito K, Tsutsui H, Yamamoto S, et al. Role of SR Ca²⁺ ATPase in contractile dysfunction of myocytes in tachycardia-induced heart failure. Am J Physiol Heart Circ Physiol. 1998;275:H31–40.

46. Hisamatsu Y, Ohkusa T, Kihara Y, et al. Early changes in the function of cardiac sarcoplasmic reticulum in volume-overloaded cardiac hypertrophy in rats. J Mol Cell Cardiol. 1997;29:1097–109.

47. Flesch M, Schiffer F, Zolk O, et al. Angiotensin receptor antagonism and angiotensin converting enzyme inhibition improve diastolic dysfunction and Ca²⁺ ATPase expression in the sarcoplasmic reticulum in hypertensive cardiomyopathy. J Hypertens. 1997;15:1001–9.

48. Sanganalmath SK, Babick AP, Barta J, et al. Antiplatelet therapy attenuates subcellular remodeling in congestive heart failure. J Cell Mol Med. 2008;12:1728–38.

49. Sallinen P, Manttari S, Leskinen H, et al. Time course of changes in the expression of DHPR, RyR(2), and SERCA2 after myocardial infarction in the rat left ventricle. Mol Cell Biochem. 2007;303:97–103.

50. Prunier F, Chen Y, Gellen B, et al. Left ventricular SERCA2a gene down-regulation does not parallel ANP gene up-regulation during post-MI remodeling in rats. Eur J Heart Fail. 2005;7:739–47.

51. Xu YJ, Chapman D, Dixon IM, et al. Differential gene expression in infarct scar and viable myocardium from rat heart following coronary ligation. J Cell Mol Med. 2004;8:85–92.

52. Guo X, Chapman D, Dhalla NS. Partial prevention of changes in SR gene expression in congestive heart failure due to myocardial infarction by enalapril or losartan. Mol Cell Biochem. 2003;254:163–72.

53. Sakai S, Miyauchi T, Yamaguchi I. Long-term endothelin receptor antagonist administration improves alterations in expression of various cardiac genes in failing myocardium of rats with heart failure. Circulation. 2000;101:2849–53.

54. Ambrose J, Pribnow DG, Giraud GD, et al. Angiotensin type 1 receptor antagonism with irbesartan inhibits ventricular hypertrophy and improves diastolic function in the remodeling post-myocardial infarction ventricle. J Cardiovasc Pharmacol. 1999; 33:433–9.

55. Shao Q, Ren B, Zarain-Herzberg A, et al. Captopril treatment improves the sarcoplasmic reticular Ca^{2+} transport in heart failure due to myocardial infarction. J Mol Cell Cardiol. 1999;31:1663–72.

56. Zhang QX, Ng YC, Moore RL, et al. In situ SR function in postinfarction myocytes. J Appl Physiol. 1999;87:2143–50.

57. Iijima K, Geshi E, Nomizo A, et al. Alterations in sarcoplasmic reticulum and angiotensin II type 1 receptor gene expression after myocardial infarction in rats. Jpn Circ J. 1998;62:449–54.

58. Münch G, Bölck B, Hoischen S, et al. Unchanged protein expression of sarcoplasmic reticulum Ca^{2+}-ATPase, phospholamban, and calsequestrin in terminally failing human myocardium. J Mol Med. 1998;76:434–41.

59. Yue P, Long CS, Austin R, et al. Post-infarction heart failure in the rat is associated with distinct alterations in cardiac myocyte molecular phenotype. J Mol Cell Cardiol. 1998;30:1615–30.

60. Zarain-Herzberg A, Afzal N, Elimban V, et al. Decreased expression of cardiac sarcoplasmic reticulum Ca^{2+}-pump ATPase in congestive heart failure due to myocardial infarction. Mol Cell Biochem. 1996;163–164:285–90.

61. Jones LR, Simmerman HKB, Wilson WW, et al. Purification and characterization of phospholamban from canine cardiac sarcoplasmic reticulum. J Biol Chem. 1985;260:7721–30.

62. Sasaki T, Inui M, Kimura Y, et al. Molecular mechanism of regulation of Ca^{2+} pump ATPase by phospholamban in cardiac sarcoplasmic reticulum. Effects of synthetic phospholamban peptides on Ca^{2+} pump ATPase. J Biol Chem. 1992;267:1674–9.

63. Luo W, Gurpp IL, Harrer J, et al. Targeted ablation of the phospholamban gene is associated with markedly enhanced myocardial contractility and loss of β-agonist stimulation. Circ Res. 1994;75:401–9.

64. Inui M, Saito A, Fleischer S. Purification of the ryanodine receptor and identity with the feet structures of functional terminal cisternae of sarcoplasmic reticulum from fast skeletal muscle. J Biol Chem. 1987; 262:1740–7.

65. Lai FA, Erickson HP, Rousseau E, et al. Purification and reconstitution of the calcium release channel from skeletal muscle. Nature. 1988;331:315–9.

66. Zorzato F, Fujii J, Otsu K, et al. Molecular cloning of cDNA encoding human and rabbit forms of the Ca^{2+} release channel (ryanodine receptor) of skeletal muscle sarcoplasmic reticulum. J Biol Chem. 1990; 265:2244–56.

67. Arai M, Otsu K, MacLennan DH, et al. Regulation of sarcoplasmic reticulum gene expression during cardiac and skeletal muscle development. Am J Physiol Cell Physiol. 1992;262:C614–20.

68. Holmberg SR, Williams AJ. The calcium-release channel from cardiac sarcoplasmic reticulum: function in the failing and acutely ischemic heart. Basic Res Cardiol. 1992;87(suppl 1):255–68.

69. Holmberg SRM, Williams AJ. Single channel recordings from human cardiac sarcoplasmic reticulum. Circ Res. 1989;65:1445–9.

70. Beucklemann DJ, Nabauer M, Erdmann E. Intracellular calcium handling in isolated ventricular myocytes from patients with terminal heart failure. Circulation. 1992;85:1046–55.

71. Cory CR, McCutcheon LJ, O'Grady M, et al. Compensatory downregulation of myocardial Ca channel in SR from dogs with heart failure. Am J Physiol. 1993;33:H926–37.

72. Pennock GD, Spooner PH, Summers CE, et al. Prevention of abnormal sarcoplasmic reticulum calcium transport and protein expression in post-infarction heart failure using 3,5-diiodothyropropionic acid (DITPA). J Mol Cell Cardiol. 2000;32:1939–53.

73. Solaro RJ, Montgomery DM, Wang L, et al. Integration of pathways that signal cardiac growth with modulation of myofilament activity. J Nucl Cardiol. 2002;9:523–33.

74. Eisenberg BR. Quantitative ultrastructure of mammalian skeletal. In: Peachey LD, Adrian RH, Geiger SR, editors. Handbook of physiology: skeletal muscle. Baltimore: American Physiological Society; 1983. p. 73–112.

75. Morano I, Hadicke K, Haase H, et al. Changes in essential myosin light chain isoform expression provide a molecular basis for isometric force regulation in the failing human heart. J Mol Cell Cardiol. 1997;29:1177–87.

76. Hart DL, Heidkamp MC, Iyengar R, et al. CRNK gene transfer improves function and reverses the myosin heavy chain isoenzyme switch during post-myocardial infarction left ventricular remodeling. J Mol Cell Cardiol. 2008;45:93–105.

77. Schwarzer M, Faerber G, Rueckauer T, et al. The metabolic modulators, Etomoxir and NVP-LAB121, fail to reverse pressure overload induced heart failure in vivo. Basic Res Cardiol. 2009;104:547–57.

78. Freire G, Ocampo C, Ilbawi N, et al. Overt expression of AP-1 reduces alpha myosin heavy chain expression and contributes to heart failure from chronic volume overload. J Mol Cell Cardiol. 2007;43:465–78.

79. Wang J, Guo X, Dhalla NS. Modification of myosin protein and gene expression in failing hearts due to myocardial infarction by enalapril or losartan. Biochim Biophys Acta. 2004;1690:177–84.

80. Wang J, Liu X, Ren B, et al. Modification of myosin gene expression by imidapril in failing heart due to

myocardial infarction. J Mol Cell Cardiol. 2002;34: 847–57.

81. Huang Y, Liu H, Li Y. Alterations in myosin heavy chain isoform gene expression during the transition from compensatory hypertrophy to congestive heart failure in rats. Chin Med J (Engl). 2001;114:183–5.

82. Chang KC, Figueredo VM, Schreur JH, et al. Thyroid hormone improves function and Ca^{2+} handling in pressure overload hypertrophy. Association with increased sarcoplasmic reticulum Ca^{2+}-ATPase and alpha-myosin heavy chain in rat heart. J Clin Invest. 1997;100:1742–9.

83. Simonini A, Massie BM, Long CS, et al. Alterations in skeletal muscle gene expression in the rat with chronic congestive heart failure. J Mol Cell Cardiol. 1996;28:1683–91.

84. Alpert NR, Gordon MS. Myofibrillar adenosine triphosphate activity in congestive heart failure. Am J Physiol. 1962;202:940–6.

85. Anderson PAW, Malouf NN, Oakeley AE, et al. Troponin T isoform expression in the normal and failing human left ventricle: a correlation with myofibrillar ATPase activity. Basic Res Cardiol. 1992;87(suppl 1):117–27.

86. Solaro RJ, Powers FM, Gao L, et al. Control of myofilament activation in heart failure. Circulation. 1993;87(suppl VII):38–43.

87. Peters TJ, Wells G, Oakley CM, et al. Enzymatic analysis of endomyocardial biopsy specimens from patients with cardiomyopathy. Br Heart J. 1977;39:1333–9.

88. Pagani ED, Alousi AA, Grant AM, et al. Changes in myofibrillar content and Mg-ATPase activity in ventricular tissues from patients with heart failure caused by coronary artery disease, cardiomyopathy, or mitral valve insufficiency. Circ Res. 1988;63:380–5.

89. Alousi AA, Grant AM, Etzler LR, et al. Reduced cardiac myofibrillar Mg-ATPase activity without changes in myosin isozymes in patients with end-stage heart failure. Mol Cell Biochem. 1990;96:79–88.

90. Lowey S, Risby D. Light chains from fast and slow muscle myosins. Nature. 1971;234:81–5.

91. Weeds AG, Pope B. Chemical studies on light chains from cardiac and skeletal muscle myosins. Nature. 1971;234:85–8.

92. Ebashi S. Ca^{2+} and the contractile proteins. J Mol Cell Cardiol. 1984;16:129–36.

93. Cooper TA, Ordahl CP. A single cardiac troponin T gene generates embryonic and adult isoforms via developmentally regulated alternative splicing. J Biol Chem. 1985;260:11140–8.

94. Dhalla NS, Das PK, Sharma GP. Concise review: subcellular basis of cardiac contractile failure. J Mol Cell Cardiol. 1978;10:363–85.

95. Hess ML. Concise review: subcellular function in the acutely failing myocardium. Circ Shock. 1979;6: 119–36.

96. Effron MB, Bhatnagar GM, Spurgeon HA, et al. Changes in myosin isoenzymes, ATPase activity, and contraction duration in rat cardiac muscle with aging can be modulated by thyroxine. Circ Res. 1987;60:238–45.

97. Dhalla NS, Pierce GN, Panagia V, et al. Calcium movements in relation to heart function. Basic Res Cardiol. 1982;77:117–39.

98. Dhalla NS, Dixon IMC, Beamish RE. Biochemical basis of heart function and contractile failure. J Appl Cardiol. 1991;6:7–30.

99. Leinwand LA, Fournier REK, Nadal-Ginard B, et al. Isolation and characterization of human myosin heavy chain gene. Proc Natl Acad Sci USA. 1983;80:3716–20.

100. Mahdavi V, Chambers AP, Nadal-Ginard B. Cardiac alpha- and beta- MHC genes are organized in tandem. Proc Natl Acad Sci USA. 1984;81:2626–30.

101. Buttrick P, Malhotra A, Factor S, et al. Effect of chronic dobutamine administration on hearts of normal and hypertensive rats. Circ Res. 1988;63:173–81.

102. Haddad F, Bodell PW, McCue SA, et al. Food restriction-induced transformations in cardiac functional and biochemical properties in rats. J Appl Physiol. 1993;74:606–12.

103. Izumo S, Lompre A, Matsuoka R, et al. Myosin heavy chain messenger RNA and protein isoform transitions during cardiac hypertrophy. J Clin Invest. 1987;79:970–7.

104. Nadal-Ginard B, Mahdavi V. Molecular basis of cardiac performance: plasticity of the myocardium generated through protein isoform switches. J Clin Invest. 1989;84:1693–700.

105. Swoap SJ, Bodell P, Baldwin KM. Interaction of hypertension and caloric restriction on cardiac mass and isomyosin expression. Am J Physiol Regul Integr Comp Physiol. 1995;268:R33–9.

106. Swoap SJ, Haddad F, Boddell P, et al. Effect of chronic energy deprivation on thyroid hormone receptor and isomyosin expression. Am J Physiol Endocrinol Metab. 1994;266:E254–60.

107. Swoap SJ, Haddad F, Bodell P, et al. Control of β-myosin heavy chain expression in systemic hypertension and caloric restriction in the rat heart. Am J Physiol Cell Physiol. 1995;269:C1025–33.

108. Eble DM, Walker JD, Mukherjee R, et al. Myosin heavy chain synthesis is increased in a rabbit model of heart failure. Am J Physiol Heart Circ Physiol. 1997;272:H969–78.

109. Imamura T, McDermott PJ, Kent RL, et al. Acute changes in myosin heavy chain synthesis rate in pressure versus volume overload. Circ Res. 1994; 75:418–25.

110. Toffolo RL, Ianuzzo CD. Myofibrillar adaptations during cardiac hypertrophy. Mol Cell Biochem. 1994;131:141–9.

Cardiomyopathy, Sarcomeropathy, and Z-diskopathy

Akinori Kimura

Abstract

Cardiomyopathy is caused by functional abnormalities of cardiac muscle, which include both extrinsic and intrinsic factors. The intrinsic factor involves mutations in genes playing roles in performance, regulation, or maintenance of cardiac function. Cardiomyopathy caused by the intrinsic factor is called idiopathic or primary cardiomyopathy, and there are several clinical types of primary cardiomyopathy including hypertrophic cardiomyopathy and dilated cardiomyopathy. Linkage studies and candidate gene approaches have deciphered the disease genes for hereditary primary cardiomyopathy: mutations in genes for components of sarcomere, sarcolemma, Z-disk, proteins of I band region, nuclear membrane, and transcriptional machinery. The most interesting findings are that mutations in different disease genes can be found in the same clinical types of cardiomyopathy and that mutations in the same disease gene can be found in different clinical types of cardiomyopathy. Functional analyses of disease-related mutations have revealed that characteristic functional alterations are associated with each clinical type of cardiomyopathy. In this review I focus on the cardiomyopathy-associated mutations found in genes for sarcomere and Z-disk elements and their functional relevance in the pathogenesis of primary cardiomyopathy.

Keywords

Calcium sensitivity • Cardiomyopathy • Mutation • Stress response • Stretch response • Z-disk

A. Kimura (✉)
Department of Molecular Pathogenesis, Medical
Research Institute, and Laboratory of Genome Diversity,
Graduate School of Biomedical Science, Tokyo Medical
and Dental University, Tokyo, Japan
e-mail: akitis@mri.tmd.ac.jp

Introduction

Cardiomyopathy is a heterogeneous disease caused by functional abnormality of cardiac muscle and classified into primary cardiomyopathy and secondary cardiomyopathy [1]. Secondary cardiomyopathy is caused by extrinsic factors including infection, ischemia, hypertension, and metabolic disorders. On the other hand, diagnosis of primary cardiomyopathy is based on the exclusion of secondary cardiomyopathy and there are several different clinical types [2, 3]. Hypertrophic cardiomyopathy (HCM) and dilated cardiomyopathy (DCM) are two major clinical types of primary cardiomyopathy. HCM, a major cause of sudden death in young and heart failure, is characterized by left ventricular hypertrophy, often asymmetric, accompanied by myofibrillar disarrays and reduced compliance (diastolic dysfunction) of cardiac ventricles. In contrast, DCM is characterized by dilated ventricular cavity with systolic dysfunction. Clinical symptom of DCM is heart failure and is often associated with sudden death. Other clinical types of cardiomyopathy include restrictive cardiomyopathy (RCM) and arrhythmogenic right ventricular cardiomyopathy (ARVC). RCM is accompanied by increased stiffness of the myocardium with diastolic dysfunction without significant hypertrophy, while ARVC is characterized by a dilated dysfunctional right ventricle (RV), ventricular arrhythmias, and fibrofatty replacement of the RV. Another cardiomyopathy is the left ventricular noncompaction (LVNC) characterized by trabeculations in the left ventricle (LV) accompanied by LV hypertrophy and/or dilation.

During the last two decades, the etiology of primary cardiomyopathy has been unraveled to be associated with genetic abnormalities at least in part of the patients [4]. More than half of HCM patients have family history of the disease consistent with autosomal dominant genetic trait. In the case of DCM, about 20–35% patients had family history of the disease, mainly consistent with the autosomal dominant inheritance, although some familial cases can be explained by autosomal recessive or X-linked recessive trait. Familial occurrence is also noted in RCM, ARVC, and LVNC. Because the presence of family history suggested the genetic etiology of the disease, linkage studies in multiplex families and subsequent candidate gene approaches have been successful in unraveling novel disease genes. As shown in Table 1 many different disease genes were identified. It should be noted here that each patient or family usually carries only one mutation in the disease gene, albeit that exceptional cases harbor mutations in two or more disease genes, demonstrating the genetic heterogeneity of cardiomyopathy. Another noteworthy issue is the overlapping of disease genes for different clinical types. The disease genes can be classified into several categories; mutations in genes for sarcomere components, Z-disk elements, sarcoplasmic proteins, sarcolemma proteins, nuclear lamina, and others. The majority of disease genes encode sarcomere components, but a considerable number of disease-associated mutations can be found in Z-disk elements (Fig. 1).

Sarcomere Mutations in Cardiomyopathy: Sarcomeropathy

The first report of the disease gene for HCM was the identification of a disease-linked missense mutation in cardiac β-myosin heavy chain gene (*MYH7*) found in a large multiplex family [5]. Subsequently, *MYH7* was analyzed for mutations in HCM patients and many different missense mutations were identified. However, frequency of *MYH7* mutations in the patients was less than half, and linkage studies in non-*MYH7*-linked HCM families have revealed disease-linked mutations in α-tropomyosin gene (*TPM1*), cardiac troponin T gene (*TNNT2*), and cardiac myosin binding protein-C gene (*MYBP3*). Because these genes encode components of sarcomere involved in muscle contraction, genes for other sarcomere components were analyzed and led to the identification of HCM-associated mutations in ventricular myosin essential light chain gene (*MYL3*), ventricular myosin regulatory light chain gene (*MYL2*), cardiac troponin I gene (*TNNI3*), cardiac

Table 1 Disease genes for hereditary cardiomyopathy

Clinical phenotype	Heredity	Gene symbol	Coding protein
HCM/DCM/RCM/LVNC	AD	MYH7	Cardiac β-myosin heavy chain
HCM/DCM/RCM/LVNC	AD	TNNT2	Cardiac troponin T
HCM/DCM	AD	TPM1	α-Tropomyosin
HCM/DCM	AD	MYBPC3	Cardiac myosin binding protein-C
HCM	AD	MYL3	Ventricular myosin essential light chain
HCM	AD	MYL2	Ventricular myosin regulatory light chain
HCM/DCM/RCM	AD	TNNI3	Cardiac troponin I
HCM/DCM/LVNC	AD	ACTC	Cardiac α-actin
HCM/DCM	AD	TTN	Titin, connectin
HCM/DCM	AD	TNNC1	Cardiac troponin C
HCM	AD	MYH6	Cardiac α-myosin heavy chain
HCM/DCM	AD	CSRP3	Muscle LIM protein, MLP
HCM	AD	CAV3	Caveolin-3
HCM/DCM	AD	TCAP	Titin-cap, Tcap, telethonin
HCM/DCM	AD	VCL	Metavinculin
HCM	AD	JPH-2	Junctophilin-2
HCM	AD	OBSCN	Obscurin
HCM	AD	MYOZ2	Myozenin, calsartin-1
HCM/DCM	AD	ANKRD1	CARP
DCM/RCM	AD	DES	Desmin
DCM/LVNC	AD	LMNA	Lamin A/C
DCM	AD	SAGD	δ-Sarcoglycan
DCM	AD	ACTN2	α-Actinin-2
DCM/LVNC	AD	LDB3	Cypher, ZASP, oracle
DCM/HCM	AD	PLB	Phospholamban
DCM	AD	ABCC9	K_{ATP} channel
DCM	AD	SCN5A	Cardiac Na channel
DCM/HCM	AD	CRYAB	αB crystallin
DCM	AD	PSEN1	Presenilin-1
DCM	AD	PSEN2	Presenilin-2
DCM	AD	FHL2	Four and half LIM protein-2, FHL2
DCM	AD	LMNA4	Laminin α4
DCM	AD	ILK	Integrin-linked kinase
DCM	AD	MYPN	Myopalladin
DCM	AD	CHRM2	Acetylcholine receptor
DCM	AD	RBM20	RNA binding motif protein 20
DCM	AD	NEXN	Nexilin
DCM	AD	NBLT	Nebulette
DCM	XR	DMD	Dystrophin
DCM	XR	EMD	Emerin
LVNC/DCM	XR	TAZ	Tafazzin, G4.5
DCM	XR	FKTN	Fuktin
ARVC/DCM	AR	DSP	Desmoplakin
ARVC/DCM	AR, AD	JUP	Plakoglobin
ARVC	AD	PKP2	Plakophilin-2
ARVC	AD	TGFB3	TGFβ3
ARVC	AD	RYR2	Ryanodine receptor 2
ARVC	AD	DSG3	Desmoglein 3
LVNC	AD	DTNA	α-Dystrobrevin

AD autosomal dominant, *AR* autosomal recessive, *XR* X-linked recessive

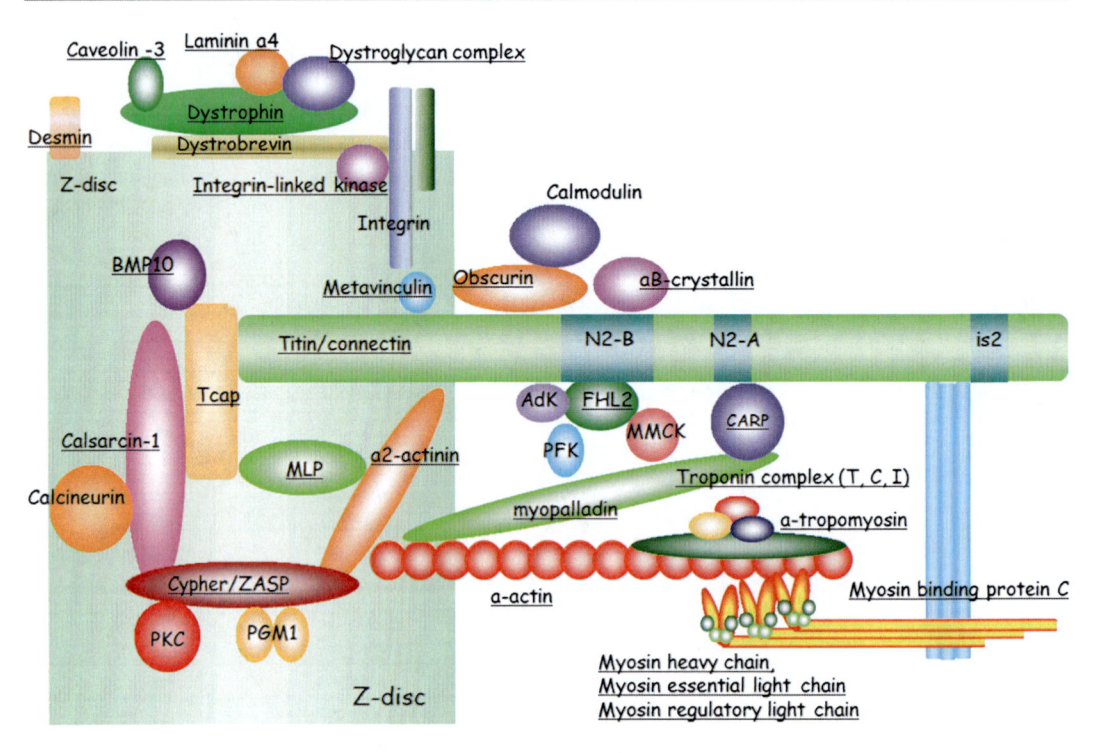

Fig. 1 Schematic representation of sarcomere components. Half sarcomere is schematically shown. Components in which cardiomyopathy-associated mutations are found are underlined

α-actin (*CACT*), and cardiac troponin C (*TNNC1*). Therefore, mutations in any components of sarcomere can result in HCM [4], suggesting that a part of cardiomyopathy can be sarcomeropathy.

Initial analysis of functional changes caused by the HCM-associated *MYH7* mutations demonstrated decreased power generation by the mutant myosin heavy chains [6], and the identification of HCM-related mutations in sarcomere components, troponin T, and α-tropomyosin led to a hypothesis that HCM is the disease of sarcomere and that cardiac hypertrophy was a compensation of decreased power generation [7]. However, we found HCM-associated *TNNI3* mutations at the contraction inhibitory domain [8], which implied that the decreased power was not a common functional change caused by the sarcomere mutations. Indeed, subsequent functional analyses of mutations in genes for other sarcomere components than *MYH7* have revealed that contractile performance was not decreased by the mutations and most HCM-associated sarcomere mutations resulted in increased Ca²⁺ sensitivity of muscle

contraction [9–14]. Because a *MYH7* mutation that caused HCM in transgenic mice also increased Ca²⁺ sensitivity at the muscle fiber level [15], a common functional alteration caused by HCM-related sarcomere mutations may be the increased Ca²⁺ sensitivity. Muscle contraction is regulated by the concentration of intracellular Ca²⁺ that is released from sarcoplasmic reticulum (SR) via ryanodine receptor (RyR2) and reuptaken to SR via sarcoplasmic reticulum Ca²⁺–ATPase (SERCA). When the concentration of Ca²⁺ is increased or decreased, muscle is contracted or relaxed, respectively. Increased Ca²⁺ sensitivity is a leftward shift of Ca²⁺-tension curve; more tension is generated by mutant sarcomere than normal sarcomere at the same Ca²⁺ concentration (hypercontraction) or muscle with mutant sarcomere is under less relaxed states (diastolic dysfunction) than normal sarcomere. This is consistent with the finding that characteristic features of HCM are hypercontraction and diastolic dysfunction.

On the other hand, mutations in the sarcomeric genes have also been found in patients with DCM.

The first demonstration of DCM-linked sarcomeric mutation was the identification of cardiac α-actin gene (*CACT*) mutations in multiplex families with autosomal dominant DCM [16]. As described above, *CACT* mutation can be found in HCM [17], which demonstrates that sarcomere mutations cause both HCM and DCM, i.e., overlapping disease genes for different cardiomyopathy. Molecular basis of different phenotypes caused by *CACT* mutations was suggested by the fact that DCM-associated mutations were found at the α-actinin interacting domain [16], while HCM-associated mutations were at the interacting domain to myosin heavy chain [17]. In addition, recent data have suggested that there is a difference in folding property between the DCM-associated mutant actin and the HCM-associated mutant actin [18]. Another example of overlapping disease gene was the identification of *TNNT2* mutation in DCM [19]. Functional study of *TNNT2* mutations clearly demonstrated the difference between DCM-associated mutation and HCM-associated mutation, i.e., the DCM-associated *TNNT2* mutation decreased Ca^{2+} sensitivity of muscle contraction, which is in clear contrast to the increased sensitivity caused by the HCM-associated mutation [20]. Therefore, sarcomere mutations can be found in both HCM and DCM, but differences in the functional alterations may determine the different phenotypes.

Z-Disk Element Mutations in Cardiomyopathy: Z-Diskopathy

Mutations in the sarcomere components could be found in only less than half of patients with hereditary cardiomyopathy, and a considerable part of the patients carried disease-associated mutations in Z-disk elements. Identification of a HCM-associated mutation in titin gene (*TTN*) was the first example of disease gene other than the sarcomere components [21], and the functional alteration due to the *TTN* mutation was an increased binding to α-actinin (Fig. 2). In addition, we demonstrated that the HCM-associated Tcap gene (*TCAP*) mutations increased the binding of Tcap to titin and calsarcin-1 [22] (Fig. 3),

leading to a hypothesis that Z-disk mutations in HCM may result in increased binding of Z-disk components and hence "stiff sarcomere" (Fig. 4). "Stiff sarcomere" would increase passive tension upon stretch of the sarcomere. Because the increased passive tension was associated with the increased Ca^{2+} sensitivity [23–25], we have speculated that HCM-associated abnormality in both Z-disk components and sarcomere components causes the increased Ca^{2+} sensitivity.

In clear contrast, several DCM-associated Z-disk protein gene mutations could be identified in *TTN*, *CSRP3*, *TCAP*, and Cypher/ZASP gene (*LDB3*) [4]. Functional analysis of the DCM-associated *TTN* mutation at the actinin-binding domain revealed a decreased binding to actinin [26] but the opposite functional change as was found with the HCM-associated *TTN* mutation [21] (Fig. 2). In addition, another DCM-associated TTN mutation at the Tcap binding domain showed decreased binding to Tcap. Furthermore, *TCAP* mutations found in DCM patients showed opposite functional alterations to that caused by the HCM-associated mutations, i.e., DCM-associated mutations decreased binding of Tcap to titin, calsarcin-1, and MLP [22] (Fig. 3). These observations led us to hypothesize that DCM was the disease of "loose sarcomere" (Fig. 4). The loose sarcomere is evident in an animal model of DCM, *CSRP3* (MLP) knockout mouse, in which the Z-disk was wide and stretch response was impaired [27]. Since the stretch response is a hypertrophic response of cardiomyocytes against passive tension and Z-disk element is suggested to be a stretch sensor of cardiomyocytes, abnormality in Z-disk elements may alter the regulation of stretch response. It should be noted here that a possible controversy exists, i.e., HCM-associated MLP gene (*CSRP3*) mutations were reported to decrease the binding to α-actinin and N-RAP [28, 29]. However, because DCM-associated mutations were found in *CSRP3* and α-actinin gene (*ACTN2*), these mutations decreased binding to each other [30]. Therefore, the decreased binding between MLP and α-actinin was associated with both HCM and DCM. This discrepancy should be resolved by further studies.

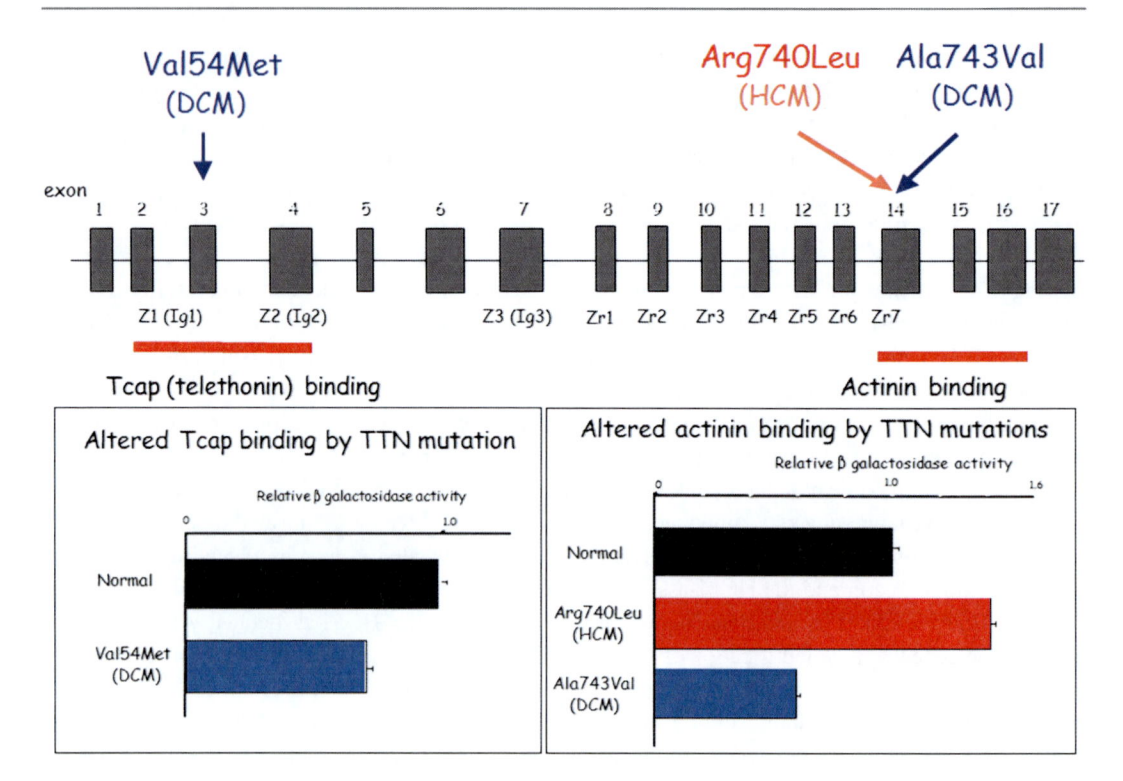

Fig. 2 Schematic representation of *TTN* mutations found in the Z-disk domain and their functional alterations. Titin in the Z-disk domain is encoded by 17 exons. One HCM-associated mutation was found in exon 14, while two DCM-associated mutations were found in exon 3 and exon 14. Functional analyses showed altered binding of titin to Tcap or actinin

Cypher/ZASP is a Z-disk element connecting calsarcin and actinin [31]. Calsarcin binds calcineurin [32], a Ser/Thr phosphatase involved in the process of hypertrophic program of cardiomyocytes [33, 34]. The functional significance of calcineurin anchorage to the Z-disk is not fully understood but it may be involved in the stress-induced calcineurin-NFAT activation, because heterozygous *MLP* knockout mice showed reduction in NFAT activation along with dislocation of calcineurin from Z-disk [35]. In addition, Cypher/ZASP is known to bind protein kinase C (PKC), [31] and a DCM-associated *LDB3* mutation in the PKC binding domain was found to increase the binding [36]; it was suggested that phosphorylation/dephosphorylation of Z-disk elements might be involved in the stretch response. The identification of target protein(s) for phosphorylation (by PKC)/dephosphorylation (by calcineurin) will unravel the molecular mechanism(s) of stretch response and/or signaling molecule(s) of cardiac hypertrophy.

Several other *LDB3* mutations not in the PKC interacting domain were reported in DCM or LVNC [37]. Because the functional changes caused by these mutations had not been demonstrated, we have searched for the binding protein to Cypher/ZASP by using yeast two-hybrid method, and found that phosphoglucomutase-1 (PGM1) is a novel binding protein [38]. PGM1 is an enzyme involved in the conversion between glucose-6-phosphate and glucose-1-phosphate, which is involved in the glucose/glycogen metabolism. Functional significance of the binding between PGM1 and the Z-disk element Cypher/ZASP was not known, but the DCM-associated mutations showed decreased binding to PGM1 [38] (Fig. 3). In addition, PGM1 was demonstrated to be localized at the Z-disk under the stressed culture conditions, low serum and low

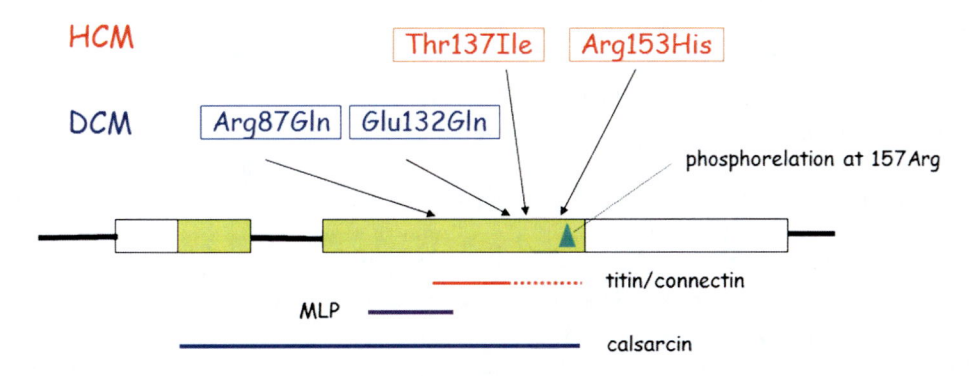

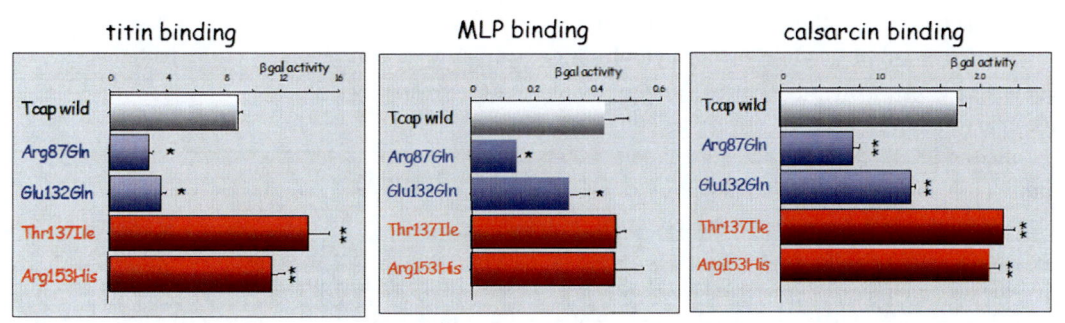

Fig. 3 Schematic representation of *TCAP* mutations and their functional alterations. Tcap is encoded by 2 exons. Two HCM-associated mutations and two DCM-associated mutations were found in exon 2. Domain structure of Tcap is schematically indicated below the exon–intron structure. Functional analyses showed altered binding of Tcap to titin, MLP, and calsarcin

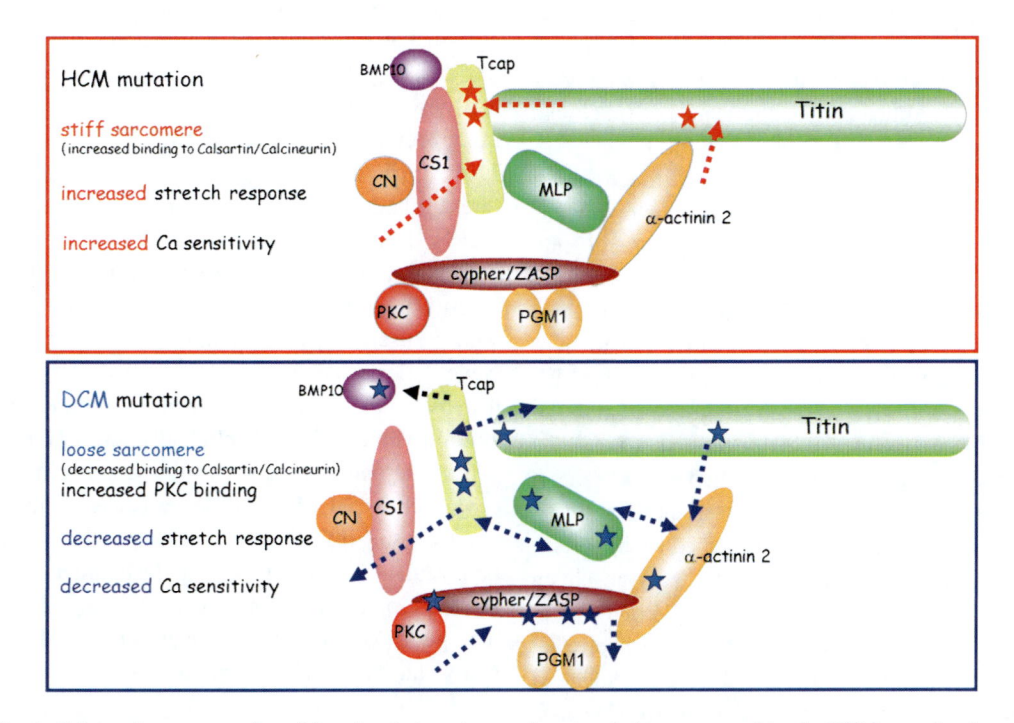

Fig. 4 Schematic representation of functional alterations caused by Z-disk mutations. Functional alterations caused by the HCM-associated mutations (*red stars*) are shown in the *upper panel*, while the *lower panel* indicated the functional changes caused by the DCM-associated mutations (*blue stars*). *Broken arrows* show the altered interactions caused by the mutations. *CN*; calcineurin, *CS1*; calsarcin-1

glucose, suggesting the role of PGM1 in the energy metabolism at the Z-disk [38]. These observations suggested that the decreased stress response due to the abnormality in Z-disk elements might be involved in the pathogenesis of DCM.

There are other DCM-associated mutations found in genes for other Z-line-associated proteins desmin (*DES*) and metavinculin (*VCL*) [4]. The *VCL* mutation was shown to impair the binding to actin [39], while the *DES* mutations resulted in a subtle change in the cytoplasmic desmin network [40]. In addition, mutations in the myopalladin gene (*MYPN*) have recently been reported in DCM. Although the molecular mechanisms of *MYPN* mutations leading to DCM remained unclear, the DCM-associated mutations impaired the myofibrinogenesis [41]. Because myopalladin binds a transcriptional cofactor, CARP [42], and CARP is involved in the regulation of gene expression associated with stretch response, cardiac remodeling, and myofibrinogenesis [43], Z-disk might be in part involved in the cardiac remodeling process related with pathogenesis of cardiomyopathy. In this regard, it is noteworthy that HCM-associated CARP mutations were reported to increase binding to myopalladin [44], although the significance of functional alterations remains to be resolved further.

Another Z-disk element, the mutation of which was associated with cardiomyopathy, is BMP10. BMP10 is a member of TGF family and is specifically expressed in the cardiomyocytes especially in fetal heart [45]. It was reported that knockout of BMP10 gene in mice led to hypoplastic heart with less trabeculation [46]. We have previously reported that expression of BMP10 is increased in the course of cardiac remodeling associated with hypertensive heart disease and found a BMP10 variant, Thr326Ile, in two DCM patients accompanied by hypertension [47]. This variant was a rare polymorphism but is a significant risk factor of DCM in the presence of hypertension. It should be noted here that this variant was also found in the father of a DCM patient and he also suffered from hypertensive heart disease. Because another TGF family, myostatin, which is specifically expressed in the skeletal muscle, is reported to bind Tcap [48], we have investigated the binding of BMP10 with Tcap and the effect of BMP10 variant on the binding, if any. It was found that BMP10 indeed bound Tcap and the variant decreased the binding, which in turn resulted in the increased secretion of BMP10 [47]. We also demonstrated that BMP10 facilitated hypertrophy and maturation of rat cardiomyocytes in primary culture [47]. These observations suggested a pivotal role of the Z-disk in cardiac remodeling through release of cardiac-specific growth factor, BMP10, and its impairment was involved in the pathogenesis of cardiomyopathy (Fig. 4).

Conclusions

In this review, cardiomyopathy-associated mutations in genes for sarcomere and Z-disk elements are summarized. Cardiomyopathy caused by sarcomere mutations may be considered as sarcomeropathy, and the functional alterations associated with sarcomeropathy can be an altered Ca^{2+} sensitivity. On the other hand, cardiomyopathy due to mutations in Z-disk element can be classified as Z-diskopathy, but the functional alterations in the Z-diskopathy may be heterogeneous abnormalities in stretch response, stress response, myofibrinogenesis, and/or cardiac remodeling. There are many other disease genes by which different functional alterations were elicited to ultimately lead to cardiomyopathy. Even though many disease genes have been deciphered, there is still a considerable proportion of patients whose disease genes remain to be unraveled. Nevertheless, each family or patient should have usually only one disease-causing mutation, and cardiomyopathy is both clinically and etiologically heterogeneous even in a specific clinical type such as HCM or DCM. Because different causes result in the same phenotype, there may be several common pathways in the pathogenesis. Intervention of these common pathways will be a therapeutic or preventive strategy for cardiomyopathy caused by different mutations.

Acknowledgments This work was supported in part by Grant-in-Aids for Scientific Research from the Ministry of Education, Culture, Sports, Science and Technology, Japan; research grant for Idiopathic Cardiomyopathy from the Ministry of Health, Labor and Welfare, Japan; grants for Basic Scientific Cooperation Program between Japan and Korea from the Japan Society for the Promotion of Science, the Korea Science and Engineering Foundation, and National Research Foundation of Korea; and research grants from the Institute of Life Science. This work was also supported by the follow-up grants provided from the Tokyo Medical and Dental University.

References

1. Maron BJ, Towbin JA, Thiene G, et al. Contemporary definitions and classification of the cardiomyopathies: an American Heart Association Scientific Statement from the Council on Clinical Cardiology, Heart Failure and Transplantation Committee; Quality of Care and Outcomes Research and Functional Genomics and Translational Biology Interdisciplinary Working Groups; and Council on Epidemiology and Prevention. Circulation. 2006;113:1807–16.
2. Towbin JA, Bowles NE. The failing heart. Nature. 2002;415:227–33.
3. Ahmad F, Seidman JG, Seidman CE. The genetic basis for cardiac remodeling. Annu Rev Genomics Hum Genet. 2006;6:185–216.
4. Kimura A. Molecular basis of hereditary cardiomyopathy: abnormalities in calcium sensitivity, stretch response, stress response and beyond. J Hum Genet. 2010;55:81–90.
5. Geisterfer-Lowrance AAT, Kass S, Tanigawa G, et al. A molecular basis for familial hypertrophic cardiomyopathy: a beta cardiac myosin heavy chain gene missense mutation. Cell. 1990;62:999–1006.
6. Sweeney HL, Straceski AJ, Leinwand LA, et al. Heterologous expression of a cardiomyopathic myosin that is defective in its actin interaction. J Biol Chem. 1994;269:1603–5.
7. Thierfelder L, Watkins H, MacRae C, et al. Alpha-tropomyosin and cardiac troponin T mutations cause familial hypertrophic cardiomyopathy: a disease of the sarcomere. Cell. 1994;77:701–12.
8. Kimura A, Harada H, Park JE, et al. Mutations in the cardiac troponin I gene associated with hypertrophic cardiomyopathy. Nat Genet. 1997;16:379–82.
9. Yanaga F, Morimoto S, Ohtsuki I. Ca^{2+} sensitization and potentiation of the maximum level of myofibrillar ATPase activity caused by mutations of troponin T found in familial hypertrophic cardiomyopathy. J Biol Chem. 1999;274:8806–12.
10. Bottinelli R, Coviello DA, Redwood CS, et al. A mutant tropomyosin that causes hypertrophic cardiomyopathy is expressed in vivo and associated with an increased calcium sensitivity. Circ Res. 1998;82:106–15.
11. Elliott K, Watkins H, Redwood CS. Altered regulatory properties of human cardiac troponin I mutants that cause hypertrophic cardiomyopathy. J Biol Chem. 2000;275:22069–74.
12. Witt CC, Gerull B, Davies MJ, et al. Hypercontractile properties of cardiac muscle fibers in a knock-in mouse model of cardiac myosin-binding protein-C. J Biol Chem. 2001;276:5353–9.
13. Roopnarine O. Mechanical defects of muscle fibers with myosin light chain mutants that cause cardiomyopathy. Biophys J. 2003;84:2440–9.
14. Pinto JR, Parvatiyar MS, Jones MA, et al. A functional and structural study of troponin C mutations related to hypertrophic cardiomyopathy. J Biol Chem. 2009;284:19090–100.
15. Tyska MJ, Hayes E, Giewat M, et al. Single-molecule mechanics of R403Q cardiac myosin isolated from the mouse model of familial hypertrophic cardiomyopathy. Circ Res. 2000;86:737–44.
16. Olson TM, Michels VV, Thibodeau SN, et al. Actin mutations in dilated cardiomyopathy, a heritable form of heart failure. Science. 1998;280:750–2.
17. Mogensen J, Klausen IC, Pedersen AK, et al. Alpha-cardiac actin is a novel disease gene in familial hypertrophic cardiomyopathy. J Clin Invest. 1999;103:R39–43.
18. Vang S, Corydon TJ, Børglum AD, et al. Actin mutations in hypertrophic and dilated cardiomyopathy cause inefficient protein folding and perturbed filament formation. FEBS J. 2005;272:2037–49.
19. Kamisago M, Sharma SD, DePalma SR, et al. Mutations in sarcomere protein genes as a cause of dilated cardiomyopathy. N Engl J Med. 2000;343:1688–96.
20. Morimoto S, Lu QW, Harada K, et al. Ca^{2+}-desensitizing effect of a deletion mutation Delta K210 in cardiac troponin T that causes familial dilated cardiomyopathy. Proc Natl Acad Sci USA. 2002;99:913–18.
21. Satoh M, Takahashi M, Sakamoto T, et al. Structural analysis of the titin gene in hypertrophic cardiomyopathy: identification of a novel disease gene. Biochem Biophys Res Commun. 1999;262:411–17.
22. Hayashi T, Arimura T, Itoh-Satoh M, et al. Tcap gene mutations in hypertrophic cardiomyopathy and dilated cardiomyopathy. J Am Coll Cardiol. 2004;44:2192–201.
23. Cazorla O, Wu Y, Irving TC, et al. Titin-based modulation of calcium sensitivity of active tension in mouse skinned cardiac myocytes. Circ Res. 2001;88:1028–35.
24. Fujita H, Labeit D, Gerull B, et al. Titin isoform-dependent effect of calcium on passive myocardial tension. Am J Physiol Heart Circ Physiol. 2004;287:H2528–34.
25. Fuchs F, Martyn DA. Length-dependent Ca^{2+} activation in cardiac muscle: some remaining questions. J Muscle Res Cell Motil. 2005;26:199–212.
26. Itoh-Satoh M, Hayashi T, Nishi H, et al. Titin mutations as the molecular basis for dilated cardiomyopathy. Biochem Biophys Res Commun. 2002;291:385–93.
27. Knöll R, Hoshijima M, Hoffman HM, et al. The cardiac mechanical stretch sensor machinery involves a Z-disk complex that is defective in a subset of human dilated cardiomyopathy. Cell. 2002;111:943–55.
28. Geier C, Perrot A, Ozcelik C, et al. Mutations in the human muscle LIM protein gene in families with hypertrophic cardiomyopathy. Circulation. 2003;107:1390–5.
29. Gehmlich K, Geier C, Osterziel KJ, et al. Decreased interactions of mutant muscle LIM protein (MLP)

with N-RAP and alpha-actinin and their implication for hypertrophic cardiomyopathy. Cell Tissue Res. 2004;317:129–36.

30. Mohapatra B, Jimenez S, Lin JH, et al. Mutations in the muscle LIM protein and alpha-actinin-2 genes in dilated cardiomyopathy and endocardial fibroelastosis. Mol Genet Metab. 2003;80:207–15.

31. Zhou Q, Ruiz-Lozano P, Martone ME, et al. Cypher, a striated muscle-restricted PDZ and LIM domain-containing protein, binds to alpha-actinin-2 and protein kinase C. J Biol Chem. 1999;274:19807–13.

32. Frey N, Richardson JA, Olson EN. Calsarcins, a novel family of sarcomeric calcineurin-binding proteins. Proc Natl Acad Sci USA. 2000;97:14632–7.

33. Wilkins BJ, Molkentin JD. Calcium-calcineurin signaling in the regulation of cardiac hypertrophy. Biochem Biophys Res Commun. 2004;322:1178–91.

34. Heineke J, Molkentin JD. Regulation of cardiac hypertrophy by intracellular signalling pathways. Nat Rev Mol Cell Biol. 2006;7:589–600.

35. Heineke J, Ruetten H, Willenbockel C, et al. Attenuation of cardiac remodeling after myocardial infarction by muscle LIM protein-calcineurin signaling at the sarcomeric Z-disk. Proc Natl Acad Sci U S A. 2005;102:1655–60.

36. Arimura T, Hayashi T, Terada H, et al. A Cypher/ZASP mutation associated with dilated cardiomyopathy alters the binding affinity to protein kinase C. J Biol Chem. 2004;279:6746–52.

37. Vatta M, Mohapatra B, Jimenez S, et al. Mutations in Cypher/ZASP in patients with dilated cardiomyopathy and left ventricular non-compaction. J Am Coll Cardiol. 2003;42:2014–27.

38. Arimura T, Inagaki N, Hayashi T, et al. Impaired binding of ZASP/Cypher with phosphoglucomutase 1 is associated with dilated cardiomyopathy. Cardiovasc Res. 2009;83:80–8.

39. Olson TM, Illenberger S, Kishimoto NY, et al. Metavinculin mutations alter actin interaction in dilated cardiomyopathy. Circulation. 2002;105:431–7.

40. Taylor MR, Slavov D, Ku L, et al. Prevalence of desmin mutations in dilated cardiomyopathy. Circulation. 2007;115:1244–51.

41. Duboscq-Bidot L, Xu P, Charron P, et al. Mutations in the Z-band protein myopalladin gene and idiopathic dilated cardiomyopathy. Cardiovasc Res. 2008;77:118–25.

42. Aihara Y, Kurabayashi M, Saito Y, et al. Cardiac ankyrin repeat protein is a novel marker of cardiac hypertrophy: role of M-CAT element within the promoter. Hypertension. 2000;36:48–53.

43. Witt SH, Labeit D, Granzier H, et al. Dimerization of the cardiac ankyrin protein CARP: implications for MARP titin-based signaling. J Muscle Res Cell Motil. 2006;262:1–8.

44. Arimura T, Bos MJ, Sato A, et al. Cardiac ankyrin repeat protein gene (ANKRD1) mutations in hypertrophic cardiomyopathy. J Am Coll Cardiol. 2009;54:334–42.

45. Neuhaus H, Rosen V, Thies R. Heart specific expression of mouse BMP-10 a novel member of the TGF-beta superfamily. Mech Dev. 1999;80:181–4.

46. Chen H, Shi S, Acosta L, et al. BMP10 is essential for maintaining cardiac growth during murine cardiogenesis. Development. 2004;131:2219–31.

47. Nakano N, Hori H, Abe M, et al. Interaction of BMP10 with Tcap may modulate the course of hypertensive cardiac hypertrophy. Am J Physiol Heart Card Physiol. 2007;293:H3396–403.

48. Nicholas G, Thomas M, Langley B, et al. Titin-cap associates with, and regulates secretion of, Myostatin. J Cell Physiol. 2002;193:120–31.

Left Ventricular Assist Device: Morphological, Molecular, and Genetic Changes After Mechanical Support

Hideo A. Baba, Atsushi Takeda, Nobuakira Takeda, and Jeremias Wohlschlaeger

Abstract

Left ventricular assist devices (LVADs) are currently used to either "bridge" patients with terminal congestive heart failure (CHF) to cardiac transplantation or optionally for patients with contraindications for transplantation ("destination therapy"). Mechanical support is associated with a marked decrease of cardiac dilation and hypertrophy as well as numerous cellular and molecular changes ("reverse cardiac remodeling"), which can be accompanied by improved cardiac function ("bridge to recovery") in a relatively small subset of patients. In these patients, heart transplantation is no longer necessary even after removal of the device ("weaning"). In the recent past, novel pharmacological strategies have been developed and are combined with mechanical support, which has increased the percentage of patients with improved clinical status and cardiac performance. Gene expression profiles have demonstrated that individuals who recover after LVADs show different gene expression compared to individuals who do not respond to unloading. This chapter focuses on signal transduction, transcriptional regulation, and aspects of neurohormonal activation in the failing human heart before and after ventricular unloading.

Keywords

Chromogranin A • Heart failure • Hypertrophy • Myocytes • Natriuretic peptides • Remodeling

H.A. Baba (⊠)
Institute of Pathology and Neuropathology,
University Hospital of Essen, University
of Duisburg-Essen, Germany
e-mail: hideo.baba@uk-essen.de

Introduction

Chronic heart failure is a major cause of morbidity and mortality in both western industrialized and developing nations and causes considerable economic burden to the medical systems. The average mortality from the time of diagnosis of heart failure is greater than 60% at 5 years and much higher when patients reach the most advanced stages [1]. Patients typically become progressively less responsive to medical therapy with the consequence of impaired heart function as well as quality of life [2].

Transplantation is currently the most established treatment for refractory heart failure [1]. However, this option is only available to fewer than 2,300 patients per year, with a relatively constant donor organ supply. As a result, the use of left ventricular assist devices (LVADs) in treating patients with end-stage heart failure has increased significantly in recent years [3]. LVADs are electrically powered either pulsatile or non-pulsatile pumps or turbines, which can be installed extracorporally or intrathoracically parallel to the circulation, i.e., they transport blood from the left ventricle to the ascending aorta and thereby provide profound volume and pressure reduction and restore systemic blood pressure and flow to near normal levels.

Regardless of the cause of myocardial injury, a clinical phenotype is recognized that is referred to as remodeling, which includes eccentric dilatation of the ventricular chamber, reduction in contractile function, and an increase in cardiac filling pressures and wall stress. These clinical phenotypic changes of heart failure are paralleled by significant histological, cellular, and molecular changes in most structural and functional components of the myocyte including alterations in myocyte geometry and size, progressive interstitial fibrosis, upregulation of cytokines and inflammation, as well as reductions in myocardial energetics, beta receptor density, and calcium-handling proteins. There is now compelling evidence that prolonged near-total unloading of the left ventricle in CHF is associated with numerous morphological and molecular changes in the myocardium ("reverse remodeling") [4, 5], which can be accompanied by functional improvement and decreased cardiac dilatation [6]. Despite encouraging data on morphological and molecular changes of the affected heart, clinical cardiac recovery sufficient to allow device removal ("weaning") is reported to occur only in a small subset of individuals [7, 8]. In general, it is accepted that cellular and molecular improvement is greater than clinical cardiac recovery [9]. The present paper mainly focuses on the major morphological and molecular changes that occur in the heart during "reverse cardiac remodeling" by ventricular unloading.

Functional Improvements in Myocytes in Response to the LVAD Linked to Molecular and Gene Expression Changes

There is evidence of early mechanical improvements in failing hearts treated with VADs [9–12]. These early findings are important in showing that contractile performance of myocytes was partially recovered in response to therapy with a VAD. Myocyte contractile performance was significantly greater in isolated myocytes of failing human hearts post VAD support compared to failing human hearts without VAD support [11]. Improvements in the magnitude of shortening were seen in response to beta-adrenergic agonists, and basal relaxation was also improved in myocytes following VAD support. This was confirmed in isolated trabecular preparations in a separate study [13].

A novel combination therapy consisting of a left ventricular assist device (LVAD) combined with pharmacological therapy including the selective beta-2-agonist clenbuterol has shown promise in restoring ventricular function in patients with heart failure [14]. Using microarray analysis of six paired human heart samples harvested at the time of LVAD implant and at the time of LVAD explant for recovery of ventricular function, the authors identified different pathways between heart failure and recovery. Significant changes in genes of the beta-adrenergic signaling pathway were observed including Rap guanine nucleotide exchange factor 4, (EPAC2), protein kinase, regulatory type I alpha (PKAr), phosphodiesterase 1A (PDE1A), phosphodiesterase 3B (PDE3B), and calcineurin A (PPP3CA/PP2B) [15].

miRNA

miRNAs constitute one of the more abundant classes of molecules regulating genes in animals. miRNAs are small, endogenous noncoding RNAs [16]. Many of these miRNAs have been shown to inhibit posttranscriptional processing [16, 17]. At least 80% of human miRNAs are conserved in fish [17]. This high degree of conservation suggests an important regulatory role for miRNA. Recent work by Matkovich and colleagues suggests that adding miRNA profiling to mRNA profiling enhances the ability of mRNA profiles to categorize the clinical status of heart failure before and after biomechanical unloading [18]. The results of this study confirmed three earlier identified miRNAs associated with heart failure (miR-24, miR-125b, and miR-195) [18, 19]. In addition, this study extended earlier work in mouse models [20] showing that miR-21, miR-23a, and miR-199a-3p were also regulated in human heart failure [18]. One important point of this study was that these miRNAs were reversible after LVAD support.

Natriuretic Peptides and Chromogranin A

Despite divergent etiologies, heart failure is characterized by activation of neurohormonal systems: catecholamines, natriuretic peptides (NP), and components of the renin-angiotensin axis are increased and were found to have pathophysiological and prognostic implications. Some of these molecules exert local paracrine activation

but their plasma levels were demonstrated to be markers of clinical outcome. Increased cardiac ANP and BNP expression in CHF patients is associated with increased expression of the NP metabolizing NPR-C receptors and blunted responsiveness of GC-A to ANP by reduced cGMP synthesis.

"Reverse remodeling" after unloading reverses these changes and reestablishes the local responsiveness of GC-A to ANP. Cardiac expression of ANP, BNP, and NPR-C mRNA correlated significantly with cardiomyocyte diameters. In contrast to the latter, the levels of the natriuretic peptides are fully reversed to the level of the controls, indicating that their expression is partly independent of cardiac hypertrophy and regulated by CHF-associated factors, such as cardiomyocyte stretch [21].

Chromogranin A is an acidic calcium-binding protein and is the major soluble constituent in secretory vesicles throughout the neuroendocrine system. Chromogranin A was found to be significantly up-regulated during CHF and is co-stored with catecholamines and NP. Chromogranin A is secreted into the circulation with a long-term plasma half-life of approximately 18 min. BNP and chromogranin A are co-stored in the myocardium of patients with dilated cardiomyopathy, whereas this co-localization was not found in healthy controls [22]. We investigated the expression of natriuretic peptides and chromogranin A by immunohistochemistry and morphometric quantification before and after VAD. In a different set of patients, chromogranin A was evaluated in the plasma. We demonstrated that in-line with ANP and BNP, chromogranin A is significantly increased in CHF compared to healthy controls and decreased by ventricular support. Moreover, sarcoplasmic co-localization of BNP and chromogranin A is diminished after unloading. However, due to its low expression the negative regulation of chromogranin A is not reflected by plasma levels; thus, chromogranin A does not appear to be an appropriate biomarker for the monitoring of "reverse cardiac remodeling" after unloading [23] (see Fig. 1).

Fig. 1 Heart failure and hypertrophy are associated with increased expression of ANP, BNP, and chromogranin A due to tensile stretch during cardiac dilatation in the heart as well as in the blood. After mechanical support, ANP and BNP levels decrease in both the heart and the blood. In contrast, chromogranin A only decreases in the heart (modified from Wohlschlaeger et al. 2008) [23]

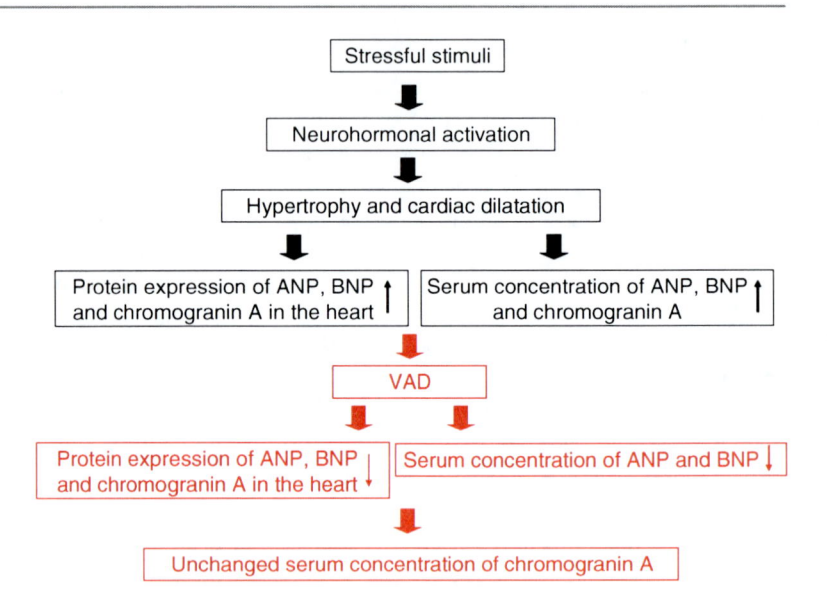

Transduction Pathways

Among others, three major signal transduction pathways have been shown to be involved in the pathogenesis of cardiac hypertrophy and "remodeling": (1) the mitogen-activated protein kinases (MAPK) with the extracellular signal-related kinases (Erks), c-jun N-terminal protein kinases (JNKs), and p38 MAPK subfamilies [24]; (2) the Ca^{2+}/calmodulin activated protein kinase (CaM kinase) and phosphatase (calcineurin) [25]; (3) the protein kinase B/Akt and its downstream target glycogen synthase kinase 3β (GSK3β) [26]. All three pathways become activated during CHF in humans. Whereas the Erks are activated by hypertrophic stimuli such as phenylephrine, angiotensin II (ATII), and endothelin-1 [24], the JNK and p38 MAPK are activated by cellular stress and seem to be involved in apoptotic cell death [27]. Apart from acting as an anti-apoptotic factor, Akt is a major repressor of cardiac hypertrophy by inhibitory phosphorylation of GSK3β [28]. The phosphatidylinositol-3-OH kinase (PI3K) is a signaling system that acts through Akt and p70S6 kinase, which is a key factor in angiotensin II (ATII) receptor-type-2-mediated cardiac hypertrophy [29]. We investigated the activity of the mitogen-activated protein kinases (MEKs), Erks, Akt,

GSK3β, p70S6 kinase, JNKs, and p38 in terminal CHF before and after unloading [30]. Western blot analysis revealed a dramatic decrease in dually phosphorylated active forms of Erk-1 and Erk-2 after mechanical support. Also the Erk-activating kinases (MEK-1/2) were shown to be significantly less phosphorylated after LVAD. After unloading, Akt is inactivated, whereas GSK3β becomes activated. Besides Akt, another kinase involved in the PI3K/Akt pathway, p70S6 kinase showed a dramatic decrease in its phosphorylation in a subset of patients. Despite the fact that p70S6 kinase and its isoform p85S6 are associated with cardiomyocyte hypertrophy mediated by angiotensin II (ATII) receptor type 2, there was no correlation between cardiomyocyte diameter reduction and phosphorylation of p70S6 kinase. In contrast, neither the JNK nor the p38-mediated signaling cascades were altered with LVAD support in this study, suggesting specific regulation of kinase signaling after mechanical support in humans in vivo. In summary, our findings underscore the emerging evidence of MEK/Erks and Akt/GSK3β in the pathogenesis and regulation of cardiac hypertrophy. The inactivation of MEK/Erks and the activation of GSK3β after LVAD are in-line with the opposing effects of these two signaling cascades with regard to cardiac "reverse remodeling" [30].

Conclusions

Numerous noxious stimuli, such as chronic ischemia, inflammation, or genetic alterations, may affect the myocardium and induce rather nonspecific compensatory and adaptive changes including cardiomyocyte hypertrophy. Although salutary at the beginning, these adaptive mechanisms may become maladaptive and deleterious over time and eventually lead to impaired cardiac function. The increased cardiac wall stress and local ischemia may be the mechanisms that activate numerous molecular and cellular responses. Protective mechanisms are overrun and the myocardium cannot further adapt to increased biomechanical stress. Neurohormonal activation, inflammatory mediators, alterations in β-adrenergic signal transduction and Ca^{2+} metabolism, and interstitial fibrosis further impair cardiac function. Despite improving medical strategies, until now cardiac transplantation remains the only curative therapeutic approach. Due to the shortage of donor organs, LVADs are currently used to maintain cardiac function in patients with terminal CHF until a donor organ is available or optionally used as a permanent therapy for patients with contraindications for transplantation. As outlined above, the use of unloading is associated with changes at cellular, molecular, and genetic levels. Although these results are encouraging, there is agreement that the clinical cardiac improvement and performance are less pronounced in the majority of cases and only a small subset of patients can be weaned from the device and live without transplantation. The approach described by Birks and coworkers consisting of combined use of mechanical support and medical treatment including clenbuterol shows promising results for the future, as the reported percentage of patients who can be weaned is considerably higher. Another important problem in this field is the absence of a suitable serum/plasma biomarker that accurately indicates cardiac recovery under LVAD therapy and possibly predicts the clinical outcome and the changes for successful weaning from the device. ANP and BNP levels are widely used but these molecules are mainly stretch-induced and their levels decrease under support because of volume and pressure reduction, but not necessarily indicate "reverse remodeling" or clinical recovery. We could not show chromogranin A serum levels to be a usable biomarker for this group of patients. Gene expression profiles, as performed by Birks et al., might serve as a possible readout frame for the future helping to identify patients who can be weaned from the device. However, the master molecular switches orchestrating the process of "reverse remodeling" are still unknown. The heterogeneity of patients with regard to the etiology of CHF, the duration of support, the type of LVAD implanted, and medication causes further difficulties, although we never found these factors to be influential on the parameters investigated. In conclusion, despite the limited clinical improvement occurring only in a subset of patients, a better understanding of the underlying biological mechanisms of cardiac "reverse remodeling" is crucial for the development of future therapeutic strategies in this still intriguing scientific field.

References

1. Hunt SA, Abraham WT, Chin MH, et al. Focused update incorporated into the ACC/AHA 2005 Guidelines for the Diagnosis and Management of Heart Failure in Adults: a report of the American College of Cardiology Foundation/American Heart Association Task Force on Practice Guidelines: developed in collaboration with the International Society for Heart and Lung Transplantation. Circulation. 2009;19:e391–479.
2. Jessup M, Brozena S. Heart failure. N Engl J Med. 2003;348:2007–18.
3. Kirklin JK, Naftel DC, Kormos RL, et al. Second INTERMACS annual report: more than 1,000 primary left ventricular assist device implants. J Heart Lung Transplant. 2010;29:1–10.
4. Wohlschlaeger J, Schmitz KJ, Schmid C, et al. Reverse remodeling following insertion of left ventricular assist devices (LVAD): a review of the morphological and molecular changes. Cardiovasc Res. 2005;68: 376–86.
5. Zafeiridis A, Jeevanandam V, Houser SR, et al. Regression of cellular hypertrophy after left ventricular assist device support. Circulation. 1998;98: 656–62.
6. Frazier OH, Benedict CR, Radovancevic B, et al. Improved left ventricular function after chronic left

ventricular unloading. Ann Thorac Surg. 1996;62: 675–81.

7. Mancini DM, Beniaminovitz A, Levin H, et al. Low incidence of myocardial recovery after left ventricular assist device implantation in patients with chronic heart failure [see comments]. Circulation. 1998;98: 2383–9.

8. Simon MA, Kormos RL, Murali S, et al. Myocardial recovery using ventricular assist devices: prevalence, clinical characteristics, and outcomes. Circulation. 2005;112(Suppl):I32–6.

9. Maybaum S, Mancini D, Xydas S, et al. Cardiac improvement during mechanical circulatory support: a prospective multicenter study of the LVAD Working Group. Circulation. 2007;115:2497–505.

10. Chaudhary KW, Rossman EI, Piacentino III V, et al. Altered myocardial Ca^{2+} cycling after left ventricular assist device support in the failing human heart. J Am Coll Cardiol. 2004;44:837–45.

11. Dipla K, Mattiello JA, Jeevanandam V, et al. Myocyte recovery after mechanical circulatory support in humans with end-stage heart failure [see comments]. Circulation. 1998;97:2316–22.

12. Heerdt PM, Holmes JW, Cai B, et al. Chronic unloading by left ventricular assist device reverses contractile dysfunction and alters gene expression in end-stage heart failure. Circulation. 2000;102:2713–19.

13. Ogletree-Hughes ML, Stull LB, Sweet WE, et al. Mechanical unloading restores beta-adrenergic responsiveness and reverses receptor downregulation in the failing human heart. Circulation. 2001;104: 881–6.

14. Birks EJ, Tansley PD, Hardy J, et al. Left ventricular assist device and drug therapy for the reversal of heart failure. N Engl J Med. 2006;355:1873–84.

15. Hall JL, Birks EJ, Grindle S, et al. Molecular signature of recovery following combination left ventricular assist device (LVAD) support and pharmacologic therapy. Eur Heart J. 2007;28:613–27.

16. Saunders MA, Liang H, Li WH. Human polymorphism at microRNAs and microRNA target sites. Proc Natl Acad Sci USA. 2007;104:3300–5.

17. Lim LP, Glasner ME, Yekta S, et al. Vertebrate microRNA genes. Science. 2003;299:1540.

18. Matkovich SJ, Van Booven DJ, Youker KA, et al. Reciprocal regulation of myocardial microRNAs and messenger RNA in human cardiomyopathy and reversal of the microRNA signature by biomechanical support. Circulation. 2009;119:1263–71.

19. van Rooij E, Sutherland LB, Liu N, et al. A signature pattern of stress-responsive microRNAs that can evoke cardiac hypertrophy and heart failure. Proc Natl Acad Sci USA. 2006;103:18255–60.

20. Tatsuguchi M, Seok HY, Callis TE, et al. Expression of microRNAs is dynamically regulated during cardiomyocyte hypertrophy. J Mol Cell Cardiol. 2007; 42:1137–41.

21. Kuhn M, Voss M, Mitko D, et al. Left ventricular assist device support reverses altered cardiac expression and function of natriuretic peptides and receptors in end-stage heart failure. Cardiovasc Res. 2004;64: 308–14.

22. Pieroni M, Corti A, Tota B, et al. Myocardial production of chromogranin A in human heart: a new regulatory peptide of cardiac function. Eur Heart J. 2007;28: 1117–27.

23. Wohlschlaeger J, von Winterfeld M, Milting H, et al. Decreased myocardial chromogranin a expression and colocalization with brain natriuretic peptide during reverse cardiac remodeling after ventricular unloading. J Heart Lung Transplant. 2008;27:442–9.

24. Michel MC, Li Y, Heusch G. Mitogen-activated protein kinases in the heart. Naunyn Schmiedebergs Arch Pharmacol. 2001;363:245–66.

25. Frey N, McKinsey TA, Olson EN. Decoding calcium signals involved in cardiac growth and function. Nat Med. 2000;6:1221–7.

26. Shioi T, McMullen JR, Kang PM, et al. Akt/protein kinase B promotes organ growth in transgenic mice. Mol Cell Biol. 2002;22:2799–809.

27. Sugden PH, Clerk A. "Stress-responsive" mitogen-activated protein kinases (c-Jun N-terminal kinases and p38 mitogen-activated protein kinases) in the myocardium. Circ Res. 1998;83:345–52.

28. Kozma SC, Thomas G. Regulation of cell size in growth, development and human disease: PI3K, PKB and S6K. Bioessays. 2002;24:65–71.

29. Senbonmatsu T, Ichihara S, Price EJ, et al. Evidence for angiotensin II type 2 receptor-mediated cardiac myocyte enlargement during in vivo pressure overload. J Clin Invest. 2000;106:R25–9.

30. Baba HA, Stypmann J, Grabellus F, et al. Dynamic regulation of MEK/Erks and Akt/GSK-3beta in human end-stage heart failure after left ventricular mechanical support: myocardial mechanotransduction-sensitivity as a possible molecular mechanism. Cardiovasc Res. 2003;59:390–9.

Vascular Ehlers–Danlos Syndrome: A Good Experimental Model Is Needed for Development of Treatment Strategies

Wilfried Briest and Mark I. Talan

Abstract

The vascular form of the Ehlers–Danlos syndrome (vEDS) is a rare inherited connective tissue disorder. Patients have a reduced life span (under 50) due to spontaneous and often fatal rupture of blood vessels and hollow organs. Until very recently no evidence-based treatment had been available. VEDS results from mutations in the *COL3A1* gene that encodes the chains of collagen type III and alters the sequence in the triple-helical domain. A mouse model of vEDS created by inactivation of the *Col3a1* gene has been of limited use as only 5% of homozygous animals survived to adulthood.

The haploinsufficiency for one *COL3A1* allele is one of the genotypes resulting in vEDS. In this review we provide evidence that haploinsufficiency for *Col3a1* in mice recapitulates features of vEDS in humans and might be used as an experimental model. There was a reduced level of aortic collagen and correspondingly reduced aortic wall strength. A spectrum of lesions was detected in the aorta similar to those observed in human patients. Lesions increased in number and age and were more common in male than in female mice.

Furthermore, potential treatment strategies are discussed including the already tested β-adrenergic receptor (AR)-blocker therapy, the inhibition of extracellular matrix degrading enzymes, and the only causative approach of selective silencing of the mutant form of *COL3A1* by allele-specific RNA interference.

Keywords

Aorta • Aortic wall strength • Beta-blocker therapy • Collagen • Connective tissue • Ehlers–Danlos syndrome • Extracellular matrix • MMP inhibition • Treatment strategies

W. Briest (✉)
Leibniz Institute for Age Research,
Fritz-Lipmann Institute, Jena, Germany
e-mail: wilfried.briest@arcor.de

Introduction

The Ehlers–Danlos syndrome (EDS) is a hetero-geneous group of inherited connective tissue dis-orders characterized by joint hypermobility, skin hyperextensibility, and tissue fragility [1–3]. The syndrome is named after Ehlers and Danlos, Danish and French dermatologists, respectively, who published their observations independently in the first decade of the twentieth century [2]. However, the pathology was first described by Tschernogobow in 1892 [2].

EDS type IV, the vascular type (vEDS, also known as Sack–Barabas syndrome, OMIM 130050), is a dominantly inherited disorder that results from mutations in the *COL3A1* gene, which encodes the constituent α1 chains of type III procollagen [4–7]. VEDS is a rare disease (prevalence 1–2:100,000) [5]. In addition to com-plications in the cardiovascular system like arte-rial dissections and ruptures, manifestations of vEDS involve the skin, joints, and hollow organs, resulting in thin/translucent skin, extensive bruis-ing, characteristic facial appearance, and intesti-nal/uterine rupture [3]. The causative gene for vEDS is *COL3A1*. Currently, nearly 200 muta-tions in the *COL3A1* gene leading to synthesis of an abnormal type III procollagen protein or hap-loinsufficiency have been identified [8]. Most of the mutations are single-nucleotide substitutions for glycine residues in the triple-helical domain of the proα1(III) chain, resulting in a regular quantity of abnormal collagen III. Haploinsuffi-ciency of collagen III (reduced quantity of nor-mal collagen III) is mostly the result of degradation of mutant transcripts due to nonsense-mediated mRNA decay. Therefore, this haploinsufficiency is a functional haploinsufficiency, not based on a complete deletion of the *COL3A1* gene on one allele. This true haploinsufficiency had been reported only once: a complete loss of one allele through hemizygous deletion of *COL3A1* and flanking genes [9].

Type III collagen is the second most abundant collagen in human tissues and occurs particularly in tissues exhibiting elastic properties, such as skin, blood vessels, and various internal organs. Several studies concerning the relative amounts of type I and III collagen have been published, all giving more or less different results, depending mainly on the tissue extraction methods used to solubilize the insoluble collagen. For example, the initial work on arterial collagens suggested a predominance of type III collagen over type I [10], but later results have suggested that type I collagen accounts for 55–88% of the total amount of these two [11, 12]. It has been suggested and this seems to be true still today that type III col-lagen predominates in tissues requiring higher levels of compliance, while type I, which forms larger fibers, predominates in denser connective tissues that are less distensible [13].

The quantitative defects or qualitative deficit of structurally normal collagen III in vEDS and corresponding changes in the wall structure are responsible for major complications observed in afflicted individual: arterial, bowel, and uterine rupture. Because of these dramatic complica-tions, life expectancy is shortened to a mean of <50 years [6, 14]. In approximately 50% affected individuals the heredity of disease cannot be established and spontaneous mutations are impli-cated. Those cases are especially deadly, because the life-threatening complication is often the first presentation of disease. Until very recently, there was no evidence-based treatment or preventive strategy available. However, in the just com-pleted first multicenter randomized trial, almost 4 years (47 months) treatment with celiprolol – a long-acting β1 antagonist with partial β2 agonist properties used for treatment of hypertension – decreased the incidence of arterial ruptures in patients with clinical diagnosis of vEDS [15]. However, positive interpretation of the results was not universally accepted.

Research directed to understanding of the pathophysiology and prevention of major compli-cations is hindered by the lack of an appropriate animal model. The *Col3a1* KO mouse (*Col3a1^{tm1Jae}*) was constructed in 1997 and proposed to serve as animal model for the vEDS [16]. However, this model was difficult to exploit because heterozygous mice, according to the authors, were phenotypically normal, while the phenotype of homozygotes was too severe. Homozygotes had an average survival rate of 5% at weaning, most dying within 48 hours of birth. Few surviving mice had a much shorter life span compared with wild-type mice. The major cause of death of mutant mice was the rupture of the major blood vessels, similar to patients with vEDS. This homozygous knockout mouse is not a suitable model for two reasons: first, human homozygosity for *COL3A1* null is statistically improbable and only a single case has ever been reported [17]. This individual did not present a typical vEDS phenotype [17]. Second, the homozygous mice have an extreme preweaning mortality, in comparison with a disease that typically manifests itself clinically in the third or fourth decade in humans. Therefore, we performed a deep evaluation of the heterozygous knockout mouse as a potential model for vEDS [18]. The results of this study will be summarized in this review and potential treatment strategies will be discussed.

Because vascular complications of large vessels are the most serious cause of morbidity and mortality in this disease, the phenotypic strategy included first of all a detailed histological assessment of pathology in the aorta across the life span in both sexes, including characterization of lesions observed. Complementary functional and biomechanical studies of the heart and large elastic (aorta) and medium muscular (gracilis) arteries were undertaken to assist in the evaluation of the vascular phenotype as well. Finally, anatomical, biomechanical, and transcriptional studies of the colon, a second major site of complications, were performed.

Histopathology of the Aorta

Different lesions were observed in the aorta of *Col3a1^{tm1Jae}* heterozygous mice. Grade 1 lesions appeared as a small break in the internal elastic lamina with no significant spindle cell proliferation (not shown). The broken ends of the laminae frequently curled under into the media. In grade 2 lesions, the distance between the fragmented

ends of the internal elastic lamina was greater and the intervening space was filled with a moderate proliferation of spindle cells and the accumulation of an abundant collagen-rich extracellular matrix (Fig. 1b). Grade 3 lesions were larger with more florid medial spindle cell proliferation and often fragmentation of one to two medial elastic laminae (Fig. 1c). In grade 4 lesions, there was a marked and abrupt attenuation of the wall thickness with abundant fibrosis and more severe fragmentation of several elastic laminae (Fig. 1d). A lack of infiltrating leukocytes as well as a relative sparing of the aortic root clearly distinguished the lesions in these mice from the recently described aortitis of BALB/c mice [19]. Grade 1 lesions were seen in 55% of analyzed aortas (93 of 170) with almost no discrimination between wild type and heterozygous mice. Because of their mild nature, as well as a high frequency in both sexes and genotypes, grade 1 lesions were excluded from statistical analysis.

Lesions were not found in female and younger male wild-type mice; however lesions were observed in a small number of older (9 months and older) male wild-type mice (Fig. 2). The number of lesions increased in number and severity with age. While there were no lesions found in 2–5-month-old mice, in older animals between 9 and 14 months of age, there were lesions found in 47% female and 88% of male *Col3a1^{tm1Jae}* heterozygous mice [18]. The lesions are similar to those reported in vEDS patients [6, 20–22]. These lesions in mice were focal to multifocal and apparently stochastic in distribution. Additionally, the nature of the lesions in haploinsufficient *Col3a1* mice overlaps with the morphologically similar, but usually milder, lesions noted in older wild-type mice, indicating that the observed lesions are themselves nonspecific. Rather, heterozygotes exhibit both a higher number and cumulative severity of lesions, suggesting that the differences between genotypes are quantitative rather than qualitative [18]. Similar quantitative rather than qualitative differences in diseased and "normal" control aortas have been noted previously in humans with vEDS as well as for other genetic and acquired aortic diseases [23–26].

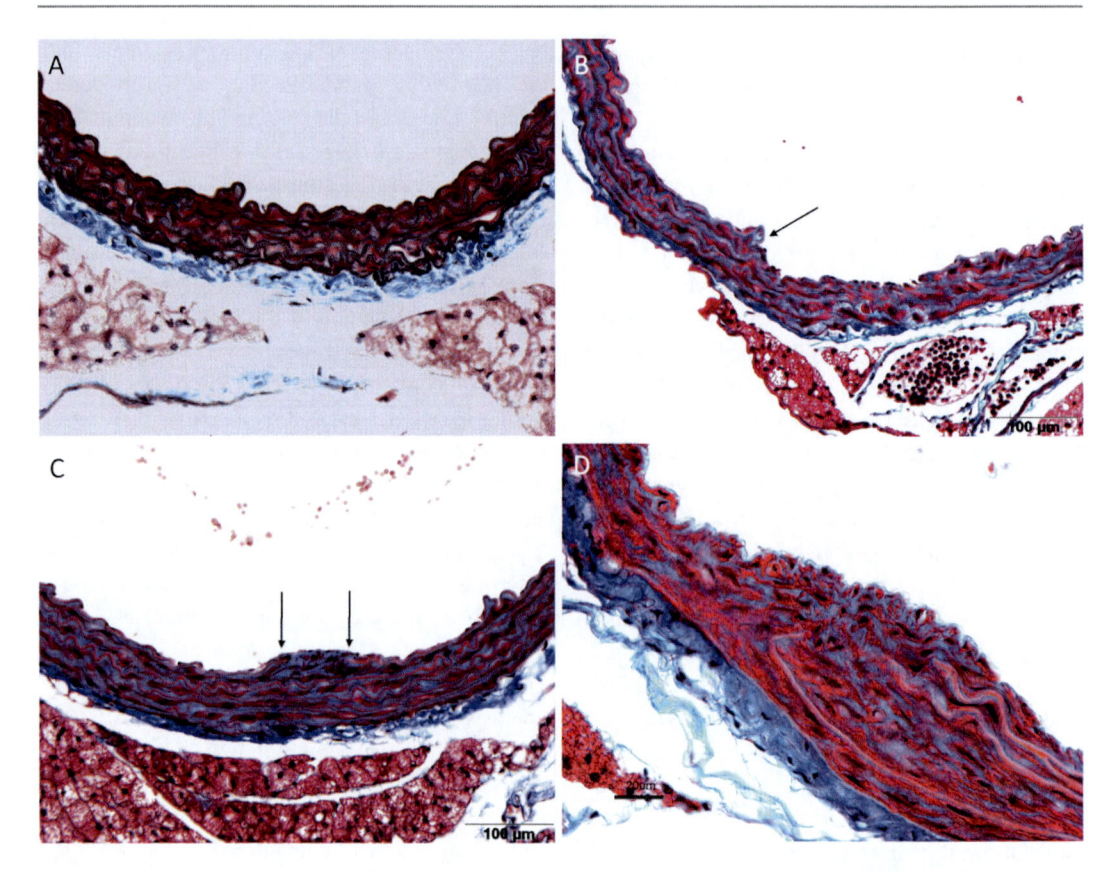

Fig. 1 Aortic lesion in the aorta. (**a**) Section of abdominal aorta from a wild-type control animal. (**b**) Aorta. Grade 2 lesion with fragmentation of the internal elastic lamina (arrow) with minimal spindle cell proliferation. (**c**) Aorta. Grade 3 lesion with fragmentation of the internal elastic lamina (arrows) with more florid spindle cell proliferation. (**d**) Aorta. Grade 4 lesion with fragmentation of the internal elastic lamina, as well as several medial laminae, with florid spindle cell proliferation and collagen-rich extracellular matrix deposition. Masson's trichrome

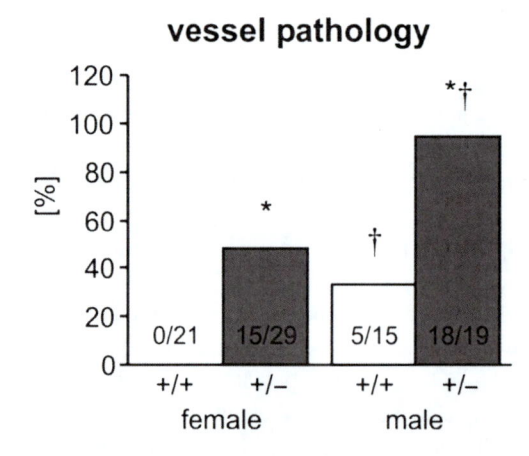

Fig. 2 Vessel pathology in the aorta [18]. Vessel pathology was quantified on the basis of lesions detected in 20 cross sections from different parts of individual aortas of 9-, 14-, and 21-month-old mice (data are summarized in the figure). *P<0.05 vs. corresponding +/+, †P<0.05 versus female. Numbers of affected and analyzed vessels were indicated

Quantification of Extracellular Matrix in the Aorta and Functional Testing

Picro-sirius red staining of the aorta sections shows diminished total collagen in heterozygotes relative to wild-type mice (Fig. 3). There was no significant difference in total collagen content of the ascending or transverse aorta between genotypes (Fig. 4). However, there was a nonsignificant decrease in total collagen in descending thoracic aorta, and a significant decrease in total collagen in the abdominal aorta of heterozygotes (Fig. 4). This could be explained by the relative higher amount of collagen and less elastin in the abdominal aorta [26, 27]. These data were in agreement with less collagen III protein

Fig. 3 Collagen accumulation in the aorta. Abdominal aorta of wild-type (**a**) and heterozygous (**b**) mice stained with picro-sirius red and viewed under polarized light demonstrates reduced adventitial and, to a lesser extent, medial total collagen in heterozygote, consistent with genotype

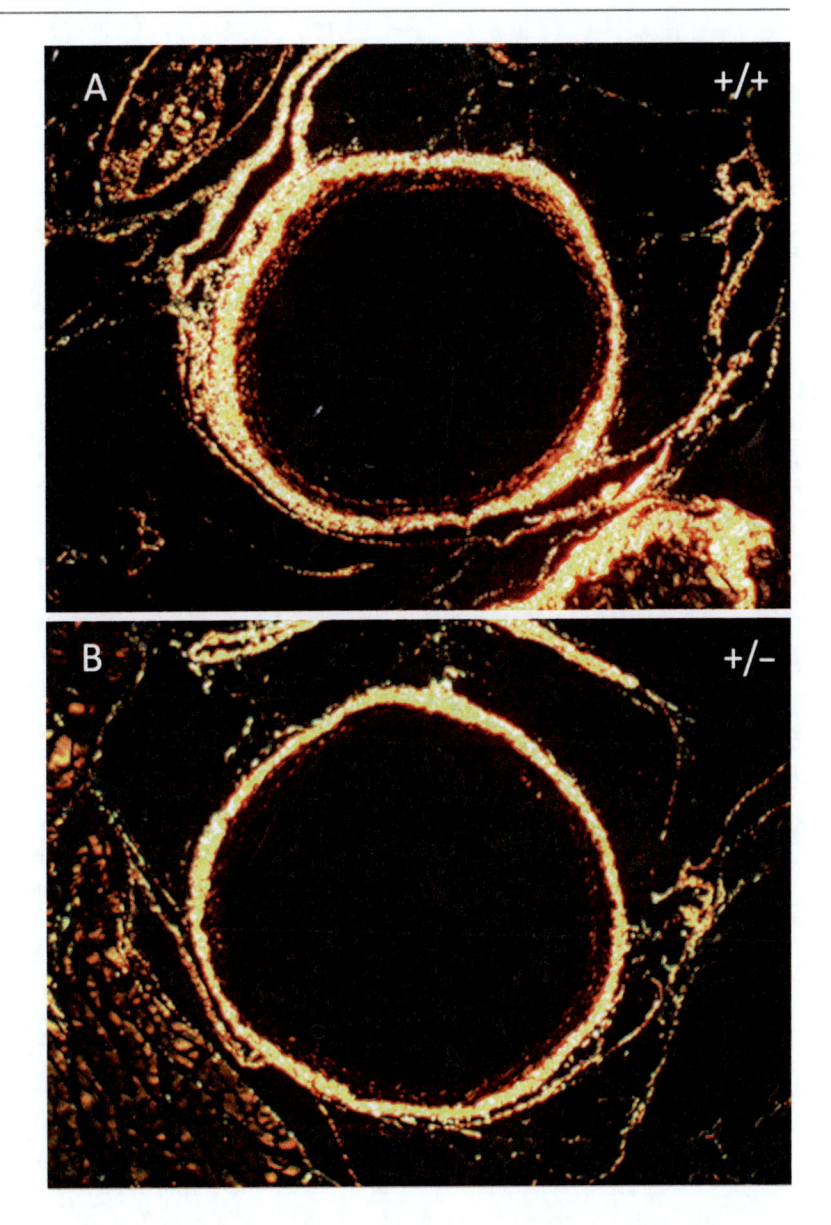

detected by Western blotting only in the abdominal aorta of heterozygotes [18]. In the descending thoracic aorta, no difference was detectable [18]. Furthermore, the data are consistent with the paradigm of a vascular wall that is structurally weakened while still apparently normal at the gross and microscopic levels of resolution.

Functional testing of the strength of the aortic wall supports this conclusion. The maximum pressure (rupture pressure) in the abdominal aorta was similar in wild-type and heterozygote mice at 14 months but significantly lower in heterozygotes at 21 months (Fig. 5). No change was detected in the distensibility of aorta of 10-month-old heterozygous animals, while higher compliance was detected in small arteries from heterozygous mice compared with the wild type [18].

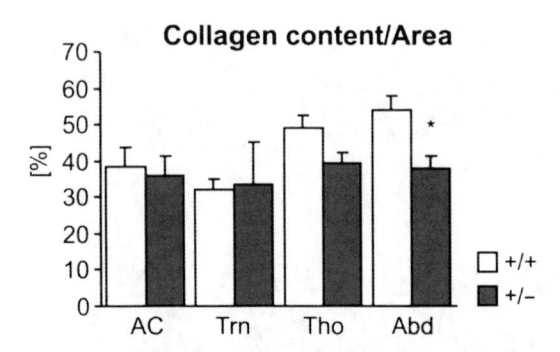

Fig. 4 Collagen accumulation in the aorta [18]. By picro-sirius red staining, wild-type (WT) mice had significantly higher collagen per unit area than heterozygotes (HT) in the abdominal aorta. AC, ascending aorta; Trn, transverse aorta; Tho, thoracic aorta; Abd, abdominal aorta (*P<0.05 vs. WT)

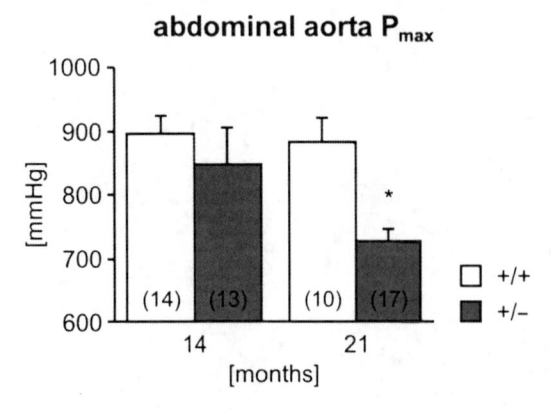

Fig. 5 Vessel function of the abdominal aorta [18]. The maximum pressure in the abdominal aorta was measured in 14- and 21-month-old wild-type (+/+) and heterozygote (+/−) mice. Number of experiments is shown in parentheses. *P<0.05 versus wild-type

Furthermore, a reduced strength and increased compliance was found in colons of heterozygous mice [18], and increased compliance was found in bladder tissue of heterozygotes as well [28]. Therefore, these findings, taken together, indicate that haploinsufficiency for *Col3a1* in mice recapitulates features of vEDS in humans and might be used as an experimental model. However, this mouse model has a number of important limitations, including the lack of spontaneous clinical signs or endpoints, which necessitate the development of a new vEDS mouse model with a knock-in of a mutation. A glycine substitution mutation would be favored since it is the most common one. Unfortunately, nobody reported a creation of this model yet.

Potential Treatments for vEDS

Clinical studies have previously addressed phenotypic characteristics and genetic features of vEDS but no randomized treatment trial has been done until the celiprolol trial [15]. Patients were often treated empirically with drugs such as β-blockers [29] or renin-angiotensin-aldosterone blockers [30] that have protective effects in Marfan's syndrome. However, the pathophysiology of Marfan's syndrome is different from that of vEDS. Marfan's syndrome is defined by a deficiency in fibrillin-1 and abnormal elastin synthesis that leads to changes in the elastic properties of the aortic wall. The ascending aorta becomes especially stiffer, which results in a higher pulse wave velocity. In contrast, vEDS is characterized by a deficiency of synthesis or structure of type III collagen. A dominant negative mechanism of pathogenesis has been inferred [31]. In this paradigm, 50% of procollagen chains are structurally abnormal, meaning that only 1 in 8 mature collagen homotrimers is structurally sound [2]. The abnormal collagen or the decreased concentration of collagen III in cases of haploinsufficiency affects the entire arterial tree, together with skin and intestine. Ultrastructural analysis of tissue from *Col3a1* knockout mice revealed that type III collagen is essential for normal collagen I fibrillogenesis in the cardiovascular system and other organs [16]. Abnormalities in the vEDS patients' vessel wall consist of decreased intima-media thickness associated with increased mechanical stress of fragile tissues [32]. These features are not present in patients with Marfan's syndrome in which dilatation of stiffened aorta predominates [33, 34].

Beta-Blocker Therapy

The rationale for treatment by β_1-AR blocker was mainly mechanical – to reduce the arterial wall stress by controlling the rate of increase of pressure over time in the pulse wave (dP/dt). The celiprolol, however, used in the successful clinical trial was not a typical β_1-AR blocker. It combines β_1-AR inhibition with some properties of β_2-AR stimulation and was proven beneficial for vEDS patients without affecting hemodynamic variables [15]. The heart rate or systolic and diastolic pressure was not decreased and pulse pressure was even elevated in patients on celiprolol. This prompts reconsideration of alternative mechanisms of celiprolol's protective effect in vEDS [35]. Celiprolol may act on molecular pathways within the arterial wall that are independent of hemodynamic stress. The key might be the transforming growth factor β (TGFβ) signaling pathway which could be activated by β_2-AR stimulation [36, 37]. It was shown that in Marfan's syndrome, one key factor in the pathogenesis of arterial lesions is an increased bioavailability of TGFβ in response to the defect in its chelation by abnormal fibrillin. The role of TGFβ in vEDS is not clear. Elevated TGFβ levels were detected in some vEDS patients as well [38], but the pathogenic relations were not shown. Raised TGFβ concentrations might be the consequence of repeated skin or arterial healing. It was proposed that the beneficial effect of losartan therapy in Marfan patients was based on TGFβ antagonism [39]. However, the causal relation between activation of TGFβ and arterial lesions might be more complex [15]. TGFβ is also an important growth factor in wound healing. TGFβ1 and 2 are necessary for collagen synthesis and TGFβ3 for organization of scar tissue [40]. Local delivery of TGFβ1 was associated with stabilization of experimental aortic aneurysms in rats [41]. On the other hand, TGFβ inhibition is not always accompanied by vascular protection: mice with angiotensin II infusion developed fatal aortic aneurysms despite exposure to neutralizing TGFβ antibodies [42]. Taken together, these studies highlight the complexity and the context-dependent roles of TGFβ in vascular disease [43].

The increased pulse pressure among the patients with celiprolol suggesting a possible increase in arterial stiffness might be a sign of induced TGFβ signaling, although the effect on

TGFβ signaling was not further analyzed [15]. There are strong associations between β-adrenergic receptors and TGFβ pathways. TGFβ2 is activated by β_2-adrenergic receptor stimulation [36, 37]. Chronic β_2 stimulation might enhance collagen synthesis through increased expression of TGFβ. This would be an opposite effect of the proposed losartan mechanism in Marfan's syndrome, based on TGFβ antagonism. Indeed, β_2 stimulation by clenbuterol in rats boosted mRNA expression of TGFβ1, 2, and 3 [36]. TGFβ could enhance the production of type I and III collagen and lead to fibrosis [44, 45]. Thus in response to celiprolol, an up-regulation of collagen synthesis might have strengthened the arterial wall, reducing its susceptibility to rupture [15, 35]. The hypothesis of a beneficial effect of β_2 stimulation through TGFβ stimulation and consequently collagen accumulation should be analyzed in the vEDS mouse model, the already existing mouse model of haploinsufficiency of *Col3a1*, or better in knock-in mouse model with a glycine mutation that is yet to be developed.

With respect to using β-AR blockers for patients with vEDS, celiprolol, while successful in the recent clinical trial, is not a universally available drug. For instance, it is not approved for use in the USA at this time. Moreover, the idea of salutary effects of β_2-AR agonist in vEDS is only a speculation, until it is proven that effectiveness of celiprolol exceeds that of other, more common, β_1-AR blockers.

MMP Inhibition

Collagen fibrils are part of the extracellular matrix. The homeostasis of extracellular matrix is equilibrated by synthesis and degradation of their components. Therefore, down-regulation of collagen-degrading enzymes would be another strategy to strengthen the arterial wall. Collagen is degraded by matrix metalloproteases (MMPs) [46].

It has been reported that in the third stage of aneurysm development, rapid expansion and increased risk of rupture are associated with accelerated degradation of collagen [47].

Doxycycline, a tetracycline antibiotic and broad spectrum MMP inhibitor, has been successfully tested in pilot clinical trials for the treatment of abdominal aortic aneurysms [48–51]. Doxycycline, given in a subantimicrobial dose, is also the only MMP inhibitor approved by the FDA. It is currently used for the treatment of periodontal disease [52, 53] and rosacea [54]. We hypothesized that MMP inhibition in the mouse experimental model of vEDS would shift the balance between collagen degradation and synthesis in the vascular wall and protect against vascular damage.

We tested this hypothesis in the $Col3a1^{tm1Jae}$ haploinsufficient mouse model [55]. Following a 3-month treatment with doxycycline, 9-month-old heterozygote mice were subjected to a surgical stressing of the aorta. While untreated heterozygote showed increased MMP-9 activity in the carotid artery and decreased collagen content in the aorta, there was normalization to wild-type levels in doxycycline-treated animals. A threefold increase in stress-induced aortic lesions found in untreated heterozygotes was fully prevented in the doxycycline dose group [55]. Since the efficacy of proposed doxycycline therapy was tested only in the haploinsufficient mouse model, it can be so far proposed as a potential treatment for only a small subset of vEDS patients with haploinsufficiency for COL3A1. Whether this treatment can be effective in the rest of vEDS patients shall be tested in the appropriate genetic mouse model yet to be developed. However, a convincing argument for doxycycline treatment was its effectiveness in the Marfan mouse model with a mutation in fibrillin-1 ($Fbn1^{C1039/+}$) [56–58]. Doxycycline delayed the aneurysm rupture [56], and was effective in secondary prevention of thoracic aortic aneurysm in combination with losartan [58].

Conclusions and Potential Treatment

Gene therapy for permanent correction of genetic mutation in COL3A1 would be an ultimate goal, but this idea is reserved for the distant future.

A defective gene cannot be replaced in dominant inherited disease such as vEDS. However, the recently developed RNA interference (RNAi) technology, which enables gene posttranscriptional expression silencing, may be applicable. Research into the treatment approach for the dominantly inherited diseases, for which cures have not yet been developed, is advancing [59–61].

Majority of the patients are heterozygous for a mutation in one copy of the COL3A1 gene. Patients that are haploinsufficient for COL3A1 have a reduced amount of non-mutated COL3A1, and seem to exhibit less severe symptoms and less subsequent complications [9, 17, 62]. Therefore, one approach to a targeted treatment of vEDS is the elimination of the mutated form of the COL3A1 gene to transform the more severe phenotype to the less severe haploinsufficient type. This would be possible by selective silencing the mutated form of the COL3A1 gene without affecting the wild-type allele of COL3A1, and thus by restoring the structural integrity of affected extracellular matrix. Allele-specific silencing of several mutant targets has been studied for diseases including osteogenesis imperfecta [63], sickle cell anemia [64], primary retinal degeneration [65], spinocerebellar ataxia [66], pachyonychia congenita [67], Huntington's disease [68], Alzheimer's disease [69], SCCMS [70], and sialuria [71].

We tested the feasibility of allele-specific knockdown of mutated COL3A1 in fibroblasts from a vEDS patient heterozygous for COL3A1 allele encoding a glycine substitution [72]. We identified one siRNA with a centered position of the mutation silencing more than 90% of the mutant allele without affecting the wild-type allele. Transmission and immunogold electron microscopy of extracellular matrices from fibroblasts of the vEDS patient revealed structurally abnormal fibrils. After siRNA treatment collagen fibers were not distinguishable from fibroblasts of normal donors [72]. Thus, a personalized siRNA therapy to replace mutated collagen condition with the condition when collagen is normal but reduced opens the possibility for consequent pharmacological stimulation of total collagen production and inhibition of its degradation.

Acknowledgments The work was mostly supported by the Intramural Research Program of the National Institutes of Health, National Institute on Aging.

References

1. Mao JR, Bristow J. The Ehlers-Danlos syndrome: on beyond collagens. J Clin Invest. 2001;107:1063–9.
2. Pyeritz RE. Ehlers-Danlos syndrome. N Engl J Med. 2000;342:730–2.
3. Beighton P, De Paepe A, Steinmann B, et al. Ehlers-Danlos syndromes: revised nosology, Villefranche, 1997. Ehlers-Danlos National Foundation (USA) and Ehlers-Danlos Support Group (UK). Am J Med Genet. 1998;77:31–7.
4. Germain DP. Clinical and genetic features of vascular Ehlers-Danlos syndrome. Ann Vasc Surg. 2002;16:391–7.
5. Germain DP. Ehlers-Danlos syndrome type IV. Orphanet J Rare Dis. 2007;2:32.
6. Pepin M, Schwarze U, Superti-Furga A, et al. Clinical and genetic features of Ehlers-Danlos syndrome type IV, the vascular type. N Engl J Med. 2000;342:673–80.
7. Pope FM, Martin GR, Lichtenstein JR, et al. Patients with Ehlers-Danlos syndrome type IV lack type III collagen. Proc Natl Acad Sci USA. 1975;72:1314–6.
8. The Human Gene Mutation Database at the Institute of Medical Genetics in Cardiff. http://www.ggmd.cf.ac.uk/ac/. Accessed Mar 9, 2010.
9. Meienberg J, Rohrbach M, Neuenschwander S, et al. Hemizygous deletion of COL3A1, COL5A2, and MSTN causes a complex phenotype with aortic dissection: a lesson for and from true haploinsufficiency. Eur J Hum Genet. 2010;18:1315–21. Epub 2010 Jul 21.
10. McCullagh KA, Balian G. Collagen characterisation and cell transformation in human atherosclerosis. Nature. 1975;258:73–5.
11. Hanson AN, Bentley JP. Quantitation of type I to type III collagen ratios in small samples of human tendon, blood vessels, and atherosclerotic plaque. Anal Biochem. 1983;130:32–40.
12. Barnes MJ. Collagens in atherosclerosis. Coll Relat Res. 1985;5:65–97.
13. Bornstein P, Sage H. Structurally distinct collagen types. Annu Rev Biochem. 1980;49:957–1003.
14. Watanabe A, Kosho T, Wada T, et al. Genetic aspects of the vascular type of Ehlers-Danlos syndrome (vEDS, EDSIV) in Japan. Circ J. 2007;71:261–5.
15. Ong KT, Perdu J, De Backer J, et al. Effect of celiprolol on prevention of cardiovascular events in vascular Ehlers-Danlos syndrome: a prospective randomised, open, blinded-endpoints trial. Lancet. 2010;376:1476–84. Epub Sep 10 2010; PMID:20825986.
16. Liu X, Wu H, Byrne M, et al. Type III collagen is crucial for collagen I fibrillogenesis and for normal cardiovascular development. Proc Natl Acad Sci USA. 1997;94:1852–6.
17. Plancke A, Holder-Espinasse M, Rigau V, et al. Homozygosity for a null allele of COL3A1 results in recessive Ehlers-Danlos syndrome. Eur J Hum Genet. 2009;17:1411–6.
18. Cooper TK, Zhong Q, Krawczyk M, et al. The haploinsufficient – Col3a1 mouse is a model for vascular Ehlers-Danlos syndrome. Vet Pathol. 2010;47:1028–39. SAGE Publications, Inc., All rights reserved. © Epub 2010 Jun 29; PMID:20587693.
19. Ramot Y, Manno RA, Okazaki Y, et al. Spontaneous aortitis in the Balb/c mouse. Toxicol Pathol. 2009;37:667–71.
20. Arteaga-Solis E, Gayraud B, Ramirez F. Elastic and collagenous networks in vascular diseases. Cell Struct Funct. 2000;25:69–72.
21. Barabas AP. Ehlers-Danlos syndrome type IV. N Engl J Med. 2000;343:366. author reply 368.
22. Stella A, Gessaroli M, Cifiello BI, et al. Sack-Barabas Syndrome (Ehlers-Danlos IV Type) (Clinic and Histopathologic Ultrastructural Correlations). Vasc Endovasc Surg. 1986;20:67–73.
23. Jain D, Dietz HC, Oswald GL, et al. Causes and histopathology of ascending aortic disease in children and young adults. Cardiovasc Pathol. 2009;20:15–25.
24. Maleszewski JJ, Miller DV, Lu J, et al. Histopathologic findings in ascending aortas from individuals with Loeys-Dietz syndrome (LDS). Am J Surg Pathol. 2009;33:194–201.
25. Schlatmann TJ, Becker AE. Pathogenesis of dissecting aneurysm of aorta. Comparative histopathologic study of significance of medial changes. Am J Cardiol. 1977;39:21–6.
26. Schlatmann TJ, Becker AE. Histologic changes in the normal aging aorta: implications for dissecting aortic aneurysm. Am J Cardiol. 1977;39:13–20.
27. Harkness ML, Harkness RD, McDonald DA. The collagen and elastin content of the arterial wall in the dog. Proc R Soc Lond B Biol Sci. 1957;146:541–51.
28. Stevenson K, Kucich U, Whitbeck C, et al. Functional changes in bladder tissue from type III collagen-deficient mice. Mol Cell Biochem. 2006;283:107–14.
29. Shores J, Berger KR, Murphy EA, et al. Progression of aortic dilatation and the benefit of long-term beta-adrenergic blockade in Marfan's syndrome. N Engl J Med. 1994;330:1335–41.
30. Ahimastos AA, Aggarwal A, D'Orsa KM, et al. Effect of perindopril on large artery stiffness and aortic root diameter in patients with Marfan syndrome: a randomized controlled trial. JAMA. 2007;298:1539–47.
31. Towbin JA, Casey B, Belmont J. The molecular basis of vascular disorders. Am J Hum Genet. 1999;64:678–84.
32. Boutouyrie P, Germain DP, Fiessinger JN, et al. Increased carotid wall stress in vascular Ehlers-Danlos syndrome. Circulation. 2004;109:1530–5.
33. Hirata K, Triposkiadis F, Sparks E, et al. The Marfan syndrome: abnormal aortic elastic properties. J Am Coll Cardiol. 1991;18:57–63.
34. Jondeau G, Boutouyrie P, Lacolley P, et al. Central pulse pressure is a major determinant of ascending

aorta dilation in Marfan syndrome. Circulation. 1999;99:2677–81.

35. Brooke BS. Celiprolol therapy for vascular Ehlers-Danlos syndrome. Lancet. 2010;376:1443–4. Epub Sep 10 2010; PMID:20825985.

36. Akutsu S, Shimada A, Yamane A. Transforming growth factor betas are upregulated in the rat masseter muscle hypertrophied by clenbuterol, a beta2 adrenergic agonist. Br J Pharmacol. 2006;147:412–21.

37. Rosenkranz S, Flesch M, Amann K, et al. Alterations of beta-adrenergic signaling and cardiac hypertrophy in transgenic mice overexpressing TGF-beta(1). Am J Physiol Heart Circ Physiol. 2002;283:H1253–62.

38. Schoenhoff FS, Griswold BF, Matt P, et al. Abstract 5095: The role of circulating transforming growth factor-{beta} in vascular Ehlers-Danlos syndrome: implications for drug therapy. Circulation. 2009; 120:S1048-b-.

39. Matt P, Habashi J, Carrel T, et al. Recent advances in understanding Marfan syndrome: should we now treat surgical patients with losartan? J Thorac Cardiovasc Surg. 2008;135:389–94.

40. Deten A, Hölzl A, Leicht M, et al. Changes in extracellular matrix and in transforming growth factor beta isoforms isoforms after coronary artery ligation in rats. J Mol Cell Cardiol. 2001;33:1191–207.

41. Dai J, Losy F, Guinault AM, et al. Overexpression of transforming growth factor-beta1 stabilizes already-formed aortic aneurysms: a first approach to induction of functional healing by endovascular gene therapy. Circulation. 2005;112:1008–15.

42. Wang Y, Ait-Oufella H, Herbin O, et al. TGF-beta activity protects against inflammatory aortic aneurysm progression and complications in angiotensin II-infused mice. J Clin Invest. 2010;120:422–32.

43. Dietz HC. TGF-beta in the pathogenesis and prevention of disease: a matter of aneurysmic proportions. J Clin Invest. 2010;120:403–7.

44. Eghbali M, Tomek R, Sukhatme VP, et al. Differential effects of transforming growth factor-beta 1 and phorbol myristate acetate on cardiac fibroblasts. Regulation of fibrillar collagen mRNAs and expression of early transcription factors. Circ Res. 1991;69:483–90.

45. Varga J, Rosenbloom J, Jimenez SA. Transforming growth factor beta (TGF beta) causes a persistent increase in steady-state amounts of type I and type III collagen and fibronectin mRNAs in normal human dermal fibroblasts. Biochem J. 1987;247:597–604.

46. Page-McCaw A, Ewald AJ, Werb Z. Matrix metalloproteinases and the regulation of tissue remodelling. Nat Rev Mol Cell Biol. 2007;8:221–33.

47. Thompson RW, Baxter BT. MMP inhibition in abdominal aortic aneurysms. Rationale for a prospective randomized clinical trial. Ann NY Acad Sci. 1999;878: 159–78.

48. Curci JA, Mao D, Bohner DG, et al. Preoperative treatment with doxycycline reduces aortic wall expression and activation of matrix metalloproteinases in patients with abdominal aortic aneurysms. J Vasc Surg. 2000;31:325–42.

49. Mosorin M, Juvonen J, Biancari F, et al. Use of doxycycline to decrease the growth rate of abdominal aortic aneurysms: a randomized, double-blind, placebo-controlled pilot study. J Vasc Surg. 2001;34: 606–10.

50. Baxter BT, Pearce WH, Waltke EA, et al. Prolonged administration of doxycycline in patients with small asymptomatic abdominal aortic aneurysms: report of a prospective (Phase II) multicenter study. J Vasc Surg. 2002;36:1–12.

51. Lindeman JH, Abdul-Hussien H, van Bockel JH, et al. Clinical trial of doxycycline for matrix metalloproteinase-9 inhibition in patients with an abdominal aneurysm: doxycycline selectively depletes aortic wall neutrophils and cytotoxic T cells. Circulation. 2009;119:2209–16.

52. Ciancio S, Ashley R. Safety and efficacy of sub-antimicrobial-dose doxycycline therapy in patients with adult periodontitis. Adv Dent Res. 1998;12:27–31.

53. Wennstrom JL, Newman HN, MacNeill SR, et al. Utilisation of locally delivered doxycycline in nonsurgical treatment of chronic periodontitis. A comparative multi-centre trial of 2 treatment approaches. J Clin Periodontol. 2001;28:753–61.

54. Del Rosso JQ, Webster GF, Jackson M, et al. Two randomized phase III clinical trials evaluating anti-inflammatory dose doxycycline (40-mg doxycycline, USP capsules) administered once daily for treatment of rosacea. J Am Acad Dermatol. 2007;56: 791–802.

55. Briest W, Cooper TK, Schubert R, et al. Doxycycline treatment attenuates the development of aortic lesions in the mouse experimental model of vascular type of the Ehlers-Danlos syndrome. Acta Physiol. 2009;195:147–8. Abstract.

56. Xiong W, Knispel RA, Dietz HC, et al. Doxycycline delays aneurysm rupture in a mouse model of Marfan syndrome. J Vasc Surg. 2008;47:166–72. discussion 172.

57. Chung AW, Yang HH, Radomski MW, et al. Long-term doxycycline is more effective than atenolol to prevent thoracic aortic aneurysm in marfan syndrome through the inhibition of matrix metalloproteinase-2 and −9. Circ Res. 2008;102:e73–85.

58. Yang HH, Kim JM, Chum E, et al. Effectiveness of combination of losartan potassium and doxycycline versus single-drug treatments in the secondary prevention of thoracic aortic aneurysm in Marfan syndrome. J Thorac Cardiovasc Surg. 2010;140(2): 305–12. e2.

59. Grimm D, Kay MA. Therapeutic application of RNAi: is mRNA targeting finally ready for prime time? J Clin Invest. 2007;117:3633–41.

60. Watanabe A, Shimada T. Vascular type of Ehlers-Danlos syndrome. J Nippon Med Sch. 2008;75: 254–61.

61. Dietz HC. New therapeutic approaches to mendelian disorders. N Engl J Med. 2010;363:852–63.

62. Khalique Z, Lyons OT, Clough RE, et al. Successful Endovascular Repair of Acute Type B Aortic Dissection in Undiagnosed Ehlers-Danlos

Syndrome Type IV. Eur J Vasc Endovasc Surg. 2009; 38: 608–9.

63. Millington-Ward S, McMahon HP, Allen D, et al. RNAi of COL1A1 in mesenchymal progenitor cells. Eur J Hum Genet. 2004;12:864–6.

64. Dykxhoorn DM, Schlehuber LD, London IM, et al. Determinants of specific RNA interference-mediated silencing of human beta-globin alleles differing by a single nucleotide polymorphism. Proc Natl Acad Sci USA. 2006;103:5953–8.

65. Palfi A, Ader M, Kiang AS, et al. RNAi-based suppression and replacement of rds-peripherin in retinal organotypic culture. Hum Mutat. 2006;27: 260–8.

66. Xia H, Mao Q, Eliason SL, et al. RNAi suppresses polyglutamine-induced neurodegeneration in a model of spinocerebellar ataxia. Nat Med. 2004;10:816–20.

67. Hickerson RP, Smith FJ, Reeves RE, et al. Single-nucleotide-specific siRNA targeting in a dominant-negative skin model. J Invest Dermatol. 2008;128: 594–605.

68. Pfister EL, Kennington L, Straubhaar J, et al. Five siRNAs targeting three SNPs may provide therapy for three-quarters of Huntington's disease patients. Curr Biol. 2009;19:774–8.

69. Miller VM, Gouvion CM, Davidson BL, et al. Targeting Alzheimer's disease genes with RNA interference: an efficient strategy for silencing mutant alleles. Nucleic Acids Res. 2004;32:661–8.

70. Abdelgany A, Wood M, Beeson D. Allele-specific silencing of a pathogenic mutant acetylcholine receptor subunit by RNA interference. Hum Mol Genet. 2003;12:2637–44.

71. Klootwijk RD, Savelkoul PJ, Ciccone C, et al. Allele-specific silencing of the dominant disease allele in sialuria by RNA interference. FASEB J. 2008;22:3846–52.

72. Briest W, Müller GA, Hansen U, et al. Selective supression of the mutated form of collagen 3A1 by siRNA in fibroblasts from a patient with the vascular form of the Ehlers-Danlos syndrome. Acta Physiol. 2010;198:129. abstract.

Multi-scale, Multi-physics Heart Simulator as a Tool to Link Bench and Bedside

S. Sugiura, T. Washio, J. Okada,
H. Watanabe, and T. Hisada

Abstract

Advances in molecular and cell biology have enabled us to identify the genes responsible for the origin of various heart diseases but, in most cases, the detailed mechanisms by which such genetic defects lead to the signs and symptoms observed at the bedside remain to be elucidated. In an attempt to investigate such problems, we have developed a multi-scale, multi-physics heart simulator, in which normal and abnormal functioning of the heart is reproduced based on the molecular mechanisms of the cardiac excitation-contraction (E-C) coupling process. This simulator, based on the finite element method, consists of solid elements representing the myocardium and fluid elements representing the blood in the heart chamber. Each solid element is implemented with a molecular model of E-C coupling and thus behaves as a virtual cardiomyocyte. Because the governing equations for the solid and fluid parts are solved by the strong coupling method, we can obtain detailed information on the blood flow as well as the electrical and mechanical states of every myocyte during the cardiac cycle. Accordingly, this simulator can be used as a tool to see whether any specific molecular abnormality would lead to the development of macroscopic findings, thus making it applicable to various fields of cardiovascular research.

Keywords

Body surface voltage map • Cardiac resynchronization therapy (CRT) • Cross-bridge kinetics • Excitation-contraction coupling • Heart 3D model • Implantable cardioverter defibrillator (ICD) • Magnetic resonance imaging (MRI) • Mathematical modeling • Pacemaker • Ultrasonic cardiogram (UCG) • Ventricular fibrillation • Ventriculoplasty • Voxel model • Windkessel

S. Sugiura (✉)
Graduate School of Frontier Sciences,
T he University of Tokyo, Tokyo,
Chiba, Japan
e-mail: sugiura@k.u-tokyo.ac.jp

B. Ostadal et al. (eds.), *Genes and Cardiovascular Function*,
DOI 10.1007/978-1-4419-7207-1_24, © Springer Science+Business Media, LLC 2011

Introduction

As in other areas of science, current cardiovascular research is facing an explosion of knowledge evidenced by the huge number of scientific journals published daily. Furthermore, since even in this limited area the research covers various subjects ranging from molecular biology to macroscopic organ physiology, it is virtually impossible for an individual doctor or researcher to understand all the subjects and memorize them in an organized manner. Quite naturally, the use of digital archives or a database has been considered, but for such databases to be useful they need to meet the specific requirements in cardiology.

Cardiac function is based on electromechanical phenomena driven by the biochemical reactions in each cell, and thus most of the clinical tests evaluate these parameters. On the other hand, knowledge at the molecular level is indispensable for the development of causal treatment. In this regard, the database required in cardiology must collect and integrate knowledge on multi-physics phenomena functioning cooperatively over multi-scale levels to facilitate our understanding of the functioning of the heart and human body under both normal and diseased conditions. This idea is now widely shared in scientific society and computer simulation is considered to be a powerful tool for its realization [1, 2].

We have developed a multi-scale, multi-physics heart simulator by applying cutting-edge techniques in computational sciences. In this simulator the propagation of excitation and contraction and relaxation of the tissue, and the resulting pressure development and blood flow, are reproduced, based on the molecular mechanisms of the cardiac excitation-contraction coupling process implemented in each element of the model representing a myocyte. This dynamic model is a functional database of the heart, retaining the 3D structure from which we can retrieve functional information of the heart from any aspect and at any level of interest. The application of the model is not limited to knowledge management or education; it can also be used as a tool for the development of novel diagnostic or therapeutic devices and strategies.

Outline of Multi-scale, Multi-physics Heart Simulator

As stated above, in the post-genome era, the integration of molecular and cellular findings to understand the functioning of organs or individuals is recognized as an important field of science [1, 2]. However, even with the advancement in computational science, this is not an easy task to accomplish because, in addition to the integration of events across the scale, description of each event involves integration of various disciplines, such as electricity, physical chemistry, solid mechanics, and fluid dynamics (in other words, a multi-physics simulation). Indeed, the simulation studies reported so far deal only with the electrophysiology [3–7] or the mechanics at either the cross-bridge kinetics [8–10] or macroscopic model [11–14]. Our heart simulator, called UT-Heart, is the only model that includes all the important physics and integrates them over the scale to reproduce clinically useful macroscopic behavior of the heart.

Framework of the Model

Cardiomyocyte Model

Since the development of the Purkinje cell model by Noble [15], studies on mathematical modeling of cardiac excitation have been reported for myocytes from various species. In this study, we adopted the human ventricular myocyte model by Ten Tusscher et al. [16], the atrial myocyte model by Courtemanche et al. [17], and the Purkinje cell model by DiFrancesco et al. [18]. All these models formulate the charge and discharge of the cell membrane as a capacitor using ion currents through channels, pumps, and transporters, while the model by Ten Tusscher includes 12 ion currents [16]. Such cell models are coupled to form the myocardial tissue in which excitation propagates through the assumed intercalated discs. We used both bi-domain and mono-domain formulations depending on the purpose of study.

In each myocyte, excitation of the cell membrane (depolarization) activates the calcium (Ca)

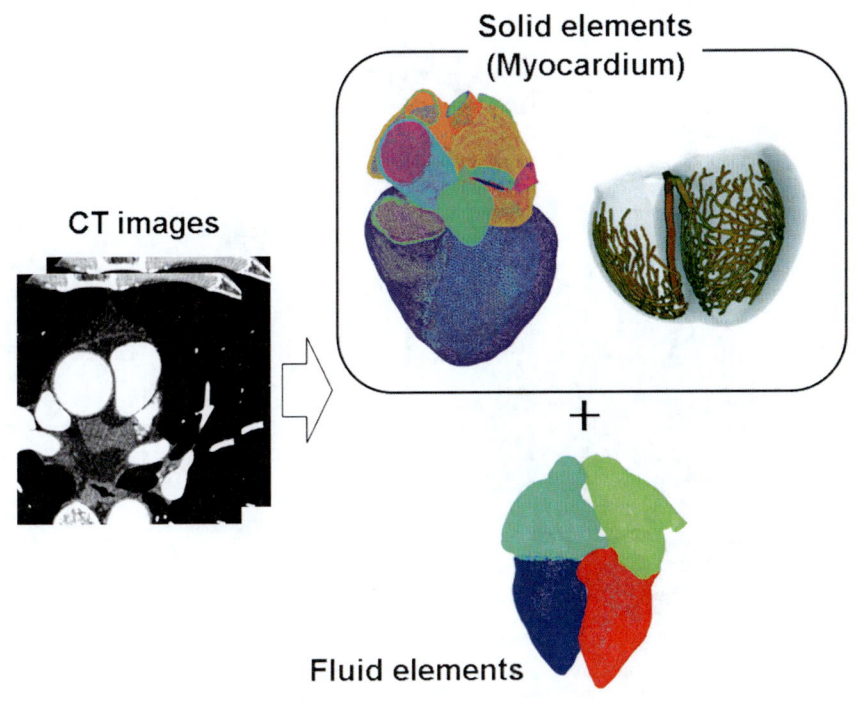

Fig. 1 Heart model. Morphology of the heart model is based on the multi-detector CT data and consists of solid and fluid parts

current through an L-type Ca-channel which, in turn, triggers the Ca release from the sarcoplasmic reticulum to produce the transient rise in cytosolic Ca concentration. Cytosolic Ca binds to troponin C on a thin filament to initiate the force generation by actomyosin interaction. This mechanism of the cardiac excitation-contraction (E-C) coupling process has also been modeled by researchers and we modified the one by Rice et al. [10] to include the co-operativity in force development. By coupling these two models for excitation and E-C coupling through the Ca signal, we were able to create the virtual myocyte model.

Heart Model

Our heart simulator is based on the finite element method and its morphology on the human multidetector CT data. The model consists of a structural part representing the myocardium (664,334 elements) and a fluid part representing the blood

in the heart chamber (435,227 elements), with the mechanics of both solved simultaneously using the strong coupling methods developed by Zhang and Hisada [19]. In the myocardial part we have reproduced the fiber and sheet structures and the conduction system has also been created as a distinct structure (Fig. 1). In addition, we have developed a voxel model of the heart with a finer mesh (20 million elements) for the electrophysiological analysis (the two models are solved simultaneously). Currently our model includes both atria and ventricles with a short segment of aortic arch, while the windkessel model of circulation with appropriate parameter values is connected to each inlet and outlet to allow physiological simulation (Fig. 2). The small dots on the heart surface correspond to the finite elements, in each of which a molecular model of the excitation-contraction coupling process is implemented. Such virtual myocytes are connected mechanically and electrically exactly as in real tissue. All the program codes were written in our laboratory and the computations were

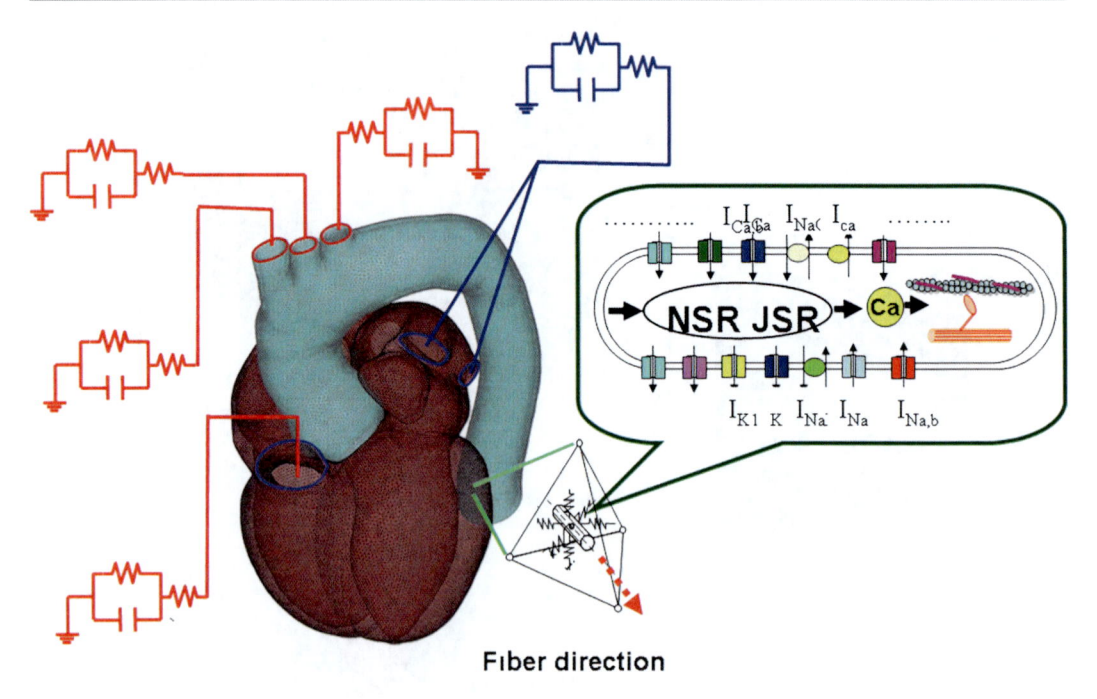

Fiber direction

Fig. 2 Multi-scale, multi-physics heart simulator based on the finite element model with a molecular model of EC coupling implemented in each element. An appropriate model of circulation is coupled to each boundary

performed using an IBM JS22 (Power6 Blade Server System) with 32 nodes/336 cores in our laboratory.

Simulation Results

Simulation of a normal heartbeat is shown as the time-lapsed images in Fig. 3. Upon stimulation applied to the sinoatrial node (pacemaker site), the excitation of the virtual myocyte propagates to the adjacent ones to spread through the atria and ventricles via the conduction system to induce the synchronous contraction of the heart (Fig. 3b). Contraction of the heart generates pressure in the atrial and ventricular cavities to drive the ejection and filling of blood (Fig. 3c). The color at the open ends of the heart models indicates the flow velocity. For simulation videos please visit our website at http://www.sml.k.u-tokyo.ac.jp/. During this process, subcellular variables, such as membrane potential, ion currents, intracellular Ca concentration, cross-bridge

states, and the developed force, are calculated in each element (Fig. 3a) at time intervals of 500 μsec. Simultaneously, regional stress/strain in the myocardial tissue and the pressure and flow distributions in the fluid (blood) part are also calculated. In other words, multi-physics phenomena including mechanics, electrical events, and fluid dynamics are solved at multi-scale levels to realize a dynamic 3D database of cardiac function.

In Silico Diagnosis

To further examine and validate our simulation results, we compared them with clinical data. As stated repeatedly, because we calculate various parameters involved in the cardiac function, we can diagnose our *in silico* heart by extracting and presenting the relevant data in the form of diagnostic modalities, such as an electrocardiogram (ECG) or ultrasonic cardiogram (UCG). First, we checked the ECG of our *in silico* heart, and for this purpose,

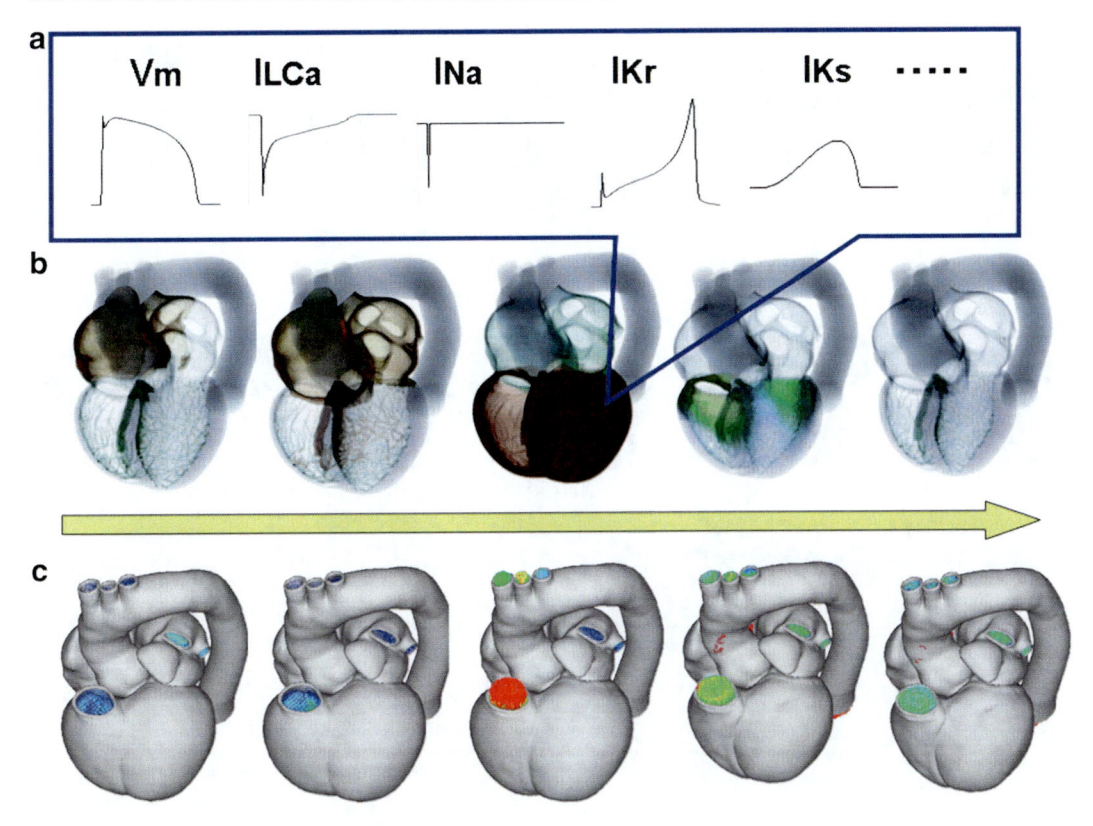

Fig. 3 Simulation of a normal heart beat: (**a**) representative ion currents in myocyte model, (**b**) propagation of excitation, (**c**) contraction and blood flow. Sequence is indicated by the arrow

we also created a torso model with the major organs in the thorax and the specific conductivity of each. By placing our heart in this torso model and calculating the electrical field using bi-domain formulation, we can obtain the body surface voltage map during the cardiac cycle (Figs. 4a, b). As the excitation of myocardial tissue propagates from the atria to ventricles (Fig. 4a), the high voltage area on the chest wall shifts to the rear side. We can find similar observations for human subjects in the literature [20]. Furthermore, if we calculate the difference between two appropriate points on the chest, we can obtain the surface ECG as shown in Fig. 4c. In this case we show only the standard limb lead II data; data in other leads including the pre-cordial leads are easily obtained in a similar way. We can apply this technique to the study of arrhythmias and have confirmed the characteristic ECGs for ventricular fibrillation, ventricular tachycardia, and bundle branch block (data not shown).

Motion of the *in silico* heart wall and/or valves in the appropriate 2D plane fixed in space corresponds to the B-mode echocardiogram and matches the clinical observations. In particular, regional strains (radial, circumferential, longitudinal) were compared with experimental data obtained by either maker technique or diffusion tensor magnetic resonance imaging (MRI) to confirm the validity of our model. In addition, because our simulator calculates the flow in 3D space at every time step (Fig. 5a), temporal changes in flow velocity at any point in the heart chambers are readily available in the form of a Doppler echocardiogram. An example of this is shown in Fig. 5b. Mitral flow (red) and aortic flow (green) reproduce the characteristic patterns recorded in human subjects.

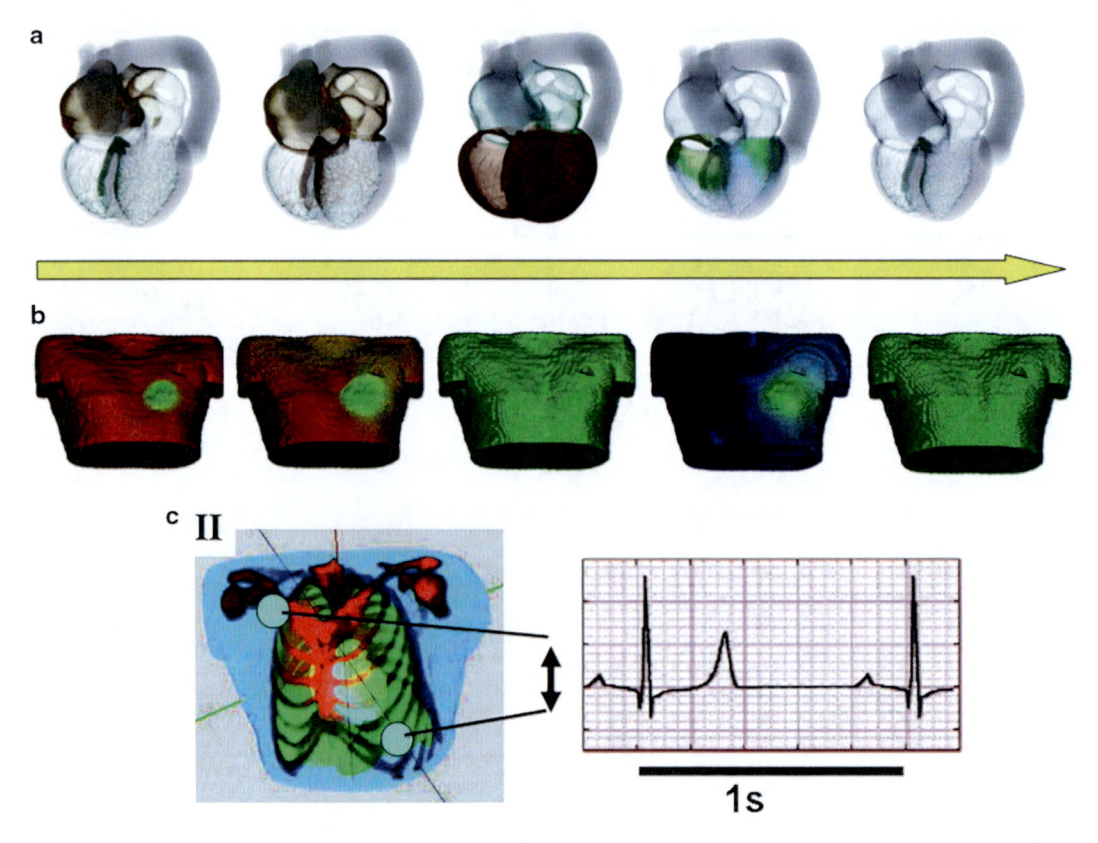

Fig. 4 ECG simulation: (**a**) propagation of excitation, (**b**) body surface voltage map, (**c**) torso model and the ECG

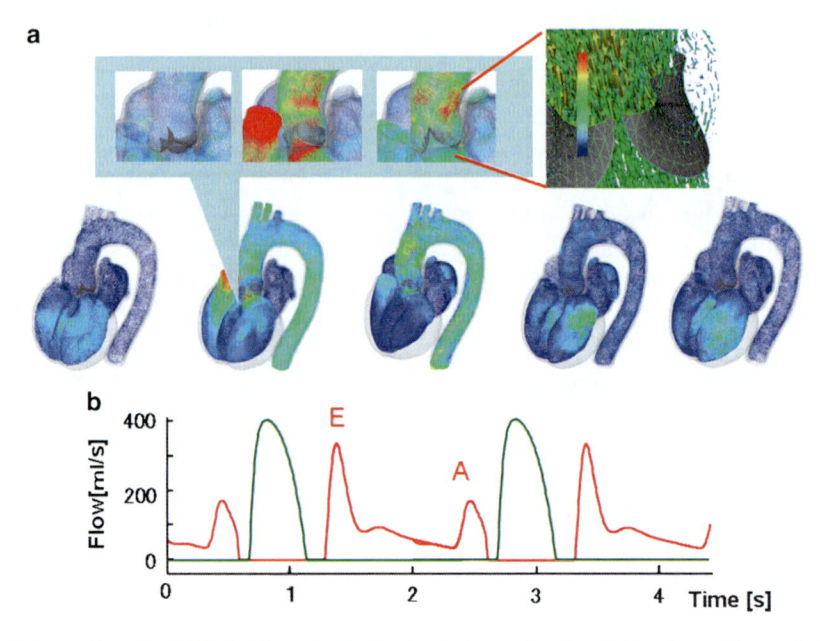

Fig. 5 Simulation of Doppler UCG: (**a**) flow distribution in the heart chamber during the cardiac cycle (upper panels show a magnified view of the aortic root), (**b**) flow patterns across the mitral valve (*red*) and aortic valve (*green*)

In Silico Treatment

This simulator is also applicable to the simulation of various types of treatments. Figure 6 shows the *in silico* treatment of ventricular fibrillation using an implantable cardioverter defibrillator (ICD) with a right ventricular electrode and generator (Fig. 6a). In this simulation, only the electrical activity in ventricles was calculated to reduce the computational cost. After ventricular fibrillation was induced by cross-field stimulation, an electrical pulse was applied at the timing indicated by the yellow thunderbolt sign to successfully terminate the spiral waves (Fig. 6b). We also found that cardioversion was successful only with the electrical power output above a certain threshold. This finding indicates that the simulator can be used to judge the efficacy of therapeutic strategies or devices.

Cardiac surgery is another area of application since reoperations should be avoided or are, in most cases, not possible. We have already attempted the simulation of ventriculoplasty for cases of intractable heart failure. Aortic root replacement surgery is another potential example [21].

Conclusions

As discussed above, the heart simulator can be used to determine both the indication and treatment strategies. Of these, development of a cardiac resynchronization therapy (CRT) device is a suitable field of application, in which the multi-physics nature of our simulator would certainly produce an innovative design with high efficiency. Finally, the application of the heart simulator is not limited to the optimization and development of therapeutic devices. The multi-scale, multi-physics

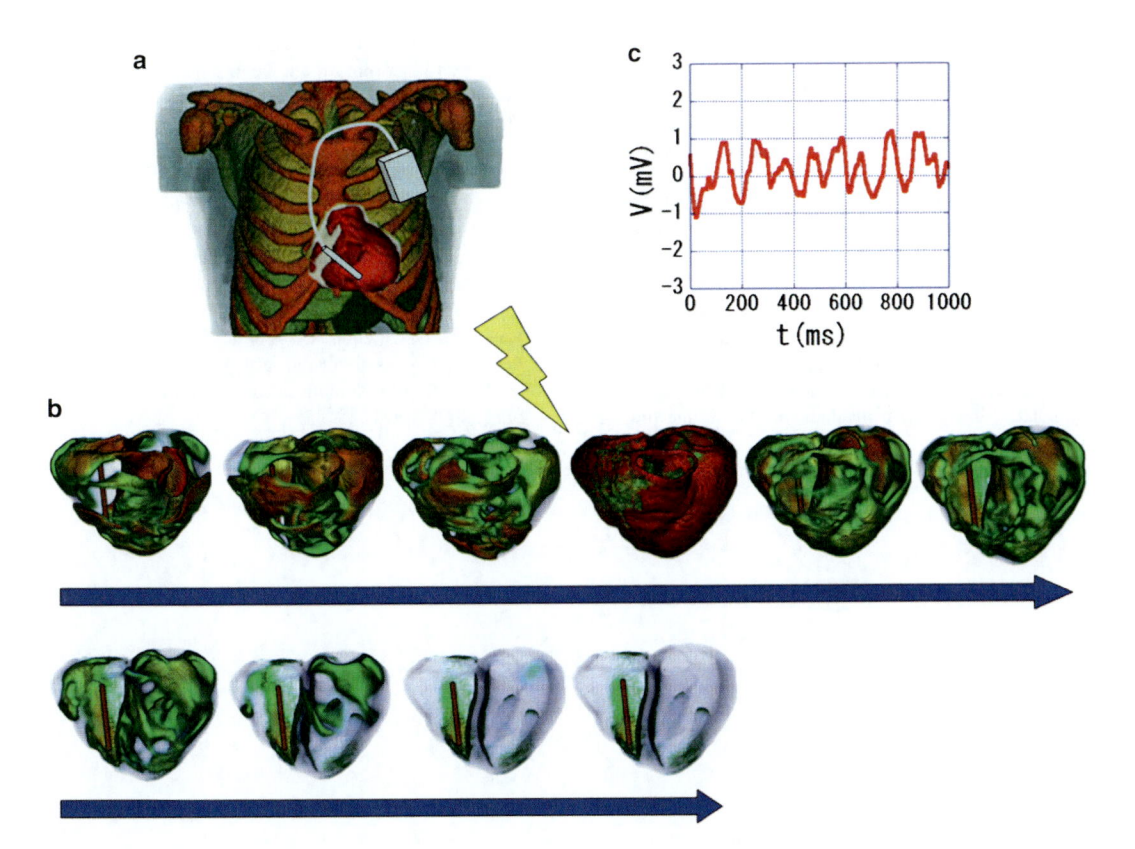

Fig. 6 Simulation of cardioversion by ICD: (**a**) diagram of the ICD system, (**b**) voltage map during the ventricular fibrillation (VF) and cardioversion, (**c**) ECG during VF

characteristics thereof allow us to use it as a tool in drug discovery and for the development of novel treatments that rely on various physics.

References

1. Noble D. Modeling the heart–from genes to cells to the whole organ. Science. 2002;295:1678–82.
2. Hunter PJ, Borg TK. Integration from proteins to organs: the physiome project. Nat Rev Mol Cell Biol. 2003;241:237–43.
3. Luo CH, Rudy Y. A model of the ventricular cardiac action potential. Depolarization, repolarization, and their interaction. Circ Res. 1991;68:1501–26.
4. Noble D, Varghese A, Kohl P, et al. Improved guinea-pig ventricular cell model incorporating a diadic space, IKr and IKs, and length- and tension-dependent processes. Can J Cardiol. 1998;14:123–34.
5. Kohl P, Noble D, Winslow RL, et al. Computational modelling of biological systems: tools and visions. Philos Trans R Soc Lond A. 2000;358:579–610.
6. Nakazawa K, Namba T. Dynamics of spiral waves in three dimensional FHN model media: a fundamental study on the mechanism of functional reentrant tachyarrhythmia by computer simulations. Biomed Eng. 1999;37:63–77.
7. Winslow RL, Scollan DF, Holmes JW, et al. Electrophysiological modeling of cardiac ventricular function: from cell to organ. Annu Rev Biomed Eng. 2000;2:119–55.
8. Negroni JA, Lascano EC. A cardiac muscle model relating sarcomere dynamics to calcium kinetics. J Mol Cell Cardiol. 1996;28:915–29.
9. Peterson JN, Hunter WC, Berman MR. Estimated time course of Ca21 bound to troponin C during relaxation in isolated cardiac muscle. Am J Physiol Heart Circ Physiol. 1991;260:H1013–24.
10. Rice JJ, Winslow RL, Hunter WC. Comparison of putative cooperative mechanisms in cardiac muscle:

11. Hunter PJ, McCulloch AD, Nielsen PMF, et al. A finite element model of passive ventricular mechanics. In: Spilker RL, Simon BR, editors. Computational Methods in Bioengineering. New York: ASME BED; 1988. p. 387–97.
12. Huyghe JM, Arts T, Van Champen DH, et al. Porous medium finite element model of the beating left ventricle. Am J Physiol Heart Circ Physiol. 1992;262:H1 256–67.
13. Kovacs SJ, McQueen DM. Modeling cardiac fluid dynamics and diastolic function. Philos Trans R Soc Lond A. 2001;359:1299–314.
14. McQueen DM. A three-dimensional computer model of the human heart for studying cardiac fluid dynamics. Comput Graph. 2000;34:57–60.
15. Noble D. Cardiac action and pacemaker potentials based on the Hodgkin-Huxley equations. Nature. 1960;188:495–7.
16. Ten Tusscher KH, Noble D, Noble PJ, et al. A model for human ventricular tissue [see comment]. Am J Physiol Heart Circ Physiol. 2004;286:H1573–89.
17. Courtemanche M, Ramirez RJ, Nattel S. Ionic mechanisms underlying human atrial action potential properties: insights from a mathematical model. Am J Physiol Heart Circ Physiol. 1998;275:H301–21.
18. DiFrancesco D, Noble D. A model of cardiac electrical activity incorporating ionic pumps and concentration changes. Philos Trans R Soc Lond B Biol Sci. 1985;307:353–98.
19. Zhang Q, Hisada T. Analysis of fluid-structure interaction problems with structural buckling and large domain changes by ALE finite element methods. Comput Methods Appl Mech Eng. 2001;190:6341–57.
20. Taccardi B. Distribution of heart potentials on the thoracic surface of normal human subjects. Circ Res. 1963;12:341–52.
21. Katayama S, Umetani N, Sugiura S, et al. The sinus of Valsalva relieves abnormal stress on aortic valve leaflets by facilitating smooth closure. J Thorac Cardiovasc Surg. 2008;136:1528–35.

10. (continued) length dependence and dynamic responses. Am J Physiol Heart Circ Physiol. 1999;276:H1734–54.

Index

B. Ostadal et al. (eds.), *Genes and Cardiovascular Function*,
DOI 10.1007/978-1-4419-7207-1, © Springer Science+Business Media, LLC 2011

Printed by Publishers' Graphics LLC
Carol Stream, IL 60188 USA